Psychiatric Consultation in Childbirth Settings

Parent- and Child-Oriented Approaches

Psychiatric Consultation in Childbirth Settings
Parent- and Child-Oriented Approaches

Richard L. Cohen, M.D.

Western Psychiatric Institute and Clinic
University of Pittsburgh
Pittsburgh, Pennsylvania

With Contributions by:

Marie D. Bloom, Ph.D.
Patricia A. Coble, R.N., B.A.
Nancy L. Day, Ph.D.
Lorraine R. Herrenkohl, Ph.D.
George A. Huber, J.D.
Margaret F. Jensvold, M.D.
Klaus K.Minde, M.D., FRCP (C)
Kathleen R. Negley, M.H.A.
James M. Perel, Ph.D.
Loren H. Roth, M.D., M.P.H.
M. Anne Spence, Ph.D.
Donna E. Stewart, M.D., D.P., FRCP (C)
Ann P. Walker, M.A.
Katherine L. Wisner, M.D., M.S.

PLENUM MEDICAL BOOK COMPANY
NEW YORK AND LONDON

Library of Congress Cataloging in Publication Data

Psychiatric consultation in childbirth settings.

Includes bibliographies and index.
1. Pregnancy—Psychological aspects. 2. Childbirth—Psychological aspects. 3. Psychiatric consultation. I. Cohen, Richard L. (Richard Lawrence), 1922-   . [DNLM: 1. Mental Disorders—psychology. 2. Pregnancy—psychology. 3. Referral and Consultation. 4. Stress, Psychological. WQ 200 P9735]
RG560.P76   1988   616.89   88-6005
ISBN-13: 978-1-4684-5441-3   e-ISBN-13: 978-1-4684-5439-0
DOI: 10.1007/978-1-4684-5439-0

© 1988 Plenum Publishing Corporation
Softcover reprint of the hardcover 1st edition 1988

233 Spring Street, New York, N.Y. 10013

Plenum Medical Book Company is an imprint of Plenum Publishing Corporation

This volume is dedicated to the hundreds of women who gave so freely of their time and energies during the past 25 years in an effort to help the author better understand the experiences of pregnancy, labor, and delivery.

Contributors

MARIE D. BLOOM, Ph.D., Research Principal, Drug and Alcohol Epidemiology, Western Psychiatric Institute and Clinic, University of Pittsburgh, Pittsburgh, Pennsylvania

PATRICIA A. COBLE, R.N., B.A., Assistant Professor of Psychiatry, Co-Director, Sleep Center, Western Psychiatric Institute and Clinic, University of Pittsburgh, Pittsburgh, Pennsylvania

RICHARD L. COHEN, M.D., Emeritus Professor of Psychiatry and Consultant, Pregnancy and Parent/Infant Program, Director of Education, Western Psychiatric Institute and Clinic, University of Pittsburgh, Pittsburgh, Pennsylvania

NANCY L. DAY, Ph.D., Associate Professor of Psychiatry, Director, Drug and Alcohol Epidemiology Program, Western Psychiatric Institute and Clinic, University of Pittsburgh, Pittsburgh, Pennsylvania

LORRAINE R. HERRENKOHL, Ph.D., Professor of Psychology, Temple University, Philadelphia, Pennsylvania

GEORGE A. HUBER, J.D., Vice President and Counsel, Medical and Health Care Division, Western Psychiatric Institute and Clinic, University of Pittsburgh, Pittsburgh, Pennsylvania

MARGARET F. JENSVOLD, M.D., Medical Staff Fellow, Biological Psychiatry Branch, National Institute of Mental Health, Bethesda, Maryland

KLAUS K. MINDE, M.D., FRCP (C), Professor and Chairman, Department of Psychiatry, Professor, Department of Pediatrics and Psychology, Queen's University, Kingston, Ontario

KATHLEEN R. NEGLEY, M.H.A., Staff Associate, Vice President for Health Sciences, Western Psychiatric Institute and Clinic, University of Pittsburgh, Pittsburgh, Pennsylvania

JAMES M. PEREL, Ph.D., Professor of Psychiatry and Pharmacology, Director, Clinical Pharmacology Program, Western Psychiatric Institute and Clinic, University of Pittsburgh, Pittsburgh, Pennsylvania

LOREN H. ROTH, M.D., M.P.H., Professor of Psychiatry, Director of Law and Psychiatry Program, Western Psychiatric Institute and Clinic, University of Pittsburgh, Pittsburgh, Pennsylvania

M. ANNE SPENCE, Ph.D., Professor, Departments of Psychiatry and Biomathematics, Division of Medical Genetics, UCLA School of Medicine, Los Angeles, California

DONNA E. STEWART, M.D., D.P., FRCP (C), Associate Professor of Psychiatry and Obstetrics and Gynecology, Chief of the Psychiatric Consultation/Liaison Service, University of Toronto, St. Michael's Hospital, Toronto, Canada

ANN P. WALKER, M.A., Assistant Professor of Pediatrics, Director, Genetic Counseling Program, University of California at Irvine, Irvine, California

KATHERINE L. WISNER, M.D., M.S., Assistant Professor of Child Psychiatry, Director, Pregnancy and Infant/Parent Program, Western Psychiatric Institute and Clinic, University of Pittsburgh, Pittsburgh, Pennsylvania

Preface

The primary purposes of this volume are:

1. To provide mental health practitioners with a current overview of our knowledge about normal parental development during pregnancy and its relation to fetal development, with particular emphasis on the impact of acute and chronic stress on these developmental processes.
2. To provide an understanding of the general state of the field of pregnancy and childbirth care both in conventional health systems and in alternative options.
3. To provide an understanding of models of consultation and liaison that are adapted to the special conditions of pregnancy and childbirth care, as contrasted to the more traditional modes that characterize these activities in medical and surgical hospitals.

If there prove to be secondary gains as a result of pursuing these goals, so much the better. The most desirable of these would be a heightening of awareness of the mental health needs of "pregnant families" and of the risks they incur in transition from nonparenthood to parenthood, and a more effective level of primary and secondary prevention of childhood mental disorders. These latter goals are more global and perhaps even a bit grandiose. Their attainment could only be documented through a series of carefully designed research projects aimed at measuring long-range developmental outcome in children and families who have experienced appropriate and early intervention during the pregnancy period.

This is quite literally a book about obstetrics and childbirth care. Obstetrics is commonly linked with gynecology and the medical and surgical diseases associated with the female pelvic region. These disorders lend themselves more easily to conventional methods of consultation and liaison approaches and are not, therefore, addressed in any special way in this volume.

ACKNOWLEDGMENT. The untiring efforts and careful attention to detail of Karen Hickey-Rhinaman in the production of this volume are gratefully acknowledged.

Richard L. Cohen, M.D.

Contents

PART I: INTRODUCTION AND BACKGROUND

1. **Purpose and Rationale** **3**
   Richard L. Cohen

   Introduction 3
   Needs of the Field of Childbirth Care 5
   Conceptual Approach 6
   Other Sources of Assistance and Information 7
   References 8
   Annotated Bibliography 8
   Consumer Bibliography 11

2. **A Brief History of the Relationship between Obstetrics and the Mental
   Health Professions** **13**
   Richard L. Cohen

   The Historical Background 13
   References 17
   Supplementary Reading Lists 17

3. **The Impact of Prenatal Stress on the Developing Fetus and Child** **21**
   Lorraine R. Herrenkohl

   Introduction 21
   Maternal Stress and Pregnancy Outcome 22
   Prenatal Stress and Fetal Outcome 24
   Maternal Stress and Neonatal Activity 27
   Mechanisms of Prenatal Stress 31
   Summary and Conclusions 33
   References 33

4. **The Epidemiology of Mental and Emotional Disorders during Pregnancy and the Postpartum Period** 37

   Patricia A. Coble and Nancy L. Day

   Introduction 37
   Review of Modern Literature 39
   Theories of Causation 39
   Normal Psychological Reactions to Pregnancy and Motherhood 41
   Subclinical States and Adjustment Disorders 41
   Psychophysiologic Conditions 42
   Psychiatric Disorders 43
   Conclusion 44
   References 44
   Selected Readings on Puerperal Mental Disturbances 46

PART II: THE BUILDING BLOCKS

5. **Developmental Tasks of Pregnancy and Transition to Parenthood: An Approach to Assessment** 51

   Richard L. Cohen

   Introduction 51
   Developmental Model of Pregnancy 54
   Other Components of the Developmental Interview 66
   Organizing and Formulating Information Gathered 67
   References 68

6. **Emotional Disorders and Mental Illness Associated with Pregnancy and the Postpartum Period** 71

   Richard L. Cohen

   Introduction 71
   Major Psychiatric Disorders 73
   Conditions in Which Stress and/or Emotional Factors May Contribute to the
     Disorder 76
   Conditions or States That May Interact Adversely with Pregnancy ... 78
   An Alternate Conceptualization 79
   References 81

7. **Current Childbirth Options and Parental Decision Making** 85

   Richard L. Cohen

   Introduction 85
   Factors Influencing Maternal Choice of Childbirth Alternatives 86
   A Comparative Study of Women Choosing Two Different Childbirth
     Alternatives 95
   Conclusions 103
   References 103

PART III: CONSULTATION PRACTICE

8. Models of Consultation and Liaison: General Principles 107

Richard L. Cohen

Introduction 107
Entrée into the System 108
Overview of Models 111
References 113

9. Direct Case Consultation 115

Richard L. Cohen and Katherine L. Wisner

Introduction 115
Case Histories 117
Conclusion 136

10. Staff Education, Liaison, and Program Consultation 137

Richard L. Cohen

Introduction 137
Educational and Liaison Activities 138
Program Consultation to Conventional or Traditional Childbirth Services ... 139
Program Consultation to Special Projects or Services 145
Program Consultation for Extramural Programs and Out-of-Hospital
   Nontraditional Services 145
Summary 146
References 146
Additional Readings of Interest to the Liaison Psychiatrist 147

11. Psychiatric Services in the Neonatal Intensive Care Unit 151

Klaus K. Minde and Donna E. Stewart

Introduction 151
Common Sources of Parental and Staff Stress in an NICU 152
The Role of the Psychiatrist in the NICU 154
Difficulties and Rewards Encountered by the Psychiatrist Working in the
   NICU 155
One Model of a Consultation-Liaison Service for an NICU 158
Services Provided by the Child Psychiatrist 161
References 163

**12. Psychopharmacologic Agents and Electroconvulsive Therapy during
   Pregnancy and the Puerperium** 165

Katherine L. Wisner and James M. Perel

Introduction 165
Antipsychotic Agents during Pregnancy 170

Antidepressant Medication 177
Lithium 182
Electroconvulsive Therapy (ECT) 188
The Benzodiazepines 191
Pregnant and Puerperal Women: Treatment Recommendations 198
References 200

13. **The Effect of Prenatal Exposure to Alcohol and Other Drugs** **207**
    Nancy L. Day, Patricia A. Coble, and Marie D. Bloom

    Alcohol Abuse 207
    The Effect of Tobacco Use during Pregnancy 212
    The Effect of Other Drug Use during Pregnancy 213
    References 215

14. **Principles of Genetic Counseling for Psychiatric Liaisons** **219**
    Ann P. Walker and M. Anne Spence

    Introduction 219
    Reasons to Refer for Genetic Counseling 220
    Prenatal Diagnosis 222
    General Genetic Counseling Issues 223
    Specific Mental Health Counseling Issues 223
    References 226

PART IV: AREAS OF SPECIAL CONCERN

15. **Variations** **231**
    Margaret F. Jensvold

    Introduction 231
    Developments Complicating Genetic, Gestational, and Social Parenting 231
    Prenatal Diagnosis and Counseling and Genetic Engineering 234
    Legal Trends in Reproductive Decision Making 236
    Implications for the Psychiatric Consultant 237
    References 239

16. **The Current Controversy in Childbirth Care: A Consultant's
    Viewpoint** **241**
    Richard L. Cohen

    Introduction 241
    Interviews with the Principal Actors 241
    References 250

17. Professional Responsibility for the Welfare of Potential Life 253

George A. Huber, Kathleen R. Negley, and Loren H. Roth

Introduction 253
Evolution of Fetal Rights 254
Competing Interests of Maternal and Fetal Rights 255
Medical Malpractice 257
Suggested Guidelines for Case Management 259
The Future 262
References 263

PART V: SUMMARY AND CONCLUSIONS

18. Conclusions and Future Directions 269

Richard L. Cohen

Index 273

I

Introduction and Background

1

Introduction and Background

1

Purpose and Rationale

RICHARD L. COHEN

Introduction

The basic principles and practices of general hospital consultation and liaison have been
laid down by several major figures in the field over the last 20 years. The reader is
assumed to be conversant with this literature. The early papers of Kaufman[1] followed by
the outstanding summary and reviews of Lipowski[2–4] are mandatory reading for all
professionals working in this field.

Reviewing the literature reminds one that it is only during more recent years that the
practice of consultation and liaison psychiatry has emerged as a more discrete entity from
that field of knowledge that we have called "psychosomatic medicine." Newer research
has marked off a territory of basic research and clinical practice that involves disorders of
psychophysiologic origin but that are not necessarily matters for the daily attention of the
consulting psychiatrist. In fact, many of them now lie well within the province of psychiatry itself, so that the primary physician is now often the psychiatrist himself. Excellent
examples of this are to be found among the eating disorders, sleeping disorders, addictive
disorders, and many of the severe developmental problems of childhood and adolescence.

The need for a book such as this has impressed several practitioners because most are
trained in conventional consultation and liaison approaches and find themselves without a
relevant paradigm to intervene when they are called upon to consult in situations in which
a women is pregnant and there is no real or suspected disease. There is only a level of
concern, even apprehension, among her childbirth caretakers that the pregnancy is at risk
for psychological reasons.

Perhaps a brief example may serve to underscore the need for a different conceptual
framework to approach childbirth interventions:

Miss A. is a 23-year-old white unmarried woman who is currently pregnant for the first time and is
estimated to be at approximately 24 weeks gestation. Currently, she demonstrates signs of a

Richard L. Cohen • Department of Psychiatry, Western Psychiatric Institute and Clinic, University of Pittsburgh, Pittsburgh, PA 15213.

progressive thought disorder. She shows evidence of a paranoid delusional system largely involving a young man by whom she became pregnant. She also claims occasional auditory hallucinations. Her affect is blunted, and she demonstrates ideas of reference that include many of her personal caretakers. Her obstetrical history to date is unremarkable. The pregnancy has progressed without problem.

Miss A. has a history of having had one acute schizophrenic episode when she was 19. This responded to neuroleptic medication, and she has been followed at a local mental health clinic near her home for the past few years. Her condition was seen as stable there prior to the current exacerbation of symptoms.

Psychiatric consultation is being sought because the maternal grandparents are very concerned about the future of the baby and want custody for it. Miss A. demands that she maintain custody. The hospital staff has involved the county children and youth service. A social worker from that organization believes the baby should be removed from the home and placed at least in temporary foster care until the mother's condition has reached a stable state.

In addition, her obstetrician is quite concerned because Miss A. was on rather large doses of depot prolixin at the time of conception and has read about the teratogenic effects of psychotropic medication during the first trimester of pregnancy.

The medical and nursing staffs are divided, concerning what is in the best interest of the mother and of the baby. The grandparents have sought legal counsel, and there is also an attorney involved in the case from the children and youth service.

The psychiatrist is asked to evaluate Miss A. to determine her potential competency to care for an infant and to predict what might be in the best interests of the baby in this situation. Miss A. claims that she was doing very well for several years and did not have any difficulties until she was deserted by her boyfriend during her pregnancy. She believes that she can once again achieve a stable condition and care for her baby quite well.

It can be observed immediately that the preceding situation requires considerable knowledge of the developmental course of pregnancy, the risks of chronic stress to the fetus, and knowledge of a repertoire of interventions that may involve additional treatment modalities beyond those found in general medical and psychiatric practices.

In fact, the need for this unique approach is simply a reflection of the fact that conception, pregnancy, and childbirth represent unique human experiences in themselves. Compressed into this brief time are forces that inexorably impact on the biological status of the female, the family homeostasis, adult family roles, the economic condition of the family, and often career aspirations of one or more family members. What other process can impinge on the family in this fashion without being a catastrophic disease or a separation by death or some other major family loss?

Yet conversely, pregnancy and childbirth are viewed by most people as being normal human events and processes. In most situations, they are seen as occasions for happy celebrations, when optimistic plans for the future are made, and an appropriate level of excitement associated with new life and new beginnings is realized.

This paradox is a crucial one. There are few experiences that carry with them such major demands for change yet are associated with such pleasurable affects. It is for this reason that pregnancy has come to be characterized as a "developmental crisis." This is particularly true of the first pregnancy which usually invokes the most demand for adaptation and shift in family equilibrium. We have learned that any process that demands major adaptational shifts in a compressed time period carries with it significant risks. These risks become greater when the process is further complicated by threats to support systems, by intercurrent family illness, or loss or by other events that add to the family's pressure for change. All such intercurrent events may not be necessarily negative in their connotations. The spouse who enjoys a major promotion at work with its attendant greater responsibility and time demands may find that economic pressures on the family are reduced but that his capacity to provide appropriate marital support may be decreased during the pregnancy.

It has been my experience that mental health professionals are not called upon often enough in situations that are at high risk for emotional decompensation during pregnancy either because childbirth professionals tend to underrate the significance of such developments or do not employ even the simplest assessment procedures to identify their presence. Part of the purpose of the liaison portion of this volume (see Chapter 10) will be to describe simple but usually effective procedures for identifying those women and families who are most at risk for adaptational failure during pregnancy and to train childbirth professionals in their use.

There is an emerging body of data, both in the animal and human literature, that should help to convince the reader that this latter effort is worth undertaking. Although this will be referenced throughout the volume, Chapter 3 will particularly highlight the data that indicate that prolonged prenatal stress may have lasting effects, not simply of a psychological, but of a biological nature on the fetus and on the child he or she becomes. These data are so significant in their import that they can no longer be dismissed. In fact, they may represent the most compelling rationale for increasing the participation of mental health personnel in the delivery of prenatal and childbirth services. It may be insufficient to state now that it is important to help new parents to deal with the stress of transition to parenthood so that they will provide more responsive child care. That has always been self-evident. It now appears that unmitigated and unrelieved stress during fetal development may so impact on various developing fetal systems (probably mediated through neurohormonal mechanisms in the mother) that carefully targeted interventions may become as important as good nutrition during pregnancy.

Needs of the Field of Childbirth Care

The underutilization of mental health consultation during pregnancy becomes even a more vexing problem in the face of the currently roiling conflict about where, how, and by whom childbirth services should be delivered. Any mental health professional who aspires to enter that complex area of the health care system without a comprehensive understanding of the nature of the current controversy, its protagonists and the fundamental issues at stake, is very likely to fail because advice will be given out of context and may not be perceived as supportive to the basic health care goals of the system involved. These issues will be addressed in Chapters 7 and 16. Very briefly and in an oversimplified version, the controversy revolves around whether pregnancy and childbirth should be viewed as normal, family-oriented life events, or conversely, whether they represent medically at-risk conditions in which care should be delivered within settings that are at the cutting edge of medical science. Some of the proponents of these views have become so polarized that the health system has become fragmented and internally uncommunicative. Any woman who moves from one component of the system to another may find derision, rejection, or even disbelief that she could have ever been gullible enough to become involved with her former caretakers.

There is probably no other component of the health care arena which is so fraught with systems problems. The sophisticated consultant needs a working knowledge of both the controversy and the childbirth options in order to be of genuine assistance to women and families in distress.

In a parallel fashion, the consumer movement and the legal and judiciary professions have become involved in the delivery of childbirth services. Perhaps for some of the same reasons that abortion has become such an emotionally charged matter at both the personal and political levels, the whole arena of childbirth care is also suffused with powerful and often opposing belief systems that pit generation against generation and sometimes even mother against fetus. The vulnerability of the fetus and the often overpowering emotional needs of young parents represent potentially all of the elements of interpersonal conflict at the most primitive levels. Mental health consultants who become involved in an effort to resolve these conflicts may find themselves quite literally in the position of King Solomon. Their own ethical, religious and family belief systems inevitably impinge on their ability to make rational and disinterested judgments. It often takes iron discipline to remove one's personal biases from the consultation process—for example, with pregnant teenage substance abusers, young parents who, in their denial of the pregnant state, are avoiding all transition to parenthood—or marriages that are dissolving during the pregnancy with heated conflict over future custody of the coming infant.

In part, for many of the previously mentioned reasons, obstetricians begin to approach their practice with a kind of siege mentality. Confronted on many sides by demands for more humanistic and individualized care, by demands for cost containment because of the mounting expense of high technology care, and by claims of liability for "wrongful births," allegedly acquired birth defects, and other iatrogenic difficulties, the entire profession needs support in thinking through newer models of service delivery. Mental health professionals can provide much of the support necessary to help in understanding and communicating more clearly with troubled families and to develop strategies for early intervention in high-risk situations. There is every reason to believe from the experience of other medical disciplines that such efforts reduce patient stress, adverserial relationships with the physician, and capricious malpractice suits.

Obstetricians now are assessed among the highest malpractice insurance premiums. Much of reason for this relates to unrealistic expectations that consumers place upon high technology care because many people still view the entire birth process as a miracle. The physician who is most associated with that process may find that miracles are expected of him. The burdensome stress imposed by such expectations in the face of a knowledge system that is incomplete and imperfect produces much anxiety, particularly in young physicians.

Appropriate liaison can be useful in helping to cope with such anxiety, not only in the physician but the delivery room nurse, the obstetric nurse practitioner, the nurse-midwife, and the entire team of health professionals who care for mother and baby.

Conceptual Approach

This volume attempts to describe and illustrate the use of an approach to consultation and liaison that recognizes the interplay of these many forces. What will be described is a conceptual model that "factors in" the developmental process of pregnancy, the significance of various stress contingencies, the setting in which childbirth care is being delivered, and the needs of the health professionals who are functioning in that setting. There is almost never a one-to-one relationship between a particular "presenting complaint" in an obstetric/psychiatric consultation and a particular type of intervention. There are too many confounding and interacting variables that must be taken into consideration and that require a kind of matrix model in which development, intercurrent stresses, family support systems, health care settings, and professional staff factors are weighed in relation to each other before any conclusions or recommendations can be formulated.

The overall plan of this book is designed to provide the mental health professional, first, with the necessary understanding of the historical process that has led to the current complex health care system in obstetrics; a basic review of maternal and fetal development in a context that is directly applicable to mental health consultation; some understanding of the impact of acute and chronic stresses (both endogenous and exogenous) on those developmental processes; an overview of the epidemiology and nosology of mental disorders in pregnancy and the postpartum period according to our present state of knowledge; a review of the present status of the field of childbirth care from high technology, tertiary care centers to home-based delivery; an intervention model that integrates the preceding information into a consultation and liaison approach with multiple case illustrations; a look at the ethical and legal issues involved in the delivery of obstetric care from the viewpoint of the mental health professional; and finally, within the limitations of available space, a description of some of the more uncommon and unusual situations encountered in mental health consultation in childbirth settings.

Other Sources of Assistance and Information

Although this work attempts to be reasonably comprehensive within its basic purpose and scope, no single volume can actually cover either the necessary background information or the many viewpoints and practices in the field as they are now described on a worldwide basis. Other texts that the reader may wish to consult for a more in-depth look at specific areas should include the following.

There are several national and international organizations that can serve as important sources of information about needs and current practices in the childbirth field. Many mental health professionals may not be familiar with these. In most instances, they have staffs or executive secretaries who are pleased to provide information about studies that have been conducted, national or international conferences where new approaches to consultation and liaison are being described, and some even have resource libraries that may be used by professionals.

The American College of Obstetrics and Gynecology, 600 Maryland Avenue, S.W., Washington, DC 20024, (202) 638-5577. The Library for History of Obstetrics and Gynecology in America – Resource Center.

The American Society for Psychosomatic Obstetrics and Gynecology, % Dennis Smith, M.D., Secretary/Treasurer, 2490 Kenilworth Road, Cleveland Heights, OH 44106. Membership includes a subscription to the *Journal of Psychosomatic Obstetrics and Gynaecology,* which is the official journal of the International Society of Psychosomatic Obstetrics and Gynaecology and the American, Australian, and Dutch Societies for Psychosomatic Obstetrics and Gynaecology.

International Childbirth Education Association, Box 20048, Minneapolis, MN 55420-0048, (612) 854-8660.

International Congress of Psychosomatic Obstetrics and Gynecology, % Professor E. V. Van Hall, Department of Obstetrics and Gynaecology, University Hospital, Rijnsburgerweg 10, 2333 AA Leiden, The Netherlands. This congress publishes proceedings every 4 years entitled *Emotion and Reproduction*.

References

1. Kaufman RM: The role of the psychiatrist in a general hospital. *Psychiatr Q* **27**:367–373, 1953.
2. Lipowski ZJ: Review of consultation psychiatry and psychosomatic medicine, I. General principles. *Psychosom Med* **29**:153–171, 1967.
3. Lipowski ZJ: Review of consultation psychiatry and psychosomatic medicine, II. Clinical Aspects. *Psychosom Med* **29**:201–224, 1967.
4. Lipowski ZJ: Review of consultation psychiatry and psychosomatic medicine, III. Theoretical Issues. *Psychosom Med* **30**:395–442, 1968.

Annotated Bibliography

Gleicher N (ed): *Principles of Medical Therapy in Pregnancy*. New York, Plenum Medical Book Company, 1985.

This is an encyclopedic reference work of almost 1,300 pages. It contains 191 chapters organized by specialty and/or organ system. It is an invaluable source book for any medical practitioner whose daily work brings him or her into contact with pregnant women. One hundred and fifty contributors presented the latest experience in assessing and managing all of the medical complications that can be associated with pregnancy. There is an especially unusual chapter (Chapter 4 and appendix) that describes the normal physiologic changes in pregnancy (not addressed in this work) and a very useful table of normal laboratory values in pregnancy. Space limitations do not allow for a major section on psychiatric disorders (10 pages). However, other areas of potential interest to the psychiatrist include problems of sterility (p. 18), endocrine disorders (p. 145), fetal growth and development (p. 320), pre-eclampsia and eclampsia (p. 765), sexual counseling (p. 894), and genetic counseling (p. 1217).

Chard T, Richards M (eds): *Benefits and Hazards of the New Obstetrics*. London, Spastics International Medical Publications, 1977.

The editors and contributors to this volume have made a good faith effort to outline the many advantages of the new high technology obstetrics and have described many of the risks and hazards of these practices. This is probably the best balanced, most objective explication of some of the dilemmas facing modern practitioners in obstetrics available.

Howells, JG (ed): *Modern Perspectives in Psycho-Obstetrics*. New York, Brunner/Mazel, 1972.

This anthology, although many of the contributions are now rather dated, represents the first significant effort to pull all of the existing knowledge about the "psychosomatic" aspects of obstetrics into one source book. It contains interesting chapters on subjects such as pseudocyesis, the couvade syndrome, childbirth in cross-cultural perspectives, the psychopathology of toxemia pregnancy, Soviet methods of psychoprophylaxis in obstetrics, the management of home confinement, infanticide, and many other subjects germane to the behavioral scientist interested in pregnancy and the childbirth process.

Blum BL: *Psychological Aspects of Pregnancy, Birthing and Bonding.* New York, Human Sciences Press, 1980.

This volume falls somewhere between the professional and the layperson in its scope and use of technical language and clinical concepts. It represents an effort on the part of several contributors to give an interdisciplinary understanding of the psychological needs and conflicts faced by contemporary women and men as they become involved in the childbirth process. It is sufficiently basic in its approach to be of use to the occasional obstetric faculty member or house officer who wishes to develop more psychological insight concerning the impact of the reproductive process.

Taylor P (ed): *Parent-Infant Relationships,* Monographs in Neonatology. New York, Grune & Stratton, 1980.

This publication is one of the prestigious monographs in the Neonatology Series and contains much of the thinking about adaptational processes in pregnancy, maladaptational to pregnancy, the impact of hospital practices, parental experiences in alternative birthing centers, and a sensible overview of the present state of our knowledge about "bonding" and attachment.

American Academy of Pediatrics and The American College of Obstetricians and Gynecologists: *Guidelines for Perinatal Care.* Authors, 1983.

This handbook was published jointly by the American College of Obstetricians and Gynecologists and the American Academy of Pediatrics. It represents the culmination of 3 years of discussion between various committees concerned with maternal and fetal medicine. It is an excellent guidebook for the professional who wants to know where organized medicine stands on acceptable practices with respect to care of the pregnant women and neonate.

Speert H: *Obstetrics and Gynecology in America: A History.* Chicago, American College of Obstetricians and Gynecologists, 1980.

This volume should be useful to the mental health professional encountering this field for the first time because it gives a perspective on the development of this specialty in American medicine that is carefully annotated from records and conferences beginning with the Colonial period in America. It discusses American Indian practices as they were encountered in the seventeenth century up to present practices and new developments in the 1980s. It is history as viewed through the eyes of organized obstetrics.

Carenza L, Zichella L (eds): *Emotion and Reproduction,* Vol. 20A. London, Academic Press, 1979.

This two-volume set constitutes the proceedings of the 5th International Congress of Psychosomatic Obstetrics and Gynecology held in Rome in 1977. The work comprises 1400 pages and consists of scores of abstracts of various presentations. Many of these are useful and provocative, but it takes a discerning reader to separate the wheat from the chaff because many of the reports involve work of questionable methodology and design and work that is in process without definitive findings. Nevertheless, a scanning of these volumes will also provide the receptive reader a dazzling overview of the international activity and attention that the "role of emotions in reproduction" is receiving.

Brown WA: *Psychological Care During Pregnancy and the Postpartum Period*. New York, Raven Press, 1979.

Consultants would do well to be aware of the presence of this volume because it represents an excellent source book for nonpsychiatric health care personnel interested in providing comprehensive psychosocial care during pregnancy. It describes a reasonable method for collecting information about the emotional status of women, for assessing that data, and for developing intervention plans. It is not a casebook as such but an approach to integrating good psychological care into obstetrics. When the occasional obstetric resident or faculty member asks for a reference written in nontechnical language and useful for obstetric nurses and other personnel, this is a commendable choice.

Brockington IF, Kumar R (eds): *Motherhood and Mental Illness*. London, Academic Press, 1982.

This volume represents a summary of the proceedings of an international conference held in June 1980, and sponsored by the University of Manchester, Department of Psychiatry. As with most conference proceedings, there is an unevenness to the work, but there are several excellent contributions particularly in the areas of epidemiologic aspects of mental illness associated with childbearing, the diagnosis and management of postpartum psychosis, and the use of illicit and psychotropic drugs during pregnancy.

Wolman BB (ed): *Psychological Aspects of Gynecology and Obstetrics*. Oradel, New Jersey, Medical Economics Company, 1978.

This volume is the result of a collaborative effort between psychiatrists, clinical psychologists, and various specialists in obstetrics and gynecology and focuses on the management of specific psychological and behavioral problems that gynecologists and obstetricians must cope with in their everyday practice. There is an interesting section on the changing psychology of women, particularly as this impacts on attitudes toward reproduction; one on various emotional problems associated with the course of pregnancy; another similar one focused on emotional problems associated with labor and childbirth; and a few additional specialized chapters on selected subjects.

Notman MT, Nadelson CC (eds): *Concepts of Femininity and the Life Cycle*. New York, Plenum Press. (Volume 1, 1978, Volumes 2 and 3, 1982)

This three-volume work attempts a comprehensive overview of later developments in the changing status of women in society and focuses on special problems in consulting, diagnosing, and treating emotional disorders particularly associated with the medical care of women, and with emotional and behavioral disorders of reproduction. Volume 1 will be of particular interest to mental health workers consulting with childbirth facilities because it focuses almost entirely on pregnancy and childbirth. The orientation is basically psychodynamic, and the authors write from broad experience in the field.

The following four volumes (all of which will be referred to later in this work) represent excellent source books for achieving better understanding of the experience of pregnancy as a step in the transition to parenthood. Each approaches developmental phenomena from a slightly different viewpoint, but all are rich with excellent illustrative material, and all are family centered in their approach to making the major shift in the family system and its attendant stresses understandable to the mental health professional.

Shereshefsky, PM, Yarrow, LJ: *Psychological Aspects of a First Pregnancy and Early Postnatal Adaptation*. New York, Raven Press, 1974.

Entwisle DR, Doering, SG: *The First Birth: A Family Turning Point*. Baltimore, The Johns Hopkins University Press, 1981.

Consumer Bibliography

It is also important for the consultant to be aware of the literature to which informed consumers are exposed. Keeping up with the popular press and media is virtually impossible because daily newspapers and weekly and monthly magazines all seem to have leaped on the bandwagon of the controversy about childbirth care, and the welter of ''expert'' opinions, feminist-oriented literature, and tape recorder journalism on the subject resembles an avalanche in its volume.

Nevertheless, there are some prominent works that have been published over the past 10 years or so with which the expert consultant should have familiarity. These range in approach and tone from the very balanced, unemotional reporting of childbirth options to strident, almost revolutionary treatises on the evils of modern obstetrics. Some of the most well-known of these works include the following:

Particularly for the male reader who wishes a first person description of a broad range of experiences with pregnancy, labor and delivery, the best choice would be:

Sorel NC: *Ever Since Eve: Personal Reflections on Childbirth.* New York, Oxford University Press, 1984.

As indicated before, this work contains scores of first-person accounts of the various experiences of pregnancy and childbirth by such famous individuals as Margaret Meade, Helen Hays, Isadora Duncan, and Golda Meir. A most revealing ''inside'' look.

The following volumes represent efforts at preparing and outlining various approaches to preparation for childbirth and the various options available for receiving professional care during childbirth:

Kramer R: *Giving Birth.* Chicago, Contemporary Books, Inc., 1978.
Hotchner T: *Pregnancy and Childbirth.* New York, Avon Books, 1979.
Walker M, Yoffe, BG, Parke H: *The Complete Book of Birth.* New York, Simon & Schuster, 1979.
Feldman S: *Choices in Childbirth.* New York, Grosset & Dunlap, 1978.

There is now an extensive literature authored by leaders in the feminist movement on the subject of pregnancy and childbirth. Because obstetrics, as with most of medicine, is a male-dominated profession and, because for the past 50 years or so, most births have taken place in large, bureaucratically operated institutions, these books make an effort to expose the evils and risks of utilizing both the medical services and the institutional environment in traditional childbirth care and tend to extol the virtues of many of the out-of-hospital choices for receiving prenatal care and for giving birth. The knowledgeable consultant should be familiar with this literature because an increasing number of young parents are being exposed to it and are strongly influenced by it in their choice of care and their subsequent reactions to physicians, nurses, and other professional attendants:

Milinaire C: *Birth,* New York, Harmony Books, 1974.
Oakley A: *Women Confined,* New York, Schocken Books, 1980.
Corea G: *The Hidden Malpractice.* New York, Jove/HBJ Books, 1977.
Arms S: *Immaculate Deception.* San Francisco, San Francisco Book Company/Houghton Mifflin Book, 1975.
Stewart D, Stewart L: *Safe Alternatives in Childbirth.* Chapel Hill, NAPSAC, Inc. 1976.
Boston Women's Health Book Collective, *New Our Bodies Our Selves.* Boston, 1971.

2

A Brief History of the Relationship between Obstetrics and the Mental Health Professions

RICHARD L. COHEN

I will greatly multiply thy sorrow and thy conception; in sorrow thou shalt bring forth children; and thy desire shall be to thy husband, and he shall rule over thee.
Genesis 3:16

They shall be in pain as a woman that travaileth.
Isaiah 13:8

The Historical Background

There is probably no subject that has fascinated mankind more during the course of history and across all cultures than that of pregnancy and childbirth.[1] Perhaps the only subject that rivals it for sustained level of interest is that of death itself. Parenthetically, it is noteworthy that these two human experiences, having been the provinces of the medical profession and of hospitals for the past 50 years, are now becoming increasing concerns for alternative health care systems. It is perhaps no coincidence that with the appearance of alternative birthing centers, one sees the simultaneous appearance of hospices in which dying is becoming more focused as a human experience and a family concern rather than as a professionalized medical "event" (see Chapter 16).

Richard L. Cohen • Department of Psychiatry, Western Psychiatric Institute and Clinic, University of Pittsburgh, Pittsburgh, PA 15213.

Indeed, it is hardly possible to leaf through a weekly news magazine or a daily newspaper or to spend an evening before the television set without being exposed either in fact or in fiction to some of the many emotionally charged questions that surround pregnancy and birth. Whether they are such age-old questions as abortion, illegitimacy, contested paternity, or pregnancy by rape, or some of the newer questions we have inherited through the blessings of modern science, such as in vitro fertilization; surrogate mothering; the birth of septuplets as a result of fertility drugs; or the risk–benefit equations surrounding amniocentesis, electronic fetal monitoring, and ultrasound, these matters bubble to the surface on a daily basis.

The most casual student of the history of childbirth care has encountered whole volumes (see Supplementary Reading List A) devoted to various aspects of the subject. Some medical libraries even have sections of books shelved with this topic as a focus. The library of the American College of Obstetricians and Gynecologists has a historical collection that occupies an entire room. We must, therefore, be very selective in the overview we consider relevant to the needs of the mental health clinician.

For the consultant who is also a history buff, additional readings beyond those sources cited in the text appear as a Supplementary Reading List at the end of this chapter.

For instance, the well-informed consultant will find it useful to know something about development of childbirth care providers (both medical and nonmedical) and some idea of their influence on the ebb and flow of popular practices over the centuries (see List A). The relationship between midwifery (almost entirely a female calling) and the emergence of the medical specialty of obstetrics (almost entirely a male profession until recently—and originally called male midwifery!) is of significance even today because of the ongoing controversy about alternative childbirth centers (see List B).

Also, some time spent understanding the evolution of societal structures and belief systems in Western and other cultures will prove of considerable value (see List C). A longitudinal view of the development of childbirth care provides a perspective for the current practitioner that often makes meaningful behavior that would otherwise be an enigma on the part of both consumer and caretaker. Invariably, these have been designed to avoid risks associated with pregnancy and childbirth and to provide protection for the mother and fetus.

Space does not permit a detailed explication of all of these areas in this brief chapter. Time spent with many of these selected references noted in the reading list should bear fruit over time.

The most relevant "history" of concern to the mental health consultant involves the relationship (or, often, lack of it) between obstetrics and psychiatry because both have emerged as medical specialties during the past century.

Although physicians have always been involved in childbirth care (note the writings of Hippocrates, Galen, Aretaeus, and Celsius, to name a few), for the most part, they were concerned with complicated or high-risk pregnancies. The ordinary, uncomplicated pregnancy and delivery was managed either by older female family members or by a female midwife.

The invention of the forceps by the Chamberlens, the work of Lister and Semmelweis on sepsis and childbirth fever, and the emergence of general anesthesia as a modality to control pain saw the gradual medicalization of childbirth care beginning in the second half of the nineteenth century. It is interesting that it was also during this same period that psychiatry emerged from its custodial role in large public asylums to become an identifiable specialty in medical practice.

The early years of both specialties demonstrate that each tended to dabble rather unscientifically in the territory of the other.

Charcot, Breuer, Freud, and Bernheim all considered the uterus to be involved in some way in the etiology of hysteria. Sexual drives and the organs of reproduction played a central role in the evolution of psychodynamic theories beginning around the turn of the century.

There is a fascinating history of the attitudes and practices of many obstetricians as they encountered various forms of mental illness among their patients and as they introduced a variety of procedures (usually surgical) to treat these.

A perusal of some of the obstetric literature of the last decade of the nineteenth and the first decade of the twentieth centuries is most revealing in this regard. King,[2] in 1890, described in great detail his understanding of the relationship between current sexual attitudes and practices, female anatomy, physiology, and the development of the clinical syndrome known as hysteria. In 1893, Rohé[3] broadened these observations to discuss the mental illnesses of the female population in general as they applied to diseased organs in the pelvis. One year later, Brown[4] described his experiences with a large population of "insane" women and his understanding of how this disorder related to pelvic disease. In 1894, Meyer[5] reported with great pride on a case of "insanity" in a young woman that he cured by removing her diseased ovaries. The subtitle of this paper is "A Phenomenal Triumph for Operative Treatment."

By 1902, nymphomania had come under consideration, and Frederick[6] gave a paper on his views about nymphomania as a cause of excessive venery.

Apparently not satisfied with explaining and treating the psychiatric disorders of women in the obstetric office, Winter[7] wrote a lengthy and complex paper entitled "Self-Abuse in Infancy and Childhood." There is a lengthy explanation of the evils of masturbation and its role in the pathogenesis of mental disorders together with a graduated regimen of interventions most of which would sound barbaric to the modern physician and parent.

As obstetrics moved more from the home to the hospital and operating room and became a specialty in which there was less "attending" to the patient and more emphasis on procedures, obstetricians appeared to become less interested in female behavior, both normal and abnormal. Since the early years of the twentieth century, there are few if any papers by obstetricians that concern themselves with a scientific understanding of, or intervention in, mental disorders in their patients.

Concurrent with this decrease in interest on the part of obstetrics, one sees the beginnings of an interest in the disorders associated with pregnancy and childbirth in some psychiatric and (later) child psychiatric pioneers. The latter group emerged largely from the mental hygiene and child guidance movements. Their orientation toward disorders of pregnancy tended to be more preventive and more concerned with reducing the risk for the future abnormal development of the offspring.

An excellent example of the first type of paper is that written by Burr,[8] reporting several cases of amnesia following childbirth. These are carefully written case reports and, although they shed little light on the pathogenesis of the disorder, they are among the earliest efforts in the modern literature documenting psychiatric disorders associated with the reproductive cycle.

An excellent example of the second type of paper is that of Hall and Mohr[9] entitled "Prenatal Attitudes of Primiparae: A Contribution to the Mental Hygiene of Pregnancy." These two writers were among the earliest child psychiatrists. This paper is remarkable because it points out many of the psychological and environmental contingencies that can occur during the pregnancy process and indicates how these may be related to the subsequent psychological maturation of the woman and to her ability to affiliate with the fetus and infant. The paper also contains interesting data about the necessity for objective counseling of young women who require reassurance during pregnancy.

Later, as the insights of crisis theory and the theoretical framework of public psychiatry became influences, an important paper by Lindemann[10] appeared. Twenty years later, Caplan[11] wrote persuasively about the importance of pregnancy in development of the family and the importance of early intervention if the precursors of disorder in family or child were discerned.

This growing interest on the part of psychiatrists was paralleled during the 1940s and 1950s by the emergence of several schools of psychoprophylaxis, beginning with the work of Grantly Dick-Read.[12] Many other obstetricians (see Supplementary List B) developed their own approaches to dealing with the fears and concerns of women about pregnancy and childbirth with the underlying considerations being (1) reduction of fear through various modalities of preparation; (2) increasing the sense of mastery by providing greater control on the part of the woman and her mate; (3) and reducing pain through appropriate exercise, nutrition, and psychological preparation.

These streams of thought proceeded on the whole, separately through the middle decades of the twentieth century. However, two apparently unrelated processes are now stimulating heightened mutual interest of both fields in the problems and contributions of the other.

Greater emphasis on research in fetal and infant development has served to heighten the awareness of psychiatrists and other mental health personnel about the importance of the pregnancy period and, therefore, of the desirable role of mental health workers in childbirth settings. Concurrently, the growth of the alternative health system, consumerism, and concerns about the dehumanizing effects of high-technology childbirth care are having the effect of directing the attention of obstetricians to the mental and emotional components of pregnancy and childbirth.

We are only at the dawn of a genuine collaboration between these two disciplines. As recently as a decade ago, there were few, if any reports of consultation and liaison programs in obstetrical services. Lately, we see preliminary reports of efforts to bring mental health expertise into childbirth care.[13-18] Admittedly, these are largely anecdotal in nature, but they are harbingers of more systematically designed programs.

As mental health workers express their legitimate interest in childbirth care because of their growing awareness of the impact of prenatal stress on family and child development, on the significance of perinatal care as a contributor to parental adaptation, and as it becomes increasingly difficult to separate, in the health care system, priorities that are concerned with biological development from those influencing behavior, new findings should inevitably move the two disciplines to a closer collaboration.

References

1. Rank O: *The Myth of the Birth of the Hero: A Psychological Interpretation of Mythology* (Authorized translation by Robbins F, Jelliffe SE). New York, Brunner, 1952.
2. King A: Psychiatric illness, deviant behavior and the reproductive system, in: Proceedings, Washington, DC, Obstetrics & Gynecology Society, April 1890.
3. Rohé GH: Further observations on the relation of pelvic disease and psychical disturbances. *Trans Am Assoc Obstet Gynecol,* **6**:249–255, 1893.
4. Brown JY: Pelvic disease and its relationship to insanity in women in: *Trans Am Assoc Obstet Gynecol* **7**:489–493, 1894.
5. Meyer J: A case of insanity caused by diseased ovaries, cured by their removal: A phenomenal triumph for operative treatment. *Trans Am Assoc Obstet Gynecol* **7**:504–504, 1894.
6. Frederick CC: Nyphomania as a cause of excessive venery. *Trans Am Assoc Obstet Gynecol* **20**:236–246, 1907.
7. Winter JT: Self-abuse in infancy and childhood, in *Proc:* Washington, DC, Obstetricians and Gynecologists Society, February, 1902.
8. Burr CW: Amnesia after childbirth, in Burr CW (ed) (authorized English ed) by Aschaffenburg G, Curschmann H et al: *Text-Book on Nervous Diseases.* Philadelphia, P. Blakiston's Son & Co, 1915, pp 271–278.
9. Hall DE, Mohr GJ: Prenatal attitudes of primipare: A contribution to the mental hygiene of pregnancy. *Ment Hyg* **17**:226–234, 1933.
10. Lindemann E: Observations on psychiatric sequelae to surgical operations in women. *Am J Psychiatry* **98**:132–137, 1941.
11. Caplan G: Emotional implications of pregnancy and influences on family relationships, in Stuart HC, Prugh DG (eds): *The Healthy Child.* Cambridge, MA, Harvard University Press, 1962, pp 72–82.
12. Dick-Read G: *Childbirth without Fear,* ed 2. New York, Harper & Row, 1959.
13. Mathis JL: Psychiatry and the obstetrician-gynecologist. *Med Clin North Am* **51**:1375–1380, 1967.
14. Pasnau RO: Psychiatry and obstetrics-gynecology: Report of a five-year experience in psychiatric liaison, in Pasnau RO (ed): *Consultation-Liaison Psychiatry.* New York, Grune & Stratton, 1975, pp 135–147.
15. Pitt B, Huntingford P: Psychiatry, obstetrics and gynaecology, in Creed F, Pfeffer JM (eds): *Medicine and Psychiatry: A Practical Approach.* Marshfield, MA, Pitman Publishing Company, 1982.
16. Padovano L: Liaison psychiatry and obstetrics-gynecology, in Finkel JB (ed): *Consultation-Liaison Psychiatry: Current Trends and New Perspectives.* New York, Grune & Stratton, 1983, pp 229–241.
17. Stotland NL: Contemporary issues in obstetrics and gynecology for the consultation-liaison psychiatrist. *Hospital & Community Psychiatry* **36**:1102–1108, 1985.
18. Bradley CF, King JF, Effer SB: Psychology in obstetrics: extinct or extant. *J Psychosom Obstet Gynaecol* **6**:49–57, 1987.

Supplementary Reading Lists

The following lists were culled from hundreds of bibliographic citations. They are representative of a vast literature on the historical roots and evolution of childbirth beliefs and practices. The mental health consultant cannot know too much about these subjects because they provide a frame of reference and a perspective about the field that enhance communication and the ability to identify with the overall purposes of those professionals directly responsible for delivering care. An interesting reference that is not included anywhere on these lists is a volume by Nancy Sorel entitled *Ever since Eve* (New York, Oxford University Press, 1984). This is a compendium, a kind of oral history, of the experiences of scores of real and fictional women as they proceeded through their pregnancies and deliveries. Direct quotations are included from such widely divergent individuals as Ann Boleyn and Golda Meir. Fascinating excerpts from the writings of Pablo Picasso, W. C. Fields, Ernest Hemingway, and Vladimir Nabokov, to name just a few of the male contributors, are also included.

A. General Historical References

The following should be useful in gaining a general overview of the development of childbirth care over the centuries:

Cianfrani T: *A Short History of Obstetrics and Gynecology.* Springfield, IL, Charles C Thomas, 1960.

Eccles A: *Obstetrics and Gynaecology in Tudor and Stuart England.* Kent, OH, Kent State University Press, 1982.

Findley P: *Priests of Lucina: The Story of Obstetrics.* Boston, Little, Brown, 1939.

Kerr JM, Johnstone RW, Phillips MH: *Historical Review of British Obstetrics and Gynecology 1800–1950.* Edinburgh and London, E & S Livingstone Ltd, 1954.

Mauriceau AM: *The Married Woman's Private Medical Companion.* New York, Joseph Frow Pub, 1850.

Mengert WF: *History of the American College of Obstetricians and Gynecologists 1950–1970.* Chicago, IL, ACOG, 1971.

Ricci JV: *Aetios of Amida: The Gynaecology and Obstetrics of the 6th Century A.D.* Philadelphia, Blackston Co, 1950.

Rowland B: *Medieval Woman's Guide to Health.* Kent, OH, Kent State University Press, 1981.

Singer S, Underwood EA: *A Short History of Medicine.* Oxford, Clarendon Press, 1962, pp 174–177.

Speert H: *Obstetrics and Gynecology in America: A History.* Chicago, American College of Obstetricians and Gynecologists, 1980.

Spencer HR: *The History of British Midwifery from 1650 to 1800.* London, John Bale, Sons and Danielsson, Ltd, 1927.

Wertz RW, Wertz DC: *Lying in: A History of Childbirth in America.* New York, Free Press, 1977.

B. Evolution of Childbirth Practices

An understanding of the shifting roles of childbirth caretakers, their approaches and skills, and their interrelationships is useful background information. During the past 40 years, the evolution of a variety of schools advocating different approaches to "prepared childbirth" is also an area of interest to the consultant.

Beck NC, Hall D: Natural childbirth: A review and analysis. *Obstet Gynecol* **52:**371–379, 1978.

Beck NC, Geden EA, Brouder GT: Preparation for labor: A historical perspective. *Psychosomatic Medicine* **41:**243–258, 1979.

Benedek T: The changing relationship between midwives and physicians during the Renaissance. *Bulletin of the History of Medicine* **51:**550–564, 1977.

Bradley RA: *Husband Coached Childbirth.* New York, Harper & Row, 1965.

Devitt N: The transition from home to hospital birth in the United States, 1930–1960. *Birth and the Family J* **4:**47–58, 1977.

Lamaze F: *Painless Childbirth* (Translated by Celestin LR). Chicago, Henry Regnery, 1970.

Odent M: The evolution of obstetrics at Pithiviers. *Birth and the Family J* **8:**7–15, 1981.

Vellay P: *Childbirth with Confidence.* New York, Macmillan Co, 1969.

Vellay P: Psychoprophylaxis and its evolution. *Birth and the Family J* **2:**19–22, 1975.

C. Belief Systems and Societal Attitudes and Practices

Concerns about the welfare of the gravid woman and the vulnerable fetus have inevitably led to the development of beliefs and practices that are designed to protect the mother and to ensure delivery of a healthy baby. Wide variations occur in these beliefs and practices both in Western and other cultures. Some understanding of these is useful in developing approaches to liaison and to counseling.

Ananth J: Hysterectomy and depression. *Obstet Gynecol* **52:**724–730, 1978.

Auerbach LS: Childbirth in Tunisia (implications of a decision-making model). *Soc Sci Med* **16:**1499–1506, 1982.

Brink PJ: Traditional birth attendants among the Annang of Nigeria (Current practices and proposed programs). *Soc Sci Med* **16:**1883–1892, 1982.

Browner C: The management of early pregnancy: Columbian folk concepts of fertility control. *Soc Sci Med* **14B:**25–32, 1980.

Chodoff P: Hysteria and women. *Am J Psychiatry* **139:**545–551, 1982.

Constantinides P: Women heal women: Spirit possession and sexual segregation in a Muslim society. *Soc Sci Med* **21:**685–692, 1985.

Delvecchio-Good MJ: Of blood and babies: The relationship of popular Islamic physiology to fertility. *Soc Sci Med* **14B:**147–156, 1980.

Firth R: Tikopia Ritual and Belief. Boston, Beacon Press, 1967, pp 36–45.

Jeffery R, Jeffery P, Lyon A: Female infanticide and amniocentesis. *Soc Sci Med* **19:**1207–1212, 1984.

Karim WJ: Malay midwives and witches. *Soc Sc Med* **18:**159–166, 1984.

Mack HC: Back to Sacajawea. *Am J Obstet Gynecol* **69:**933–949, 1955.

Merskey H: Hysteria: The history of an idea. *Can J Psychiatry* **28:**428–433, 1983.

Morsback G: Attitudes and experiences of Japanese mothers concerning the period of childbirth. *Psychologia: An International Journal of Psychology in the Orient* **26:**73–85, June 1983.

Sargent C: The implications of role expectations for birth assistance among Bariba women. *Soc Sci Med* **16:**1483–1489, 1982.

Sargent C: Obstetrical choice among urban women in Benin. *Soc Sci Med* **20:**287–292, 1985.

Weisberg DH: Northern Thai health care alternatives (patient control and the structure of medical pluralism). *Soc Sci and Med* **16:**1507–1517, 1982.

The Impact of Prenatal Stress on the Developing Fetus and Child

LORRAINE R. HERRENKOHL

Introduction

Organization of the central nervous system (CNS) and dependent behaviors are vulnerable to teratological disturbances during fetal ontogeny. The most characteristically studied agents taken by the pregnant mother have included nicotine, caffeine, alcohol, and drugs.[1,2] Depending on the kind and quantity of the agent, the range of effects on the offspring has spanned from shorter gestation, smaller birth size, poorer neuromuscular development, slower reflex functioning, and greater placidity to severe life-threatening symptoms of withdrawal, congenital deformity, intellectual retardation, and death. To the list of disruptive prenatal influences must now be added the teratological behavior of maternal stress.[3-5] In previous reviews[3-5] I have formulated premises and presented evidence that (1) stress affects the developing organism at any stage of life but that (2) prenatal stress has a particularly potent and lasting impact on the developing fetus, when the neural circuitry underlying later biochemical-behavioral events is being laid down.

Stress is defined as any real or imagined trauma, physical or psychological, that leads to the release of stress hormones.[3,5] The range of stressful stimuli is quite varied. In animal models, stressors have included discrete changes in environmental temperature or exogenously administered stress hormones. In human models, life situational stress such as death of loved ones, marital discord, and relocation have impacted negatively on health and behavior. Stress differs from organism to organism, and not uncommonly within the same organism, depending upon circumstances and time. The present review evaluates

---

Lorraine R. Herrenkohl • Department of Psychology, Temple University, Philadelphia, PA 19122.

the current status of representative studies of maternal stress on (1) pregnancy outcome, (2) fetal development, and (3) neonatal activity. Fourth, the review documents recent advances in the quest for underlying mechanisms of prenatal stress. The orientation is interdisciplinary: It takes into account psychodynamic, clinical, psychobiological, biopsychosocial, neurological, and endocrinological findings among others.

Maternal Stress and Pregnancy Outcome

There is strong evidence that pregnant mothers under stress are more likely than mothers who are unstressed to experience complications during birth, pregnancy, and labor. In reviewing the role of emotional factors in obstetrical complications, McDonald[6] examined articles that appeared in the preceding 15 years. He concluded that when findings are presented psychodynamically (i.e., when pseudocyesis is considered a hysterical symptom arising from conflict between fear of pregnancy and a wish for pregnancy to avoid abandonment by the husband), there is essentially no correlation between emotional factors and obstetrical difficulties. However, the most consistent finding was that women who subsequently experienced obstetric complications had higher anxiety levels and used fewer repressive types of defenses than did women who experienced normal pregnancies and deliveries. According to Leifer,[7] high anxiety is a characteristic affect during pregnancy. Few women remain unworried throughout this period. In her research, Leifer[7] found that women who were emotionally invested in the fetus focused their anxiety on the fetus, whereas women who were only moderately attached to the fetus expressed anxiety about both the self and the fetus. Women with minimal attachment to the fetus focused on the self or manifested low anxiety during pregnancy. Anxiety directed toward the fetus appeared to be a reflection of the developing maternal bond, whereas anxiety toward the self had regressive overtones.

Slow progress in labor appears to be related to "deep-seated conflicts" regarding reproduction and motherhood. Women having difficulty handling and communicating anxiety during the last part of pregnancy had dream content with themes of anxiety and threat and shorter labors than women reporting dreams without anxiety. The conclusion derived from the literature is that psychosomatic studies of labor should include both an evaluation of conflicts regarding reproduction and motherhood and an attempt to record the woman's way of handling such conflicts.

Women sampled by Uddenberg et al.[8] were 101 primigravidae randomly selected from the clinic of the University of Lund, Sweden. Semistructured interviews and tests were used to study the women during pregnancy and the puerperium. Interviews were conducted during the first half of pregnancy, 1 or 2 days postpartum and 4 months postpartum. During the interviews, a number of psychological tests were administered. The woman's willingness to admit and communicate anxiety was evaluated according to the presence of mental symptoms. Time in labor was estimated by measuring the time from the first painful uterine contraction until the birth of the child. Data indicated that time in labor was not related to the degree of mental handicap postpartum. Nor did results of a projective test administered during pregnancy correlate with labor duration. However, women who reported psychological symptoms during pregnancy generally experienced a short labor, whereas those with a greater number of reported mental symptoms had lengthy labors. This trend was particularly noticeable in women who became mentally handicapped postpartum. In women who had few difficulties postpartum, mental symptoms admitted during pregnancy were unrelated to time in labor.

Uddenberg et al.[8] believe their findings indicate that denial and repression of conflicts in the reproductive sphere are correlated with inhibition of psychophysiological processes involved in childbirth. Anxiety during pregnancy appears to facilitate these processes. They suggest that tendencies to control intense emotions are associated with slow and inefficient labor. Helping the pregnant woman to communicate her anxiety may possibly reduce the incidence of prolonged labor.

Standley et al.[9] addressed the question of whether prenatal anxiety is a unitary construct or a composite of concerns of pregnant women. The data were from a longitudinal study of parent–infant interaction conducted at the National Institute of Child Health and Human Development. Subjects were 73 married white women, all of whom were primigravidae with normal pregnancies. Women were interviewed about pregnancy, marital and social relationships, and expectations and preparation for childbirth and parenthood. Prenatal anxiety measures were included in the interviews. Information from hospital records after labor and birth included the following: duration of labor, dosage and time of administration of analgesic drugs, administration of regional block anesthesia, infant birth weight, and 1-minute Apgar score. The Neonatal Behavioral Assessment Scale was used at 48 to 72 hours after birth to assess behavioral outcome. All data collected were from normal, healthy mothers and infants.

Pregnant women expressed the most anxiety about the well-being of the child and the approaching labor and birth. Less anxiety was revealed concerning physical aspects of pregnancy, feeding of the infant, and other baby care. Thirty-five percent of the women admitted to at least one psychiatric symptom such as unexplained insomnia, fearfulness, strange ideas, and racing thoughts. Women reported anxieties about pregnancy and childbirth, parenting, and psychiatric symptoms. Younger, less educated, and unprepared women were more likely to be anxious, particularly about pregnancy and childbirth, and they evidenced more psychiatric symptomatology.

Correlations between prenatal anxiety and the course of labor, birth, and the newborn infant suggested that emotional states of pregnancy could impact on prenatal events and infant functioning. Maternal anxiety in the ninth month of pregnancy was found to be significantly related to administration of regional anesthesia during childbirth and to the infant's motor maturity 3 days after birth. The factor that showed the strongest association with anxiety of pregnancy and childbirth was preparation for childbirth. The authors observe that preparation for childbirth in the form of instructional classes seems to provide the expectant mother with skills of physiological and/or psychological coping to combat anxiety.

The degree of maternal anxiety related to childbirth was the focus of Crandon's[10] investigation. The IPAT Anxiety Self-Analysis Form was given to 146 women, ranging in age from 15 to 35 years during their third trimester of pregnancy. Anxiety scores were derived for each woman. An anxiety score of 7 or over defined the woman with ''anxiety hysteria'' or ''anxiety neurosis.'' The scores obtained were correlated with the incidence of preeclampsia, precipitate labor, prolonged labor, forceps delivery, primary postpartum hemorrhage, manual removal of the placenta, and clinical fetal distress. Thirty-four women were classified as high anxiety, and the remaining 112 were considered normal. Women in the high-anxiety group had a significantly higher incidence of preeclampsia than the normal group. Only two of 11 cases of preeclampsia occurred in the ''normal'' group. Forceps deliveries were also significantly more common among women with high-anxiety scores. All 8 women with prolonged labor were in the high-anxiety group. Nine of 13 women with precipitate labors were from the high-anxiety group. Three of 4 women who suffered primary postpartum hemorrhage were in the high-anxiety group. Two of these 3 women had a retained placenta, requiring manual removal. Clinical fetal distress in the forms of fetal tachycardia, bradycardia, or meconium-stained amniotic fluid occurred nine times, all in the high-anxiety group. Crandon[10] concluded that high anxiety during pregnancy could be a predisposing cause for maternal and prenatal mortality and morbidity. An objective measure of anxiety levels in pregnancy is recommended as a useful aid in identifying women at risk for emotionally related obstetrical difficulties.

Despite the striking technological improvements that have taken place in antenatal diagnosis and management during the last decade, the incidence of premature delivery has remained virtually unchanged in the United States. Although it has been estimated that perhaps 50% of premature births may have an obstetrical cause, social factors, including psychosocial stress, are also of etiologic significance. Nevertheless, most epidemiologic investigations have continued to emphasize medical and demographic factors, and the role of psychosocial factors in premature delivery has yet to be established. Berkowitz and Kasl[11] examined the relationships between life events and expression of pregnancy desirability and partner support to the risk of preterm delivery. The data were drawn from a case-control study that considered a large number of sociodemographic (i.e., parity, race), medico-obstetrical (hospital, delivery, neonatal records) and life situational events (desire to be pregnant, marital support) in an attempt to identify possible psychosocial risk factors of premature delivery. The authors assessed 166 mothers of preterm infants and 299 mothers of term infants. White women with preterm delivery reported higher numbers of life events and more negative attitudes toward the pregnancy than white women with term delivery. No substantial differences in these variables were found among black women. However, when level of life events was stratified by pregnancy desirability score, both white and black women with high pregnancy desirability scores were found to be at increased risk for a preterm delivery when exposed to high as compared to low levels of life events.

Laukaran and van den Berg[12] tapped a data bank of over 8,000 women at the Kaiser Foundation Health Plan in San Francisco to examine the relationship of maternal attitude to pregnancy outcome and obstetrical complications. Because maternal health, socioeconomic class, nutrition, and other factors were examined and controlled, it was possible to focus the report on maternal attitude. Negative maternal attitude toward having the baby was the single most prominent factor associated with postpartum infection and hemorrhages in the mother and congenital abnormalities and death in newborns. The mechanism whereby maternal attitude affected pregnancy outcome and health and survival of the young is unknown. However the authors favor a "stress-mediated-change-in-hormones" hypothesis.

Prenatal Stress and Fetal Outcome

Studies have demonstrated that the fetus can be affected by maternal stress. A prospective study of 146 women was undertaken to determine whether degree of maternal anxiety was related to the physical status of the newborn infant. Crandon[13] administered the IPAT Anxiety Self Analysis Form during the third trimester of pregnancy to estimate degree of anxiety. Data from the form were computed as an anxiety score for each woman. Of 146 women, 34 were high anxious, and the remaining 112 women were normal. Results were correlated with infants' 5-minute Apgar scores. The mean Apgar score was found to be significantly lower in the high-anxiety group; the mean was 5.83 compared with a mean of 9 for the normal group. Apgar scores equal to or less than 7 were found in the high-anxiety group. Crandon comments that the mechanism by which maternal anxiety and Apgar scores are related is unknown but speculates that anxiety via some chemical process may affect the Apgar score.

People who exercise regularly report fewer feelings of anxiety and stress as well as greater self-esteem, self-confidence, and self-control than those who are sedentary. Motives for exercising routinely relate directly to the physical and psychologic benefits. Psychologic adaptation to pregnancy includes understanding ambivalent feelings typical of the first trimester, even in a planned pregnancy. Altered body image, physical discomfort, and fear of personal safety contribute to this conflict. Exercise may help the pregnant woman feel physically and psychologically healthy, especially if she exercised routinely before the pregnancy. Exercise may help reduce the pregnant woman's anxiety and help her exercise control over her body and mind. Non-weight-bearing activities such as swimming, cycling, or stretching are presumed most beneficial during pregnancy.[14] Because clinical data vary, it is difficult to evaluate the effects of exercise on pregnancy and fetal outcome. Several studies report no relationship between maternal exercise habits and obstetric complications, infant birth weight, or Apgar scores.[14] However, investigators have noted more major obstetric complications in runners compared with women who do not run. There was also a trend toward failure to progress during labor. Runners had more cesarean sections than nonrunners. Another study showed that women who continued endurance exercise into the third trimester delivered earlier (mean, 8 days). Their infants were 500 g lower than those whose mothers had stopped exercising before the twenty-eighth week.[14] Birth weights of infants of those who stopped were similar to those of sedentary controls.

Elevated maternal core temperature during the first trimester is a major risk of teratogenesis. Researchers who studied 28 cases of offspring whose dysmorphism was of unknown cause found histories of first-trimester maternal hyperthermia. This CNS dysgenesis was similar to changes in offspring of guinea pigs whose deep-body temperature was artificially increased for 1 hour on gestational days 18 to 25, equivalent to 4 to 6 weeks in humans.[14] The critical deep-body temperature that increases risk of teratogenic events in both animal and human studies was 38.9 °C (102 °F).

Paolone and Worthington[14] increased body-core temperatures in five nonpregnant women of childbearing age by exercise for 40 minutes in a hot, humid environment or for 1 hour in a comfortable climate before immersion in a hot tub for 14 minutes. Vaginal temperature rose and exceeded rectal temperature. Exercise equivalent to brisk walking, jogging, or running during hot weather and to exercising vigorously in an aerobic dance class for an hour followed by a session in a whirlpool, sauna, or hot tub may put pregnant women at risk. The authors concluded that "prolonged, heavy exercise produces a compensatory fetal tachycardia that suggests a reactive hemodynamic response to temporary hypoxia" (p. 153).

Stress has been linked to hypertension in men and women, independent of reproductive state. Dalton and Shepherd[15] investigated fetal heart rate with particular reference to maternal hypertension. They found relative tachycardia during the third trimester in hypertensive pregnancies that appeared even before maternal blood pressure became abnormal. Two alternative hypotheses were advanced: Either tachycardia was a consistent response to a failing placenta, or it was a transient response to abdominal palpation or to maternal anxiety. However the methodology of the study was such that much longer periods of observation were needed to determine whether tachycardia observed was transient or at which gestational age it appeared. In a second study[16] to determine whether the fetal heart behaved differently in normotensive and hypertensive pregnancies, changes in baseline fetal heart rate were investigated prospectively from 15 to 38 weeks gestation in 16 women who were normotensive at the time of booking in the antenatal clinic. Fetal heart rate recordings were made ultrasonically and were computer processed by TELE-PLOT and BASELINE. Those women who remained normotensive were found to exhibit decreases of fetal heart rate with advancing gestational age. This did not occur in the 6 women who eventually developed hypertension.

Under what conditions might maternal blood pressure be elevated during pregnancy? Any number of conditions may suffice (i.e., salt intake, moderate anxiety, and stress), but certainly exposure to threat of war should be critical. Results of studies on animals and humans suggest that one of the most important variables in the development of high blood pressure is the exposure to stressful contingencies. Stressful events include situations such as loss of jobs, disaster, and conditions of war. Thus, Kasl and Cobb[17] reported that blood pressure of men was higher during anticipation of job loss, unemployment, or probationary reemployment than during stable employment. Men whose unemployment experience was severe had the longest period of high blood pressure. Ruskin et al.[18] found that diastolic blood pressures of more than one-half of the survivors of an earthquake in Texas City were markedly elevated for 2 weeks after the event. Graham[19] found that the diastolic blood pressure of 27% of soldiers who experienced combat in the African desert campaign in World War II remained high for several months afterwards. The effects on blood pressure was examined in pregnant women living in an area that had been a target of terrorist activities for a long period, as well as the effects of war.[20] The blood pressures of 5804 Israeli pregnant women, birthing between 1973 and 1975, who had lived in either high, medium, or low military stress environments were compared. Blood pressures that were measured immediately before delivery were taken from hospital records. Results showed that women in high-stress environments displayed significantly higher systolic and diastolic blood pressure, both during relatively calm periods and the period of the Yom Kippur War, than did women who lived in low-stress environments. Women who lived in the medium stress area were in between the two groups. War increased blood pressure in all environments. One wonders about the impact of elevated blood pressure on the 5804 fetuses and newborn.

Data compiled from a massive collaborative perinatal study at the National Institute of Neurological Diseases and Stroke provides a clue.[21] Over 10,000 pregnant women were studied in a longitudinal investigation of the effects of numerous conditions including prenatal life events, drugs, and health on offspring outcome (i.e., health, neurological development, school performance). The incidence of congenital deformity and neonatal deaths was extremely high among widows compared to nonwidows, suggesting that prenatal loss of husband is also a severe fetal shock.

Some insight into the mechanism of maternal stress as well as some precautionary measures can be found in Ascher's fine review.[22] Anxiety during pregnancy can result from factors such as alterations in body image, changes in life-style, concern over having a normal baby, family and financial stresses, and fears related to childbirth. Emotions of pregnancy can result in physiological effects such as motor tension, restlessness, tachycardia, sweating, and flushing. These symptoms are mediated by the sympathetic nervous system through the release of catecholamines and circulating levels of adrenocortical and other stress hormones.

Ascher[22] reviewed the effects of anxiety on pregnant animals. Intravenous administration of epinephrine and norepinephrine resulted in increased maternal blood pressure and markedly decreased uterine blood flow. The decrease was sustained and lasted long after maternal blood pressure had returned to preinfusion levels. Ascher[22] cites one study in which catecholamines in maternal circulation cause greater decrease in uterine blood flow and more fetal stress than strong uterine contractions induced by oxytocin. Another study found that fear associated with strange conditions, loud noises, and startling stimuli reduced uterine blood flow by 25% to 33%. Fetal changes included drops in fetal heart rate and blood pressure, fetal hypoxia and acidosis, and electrocardiographic changes, all of which may be due to decreased uterine blood flow and consequent fetal asphyxia. Other studies have found that greater levels of conditioned stress in pregnancy are associated with more emotionality, lower birth weights, and death in animal offspring.

Studies of human fetuses have suggested that high anxiety or psychological stress results in higher number of fetal abnormalities and maternal obstetric complications, lower infant birth weight, and poorer juvenile health. Primiparae are significantly more anxious during pregnancy than multiparae. Ascher[22] recommends that providers of maternity care increase awareness of possible consequences of anxiety or emotional stress on the outcome of pregnancy. Identification of women most at risk from anxiety is the first step. Health professionals should be utilized when a woman needs more psychological assistance. Parent education classes also are important in reducing anxiety levels. An increased emphasis on pregnancy as a normal physiological event may help eliminate prenatal anxiety. Continued effort can increase the use of birthing rooms and maternity homes to provide a comfortable and more familiar atmosphere in which to give birth.

Maternal Stress and Neonatal Activity

Lester Sontag, a pioneer in the study of neonatal development and maternal stress, presented the findings of the Fels Research Institute from 1936 to 1966.[23-25] Sontag described findings and procedures in great detail in the 1966 report.[24] Fetal movement was assessed by measuring pressure changes recorded from inflated bags specially laid over quadrants of the mother's abdomen. At the same time, the mother was instructed to record reactions by pressing buttons that activated kymographic records during the period she felt fetal activity. It was possible therefore to establish correlations between maternal reports and mechanically recorded fetal movements. Sontag described three different types of fetal activities: sharp kicking or pumping movement of the extremities that increased steadily from 6 months to birth; squirming or writhing slow movements that were at greatest frequency during the third to fourth month before birth and declined until birth; and sharp, convulsive movements that could be fetal hiccups or spasms of the diaphragm. Differences in fetal activity were found to be predictive of the degree of activity, restlessness, and resistance to handling infants during the first year of life. Sontag also examined reactions of fetuses to sound. In the 1920s, a German physician had reported a number of cases of expectant mothers who complained they could not go to symphony concerts because of intensified fetal kicking. Until Sontag, there had been no adequate explanation of the ability of the fetus to perceive sound. Sontag and his associates placed a small block of wood over the abdomen of 8 months pregnant women. They struck a doorbell clapper at the rate of 120 vibrations per second. In 90% of the cases, there was an immediate convulsive response by the fetus, which was believed to be a startle response similar to the Moro reflex after birth. Sontag considered that maternal variations in endocrine function helped determine the psychic and physiological progress of the fetus. It was self-evident that the physical and physiological adequacy of the fetus in turn were critical factors in its emotional and social adaptation after birth.

Sontag was able also to collect information on fetal responses to maternal stress. A case is given here:

> In one instance a young woman carrying her baby, which we had been studying weekly in terms of activity and heart rate level, took refuge at the Fels Institute building one evening because her husband had just suffered a psychotic break and was threatening to kill her. She was terrified, felt alone and did not know where to turn for help. She came to the Institute, and we gave her a bed and room for the night. When she complained after a few minutes conversation that the kicking of her fetus was so violent as to be painful, we proceeded to record the activity level. It was more than 10-fold what it had been in the weekly sessions prior to this incident. Another case came to our attention when a woman we had been studying lost her husband in an automobile accident. Again, the violence of the activity and the frequency of movement of the fetus increased by a factor of more than 10. During the period of 10 years, we managed to collect 8 such dramatic incidences, all showing the same phenomena of extreme increase in fetal activity in response to grief, fear and anxiety. Children of such mothers, who suffered their emotional trauma late in pregnancy and not early, showed, of course, no congenital defect. In general, they were, however, irritable, hyperactive, tended to have frequent stools and 3 of them had marked feeding problems (24, p. 784).

Davids et al.[26] reported that maternal anxiety during pregnancy affects mother–child adjustment as long as 8 months postpartum. The study was an outgrowth of a national collaborative project by the then-National Institute of Neurological Diseases and Blindness. Fifty pregnant women were examined at the Providence Lying-In Hospital. They were given a psychological test battery during the third trimester of pregnancy and when the babies were 8 months old. Pregnant women were examined by clinical psychologists who administered intelligence tests, self-ratings, questionnaires on psychodynamics, and projective techniques designed to reveal unconscious motivations. Eight months after birth, there was a psychological evaluation of the child's behavior and performance as judged by the Bailey Infant Mental Scale and Motor Test. The mother completed the Parental Attitude Research Instrument (PARI) to assess maternal attitudes toward family relations and childbearing practices. The examiner also observed the mother–child interaction. Pregnant women were dichotomized into high-anxiety and low-anxiety groups on the basis of the tests. Eight months later, the high-anxiety group evidenced significantly more negative child-rearing attitudes as measured by the PARI. They also received less favorable ratings by the interviewers at 8 months. The children of low-anxiety mothers had significantly higher developmental quotients on the Infant Mental Scale and higher developmental quotients on the Motor Scale. Children from low-anxiety mothers also tended to receive a more favorable general emotional-tone score than did those of high-anxiety mothers.

Ottinger and Simmons[27] examined the relationship between the behavior of human neonates and prenatal maternal anxiety. A group of obstetrical patients were administered an anxiety scale during each trimester of pregnancy. Women representing extreme scores were selected to test the hypothesis that there would be a positive relationship between maternal anxiety scores during gestation and neonatal behavior. Neonatal bodily activity, measured by a stabilimeter placed under the bassinette of the baby as well as crying behavior recorded on a microphone were assessed on the first few days of life. The data confirmed the hypothesis of a positive relationship between the mother's anxiety level and the amount of neonatal activity.

Spezzano[28] has reported an extreme example from the pediatric literature:

> A healthy 17-year-old girl gave birth to an apparently normal baby boy after a medically uncomplicated pregnancy. Twenty hours of normal infant care followed, with mother and child side by side. Then the baby vomited fresh blood. He was examined and still appeared healthy and vigorous, but his vomiting continued, and one hour later, the baby died. Postmortem examination revealed three peptic ulcers. Since peptic ulcers usually develop in adults who are chronically tense and anxious, the physicians wondered whether the mother could have been under enough stress during pregnancy to pass ulcer-causing hormones across the placenta. In fact, her pregnancy—especially in the last trimester—was extraordinarily stressful. Coerced by her parents into marrying the father of her child, she found herself living with an alcoholic wife-batterer. She went back to live with her parents, but her husband paid her frequent and distressing visits in an effort to persuade her to return to him. Not long before the day of birth he threw a brick through her window, and the police were called in.
>
> A single case certainly does not prove that maternal stress can cause gastric ulcers in a newborn, but the possibility would seem to warrant some kind of counseling for pregnant women who are exceptionally tense, anxious, or unhappy (28, p. 51).

Stott,[29] in Scotland, reported the findings of a follow-up study from birth to the fourth year of life of the effects of prenatal stress on a sample of 200 infants. By using medical records and interviews by health nurses in the home, Stott[29] drew impressive profiles of the impact of prenatal stress on health and behavioral development.

The types of child morbidities Stott[29] associated with personal tensions in pregnancy included physical illness (twice as much eczema and middle ear infections, somewhat more bronchitis, and severe respiratory trouble); minor physical and functional abnormalities (small size, profuse sweating, flushing, or choking); developmental difficulties (twice the incidence of late walking or poor walking such as flat-footed or clumsy, some speech defects); and behavioral abnormalities (twice as many entries for fretful, whimpering, restless, or clinging behaviors). Ten of 14 cases had one or more indications of behavioral disturbances characteristically associated with congenital hyperactivity.

Stott's[29] most striking finding was that marital crisis during pregnancy produced the highest child morbidity scores. A case involving marital discord during pregnancy that produced a high child morbidity score is given here:

> Marital relationship is not good. There has been frequent quarreling all through the marriage. The husband is reputed to be a heavy drinker, particularly on weekends when he is very abusive and often puts the wife out of the home. He is, however, a good worker (on constant night shift) and supports his wife and family fairly well. There is nevertheless, signs that the family may break

down completely. The night before the birth there had been a violent quarrel with husband (29, p. 776).

Stress and anxiety have been found to be factors in the course of childbearing. Their contributions to the experience of pregnancy, to birth complications, to emotional states of pregnancy, or to personality traits are all important issues. What is more important is that these are clinical problems that bear on the emotional and physical well-being of parents and their young. The research almost unanimously documents the detrimental "effects" of anxiety during pregnancy. Such external stressors as life events change and internal states, such as anxiety, have been implicated in obstetrical and neonatal complications. However, scientific understanding of the role of stress and anxiety in the course of childbearing is still new. Many questions are yet to be resolved.

1. The perinatal outcomes of anxiety are important. But it is easy to lose sight of present emotional states and interventions that may contribute to satisfaction with the pregnancy and a positive experience for both mother and father.

2. One speaks of the "effects" of anxiety on complications. The implication is that "anxiety" has caused the problem. There are alternatives to this model that cannot be ruled out. First, the subsequent complication may in fact be causing the antecedent anxiety. For example, a subclinical physical problem may exist prenatally and influence the woman's emotional state. Later this problem is manifested as an obstetrical problem, and then it is assumed that the anxiety has caused the problem. Another possibility is that positive and negative feedback interact to modulate and regulate the amount of stress hormones that the mother produces. In addition, the fetal system has a life and dynamic of its own. Its brain-pituitary-adrenal axis is active early in ontogeny. The fetal system also undergoes positive and negative feedback. Because the mother hosts the fetus and because they share a common blood supply via the placenta, a dynamic interplay exists between them. One responds to the other. The fetus therefore can be responder to changes in the mother's hormonal milieu and can be exposed to maternal stress hormones as well as its own.

A complex feedback relationship exists between and within the mother and fetus. On the one hand, the maternal stress system has a stress stimulus that triggers the release of corticotropin-releasing factor from her hypothalamus, which in turn triggers the release of adrenocorticotropin hormone (ACTH) from the anterior pituitary. This leads to the release of glucocorticoid hormones (corticosteroids, or corticoids) from the adrenal gland. A given tropic hormone may be released in response to a variety of stimuli. ACTH may be triggered by emotional stress, physical stress, low plasma corticosteroids, or merely during the course of sleep. When the glucocorticoid hormones reach the brain, their effect is inhibitory. Similar feedback relationships exist in the fetal system. A complex possibility is that both the anxiety and later complication are due to a third factor.

3. What is prenatal anxiety? Is it an enduring characteristic of the personality, relatively consistent across the life span and expressed in different ways under various conditions? Or is it an emotional state that is common to pregnancy? Studies should consider demographic variables in research designs so that intervention can be applied where they are most relevant and welcome.

4. Finally, if the effort is to avoid anxiety, then it is especially important to identify

those populations that are at risk for anxiety during pregnancy. If such anxiety is proven to be a powerful precursor of problems for mother and child, then prevention must include counseling.

Mechanisms of Prenatal Stress

Teratological agents such as nicotine and alcohol disrupt many organ and behavior systems in the developing young, including the brain-pituitary-gonadal axis.[30,31] All axes, including the adrenal glands, are influenced by stress. Prenatally, the mother is the host-mediator between the fetus and the outside environment. There is an interplay between her system and that of the fetus she bears. An adult under stress undergoes an interplay of brain, pituitary, and adrenal hormones, which feedback relationships occur when the fetus is in utero. It is possible, for example, for a stress stimulus such as increased ACTH in the mother to be a stress stimulus that in turn triggers hypothalamic and pituitary secretions in the fetus. Release of neurohormones occurs under the influence of neurotransmitters such as the catecholamines norepinephrine (NE) or dopamine (DA).

One current model of prenatal-stress animal research employs sexual differentiation of the brain. The sexual differentiation model of the brain states that the hormonal milieu, not the genome, determines sexual dimorphism in an inherently female brain.[32] Normal sexual behavior and gonadotropin secretion are established by adulthood as a function of androgens during critical perinatal sexual differentiation stages. Two lines of evidence support this view: Chemical or surgical castration of genetic males during perinatal life feminizes and demasculinizes reproductive functions, and exposure of genetic females to androgens during a critical developmental stage masculinizes and defeminizes reproductive physiology, morphology, and behavior. The severity of the masculinizing and defeminizing actions of perinatal androgens (particularly the potent metabolite estradiol) depends upon the amount and timing of the hormone.[32]

The possibility that maternal stress can influence sexual differentiation was demonstrated by Ward's[33] discovery that prenatal stress feminizes and demasculinizes sexual behavior in males. She exposed late-pregnant rats to the stresses of heat, restraint, and bright lights three times daily during the last trimester. By adulthood, the offspring showed a significant reduction in the percentage of stressed males that copulated and ejaculated compared to control males and a significant increase in lordotic performance. She believed that the prenatal stress syndrome in males, characterized by diminished copulatory patterns and increased lordotic behavior potentials, developed from diminished exposure of fetal males to gonadal androgens, presumably as a result to increased exposure to stress steroids. She also believed that parallel influences might be a cause for homosexuality in men.[34]

In an experiment with the endocrinologist Weisz, Ward found that maternal stress altered plasma testosterone in fetal male rats.[35] Ward and Weisz employed radioimmunoassay and measured plasma testosterone in cesarean-delivered normal and stressed fetal males during the last trimester of pregnancy. In normal males, a surge of plasma testosterone characteristically occurred on the eighteenth or nineteenth gestational day. This testosterone surge occurred prematurely in the stressed male, on day 17. On this basis, Ward and Weisz[35] concluded that the CNS of fetal males demasculinized and feminized, not as a result of decreased exposure in absolute amount of circulating testosterone during the late gestation, but because there is a desynchrony between the maturational stage of the CNS and patterns of testosterone secretion during fetal life.

Moyer et al.[36,37] have suggested that prenatal stress modifies the neuroanatomical and biochemical organization of the brains of both males and females. They combined the microdissection procedure of Palkovits for removing individual brain nuclei with sensitive radioisotopic enzymatic assays for norepinephrine (NE) and dopamine (DA). Moyer et al.[36] discovered that stress during pregnancy reduced steady-state levels of NE in brain regions of pregnant mothers associated with gonadotropic secretion. The major noradrenergic pathway that underwent change during maternal stress was the ventral ascending bundle (i.e., the medial preoptic nucleus, anterior hypothalamus, and median forebrain bundle). Locations of DA decreased as a function of prepartal stress and overlapped with those brain regions in which CA depletions have been implicated in functional affective disorders in humans. They postulated that the high incidence of certain mental disorders when sex steroids and CA fluctuate widely (as during diestrus, the postpartum period, and at menopause) suggests an interrelationship of female hormones, CA, and psychological state. Stress during pregnancy with corresponding changes in brain CA may set the stage for postpartum disorders.

Moyer et al.[37] also examined the effects of prenatal stress on CA concentrations in the brains of male and female offspring as adults. The major pattern of brain change in the male offspring was similar to that in stressed mothers. The major system that underwent change involved NE; the major direction of change was a decrease. The major brain regions that underwent change were those associated with gonadotropic secretion from the anterior pituitary gland and with the regulation of sexual behavior. They postulated that decreases in brain NE may be the basis for the feminized and demasculinized sexual behavior of males.

Among the interesting findings was that prenatal stress markedly affected CA concentrations in female offspring. Prenatal stress increased DA in the hypothalamic arcuate nucleus of stressed female offspring by 153%. Because marked alterations in arcuate DA have been associated with abnormalities in gonadotropic hormones from the anterior pituitary gland, it was predicted and ultimately observed that prenatal stress would produce reproductive dysfunctions in female offspring.[38]

Herrenkohl[38] exposed pregnant rats to restraint–heat stress during the last trimester and examined female offspring for reproductive function in adulthood. Pregnant rats were restrained in 18 × 8-cm semicircular Plexiglas cages under four bright lights. The procedure caused surface illumination of 400 ft-cd and surface temperature of 34 °C. Nonstressed mothers remained unhandled. When compared to nonstressed female offspring, stressed female offspring exhibited higher incidences of estrous cycle disorders, spontaneous abortions, and vaginal hemorrhages. They had higher incidences of stillbirths and neonatal mortalities in a subsequent generation of progeny. Cross-fostering procedures between and within treatment groups ruled out the possibility that prepartal-stress-induced disturbances during the postnatal period caused reproductive deficits in the offspring. Prenatal stress by itself markedly reduced fertility and fecundity in female offspring.[38,39]

Recent experiments report that maternal stress changes testicular (Leydig cell) and brain steroid aromatase activity in rat fetuses in patterns similar to alterations in fetal testosterone levels.[40,41] It has also been reported that maternal stress differentially alters pituitary, gonadal, and adrenal functions in rats and mice[42–45] and changes cellular morphology in the medial preoptic region (a reproductive-regulating region of the brain).[4,46]

Summary and Conclusions

Maternal stress has been related to neonatal activity and irritability in both lower animals and humans in documented research for at least the past 30 years. Contemporary animal research demonstrates that prenatal stress feminizes and demasculinizes the sexual behavior of males and reduces fertility and fecundity in females (i.e., in estrous cycle disorders, spontaneous abortions, vaginal hemorrhaging, and high neonatal mortality). Mechanisms of stress are being sought in the maternal-fetal blood exchange, hormonal alterations in the hypothalamus–pituitary–gonads and adrenals, and in brain catecholamines.

Human research demonstrates that negative maternal attitudes toward pregnancy are related to high incidences of congenital abnormalities and infant deaths. Severe psychosocial stress is related to pregnancy complications, neurological impairments in infants, and neonatal deaths. Data derived from both animal and human research may explain the etiology and mechanisms of prenatal-stress-induced reproductive dysfunctions as well as the impact of psychopathology on reproduction and well-being of young.

References

1. Jacobson SW, Fein GG, Jacobson JL: Neonatal correlates of prenatal exposure to smoking, caffeine and alcohol. *Infant Beh Dev* **7**:253–265, 1984.
2. Kandall SR: The newborn of the drug-dependent mother, in Marx GF (ed): *Clinical Management of Mother and Newborn*. New York, Springer-Verlag, 1979, p 221.
3. Herrenkohl LR: The anxiety-prone personality: Effects of prenatal stress on the infant, in Mathew RJ (ed): *The Biology of Anxiety*. New York, Brunner-Mazel, 1982, p. 51.
4. Herrenkohl, LR: Prenatal stress may alter sexual differentiation in male and female offspring, in Schlumpf M, Lichensteiger W (eds): *Drugs and Hormones in Brain Development*. Basel, Karger, 1983, p. 176.
5. Herrenkohl LR: Prenatal stress disrupts reproductive behavior and physiology in offspring, in Komisaruk BR, Siegel HI, Cheng M-F, Feder HH (eds): *Reproduction: A Behavioral and Neuroendocrine Prospective*. New York, New York Academy of Sciences, 1986, p. 120.
6. McDonald RL: The role of emotional factors in obstetrics: A review. *Psychosom Med* **30**:222–237, 1968.
7. Leifer M: Psychological changes accompanying pregnancy and motherhood. *Genet Psych Mono* **95**:73, 1977.
8. Uddenberg N, Fagerstrom C-F, Hakason-Zaunders M: Reproductive conflicts, mental symptoms during pregnancy and time in labor. *J Psych Res* **20**:575–581, 1976.
9. Standley K, Soule B, Copans SA: Dimension of prenatal anxiety and their influence on pregnancy outcome. *Am J Obstet Gynecol* **135**:22–26, 1979.
10. Crandon AJ: Maternal anxiety and obstetrical complications. *J Psych Res* **23**:109–111, 1979.
11. Berkowitz CS, Kasl SV: The role of psychosocial factors in spontaneous preterm delivery. *J Psychosom Res* **27**:283–290, 1983.
12. Laukaran VH, van den Berg BJ: The relationship of maternal attitude to pregnancy outcomes and obstetric complications. *Am J Obstet Gynecol* **136**:374–379, 1980.
13. Crandon AJ: Maternal anxiety and neonatal wellbeing. *J Psych Res* **23**:113–115, 1979.

14. Paolone AM, Worthington S: Cautions and advice on exercise during pregnancy. *The Active Human:* 150–163, October 1985.
15. Dalton KJ, Shepherd JH: Fetal tachycardia and pregnancy hypertension, in Sammour MB, Symonds EM, Zuspan FP et al (eds): *Pregnancy Hypertension.* Cairo, Ain Shams University Press, 1982, p. 151.
16. Dawson AJ, Dalton KJ, Newcombe RG: Baseline fetal heart rates from 15 to 38 weeks gestation in normotensive and hypertensive pregnancies. *Br J Obstet Gynecol* **92:**60–64, 1985.
17. Kasl SV, Cobb S: Blood pressure changes in men undergoing job loss: A preliminary report. *Psychosom Med* **32:**19–38, 1970.
18. Ruskin A, Beard OW, Schaffer RL: Blast hypertension: Elevated arterial pressure and victims of Texas City disaster. *Am J Med* **4:**228–236, 1948.
19. Graham JDP: High blood pressure after battle. *Lancet* **1:**239–240, 1945.
20. Rofé Y, Goldberg J: Prolonged exposure to a war environment and its effects on the blood pressure of pregnant women. *Br J Med Psych* **56:**305–311, 1983.
21. Niswander KR, Gordon M: *The Women and Their Pregnancies.* Washington, DC, US Dept. Health, Ed, Welfare, 1972.
22. Ascher BH: Maternal anxiety in pregnancy and fetal homeostasis. *J Obstet Gynecol Nurs* **7:**18–21, 1978.
23. Sontag LW: Differences in modifiability of fetal behavior and physiology. *Psychosom Med* **6:**151–154, 1944.
24. Sontag LW: Implications of fetal behavior and environment for adult personalities. *Ann NY Acad Sci* **134:**782–786, 1966.
25. Sontag LW, Reynolds EL, Torbet V: Status of infant at birth as related to basal metabolism of mothers in pregnancy. *Am J Obstet Gynecol* **48:**208–214, 1944.
26. Davids A, Holden RH, Gray GB: Maternal anxiety during pregnancy and adequacy of mother and child adjustment eight months following childbirth. *Child Dev* **34:**993–1002, 1963.
27. Ottinger DR, Simmons JE: Behavior of human neonates and prenatal maternal anxiety. *Psychol Rep* **14:**391–394, 1964.
28. Spezzano C: Prenatal psychology: Pregnant with questions. *Psychology Today,* May 1981, pp 49–57.
29. Stott DH: Follow-up study from birth of the effects of prenatal stress. *Dev Med Child Neurol* **15:**770–787, 1973.
30. Lichtensteiger W, Schlumpf M, Ribary U: Effects of nicotine on the developing gonadal axis and on central catecholamine systems of the male rat fetus, in Caciagli F, Giacobini E, Paoletti, R (eds): *Developmental Neuroscience: Physiological, Pharmacological and Clinical Aspects.* Rome, Elsevier, 1984, p 131.
31. Sparber S: Androgens and prenatal alcohol exposure. *Science* **229:**195, 1985.
32. Gorski RA: Sexual differentiation of the brain, in Krieger DT, Hughes JC (eds): *Neuroendocrinology.* Sunderland MA, Sinauer Associates, 1980, p. 215.
33. Ward IL: Prenatal stress feminizes and demasculinizes the behavior of males. *Science* **175:**82–84, 1972.
34. Ward IL: Sexual diversity, in Masur JD, Seligman MEP (eds): *Psychopathology: Experimental Models.* San Francisco, Freeman & Co, 1977, p. 387.
35. Ward IL, Weisz J: Maternal stress alters plasma testosterone in fetal males. *Science* **175:**82–84, 1980.
36. Moyer JA, Herrenkohl LR, Jacobowitz DM: Effects of stress during pregnancy on catecholamines in discrete brain regions. *Brain Res* **121:**385–393, 1977.
37. Moyer JA, Herrenkohl LR, Jacobowitz DM: Stress during pregnancy: Effects on catecholamines in discrete brain regions of offspring as adults. *Brain Res* **144:**173–178, 1978.
38. Herrenkohl LR: Prenatal stress reduces fertility and fecundity in female offspring. *Science* **206:**1097–1099, 1979.
39. Herrenkohl LR, Whitney JB: Effects of prepartal stress on postnatal nursing behavior, litter development and adult sexual behavior. *Physiol Beh* **17:**1019–1021, 1976.
40. Weisz J: Influence of maternal stress on the developmental pattern of the steroidogenic function in Leydig cells and steroid aromatose activity in the brain of rat fetuses, in Schlumpf M, Lichtensteiger W (eds): *Drugs and Hormones in Brain Development.* New York, Karger, 1983, p. 184.
41. Ward IL: The prenatal stress syndrome: Current status. *Psychoneuroendocrinol* **9:**3–11, 1984.
42. Politch JA, Herrenkohl LR: Effects of prenatal stress on reproduction in male and female mice. *Physiol Beh* **32:**95–99, 1984.
43. Politch JA, Herrenkohl LR: Prenatal ACTH and corticosterone: Effects on reproduction in male mice. *Physiol Beh* **32:**135–137, 1984.

44. Politch JA, Herrenkohl LR: Postnatal ACTH and corticosterone: Effects on reproduction in mice. *Physiol Behav* **32:**447–452, 1984.
45. Herrenkohl LR, Scott S: Prenatal stress and postnatal androgen: Effects on reproduction in female rats. *Experientia* **40:**101–103, 1984.
46. Anderson DK, Rhees RW, Fleming DE: Effects of prenatal stress on differentiation of the sexually dimorphic nucleus of the preoptic area (SDN-POA) of the rat brain. *Brain Res* **332:**113–118, 1985.

The Epidemiology of Mental and Emotional Disorders during Pregnancy and the Postpartum Period

PATRICIA A. COBLE AND NANCY L. DAY

Introduction

References to mental disturbances arising in association with the period of childbirth in women date back many centuries. Early, detailed clinical descriptions can be found in Hippocrates' *Third Book of Epidemics*[1] written in about the fourth century B.C., in a chapter entitled "Mental Alienation of Those Recently Confined and of Nursing Women" in Esquirol's *Treatise on Insanity* written in 1845,[2] and in what is perhaps the most frequently cited work among those in this field: *Treatise on Insanity in Pregnant, Puerperal and Lactating Women,*[3] written by Louis Marcé and published in 1858. In these early writings and in many following reports through about the middle of the twentieth century, these disorders were considered to be etiologically linked to the puerperium and to represent a discrete disease entity. Among the more distinctive features noted in many of these reports was the finding of very high rates of the presence of a toxic-confusional or delirious picture. Hence, terms such as *puerperal fever* or *milk fever* were frequently invoked in reference to these puerperal mental states. In an excellent review of the literature in this regard, Seager notes that, with the introduction and extensive use of antibiotics, these symptoms became much less frequently reported. Indeed, Seager indicates that reports published after the middle of the twentieth century typically note a very low incidence of infection and/or delirious reactions.[4]

Patricia A. Coble and Nancy L. Day • Department of Psychiatry, Western Psychiatric Institute and Clinic, University of Pittsburgh, Pittsburgh, PA 15213.

During the first half of the twentieth century, an important change occurred with respect to approaches used for the diagnostic classification of psychiatric disorders. This change also had a significant impact on earlier views of the puerperal mental disorders. Generally credited to the work of Adolph Meyer and his followers,[5] earlier nosological systems, which had highlighted classification by etiological association, were ultimately abandoned in favor of a more symptom-oriented approach. This new approach to psychiatric classification was well established by the mid-1950s, particularly in the United States. Using this nosological system, a growing number of investigators claimed to be unable to demonstrate significant evidence for a unique pattern of illness in puerperal as compared to nonpuerperal psychiatric disorders.[4,6-8] Such findings have led to prevailing views that, whereas the period of childbearing might render certain predisposed women more "vulnerable" to psychiatric breakdown, the pattern of illness among puerperally affected women, that is, its symptomatology, course, and outcome, does not differ significantly from that observed among nonpuerperal women and males. These views are reflected in our current psychiatric nomenclature in which the previously designated "puerperal disorders" or "postpartum psychoses" no longer appear as distinct diagnostic entities.[9] Nevertheless, these disorders continue to generate considerable controversy among nosologists and remain elusive with regard to etiology.[10]

Over the past two decades, there has been growing evidence of a renewed interest in disorders arising in women in temporal relationship to the periods of pregnancy and postpartum. This interest has been fueled largely by epidemiological studies that have challenged this nosologic decision based on the consistency with which they have found these periods to be associated with a differential risk for serious psychiatric impairment.

In general, psychiatric contacts and/or hospitalization during the period of pregnancy have been demonstrated to be lower than those in both postpartum and nonchildbearing periods, whereas rates in the postpartum period greatly exceed those in nonpuerperal women. In a population-based epidemiological study of public and private hospital admissions among women 15 to 44 years of age in Massachusetts in 1950, Pugh et al.[11] found admissions during pregnancy to be actually lower than expected for age-adjusted rates in the general population. Further examination of these cases indicated that this deficit could not be adequately accounted for by a delay in admission due to pregnancy. There was, however, a clear-cut and marked increase in the rate of psychiatric admissions within the first month or two postpartum followed by a gradual decline to population-based rates at about 8 or 9 months postpartum. Paffenbarger,[12] in a hospital record review of 15 to 44-year-old women admitted to psychiatric facilities in Hamilton County, Ohio, during the 1940–1958 period, likewise found the frequency of admissions during pregnancy to be low and demonstrated that up to 18 times as many women were admitted to psychiatric units in the first month postpartum as in each month of pregnancy. These patterns for lower psychiatric contact during pregnancy as compared to the postpartum period have been confirmed in more recent studies conducted in Great Britain.[13,14]

The relative risk of serious psychiatric illness when it is immediately preceded by the event of childbirth has been estimated to be 15-fold.[13] This risk estimate is striking, particularly when compared to estimates for the role played by most other major psychological stressors or life events in the genesis of psychiatric disorders. These are reported to vary from 2 to 7.[15] Although a number of risk factors have been proposed, the surest predictors of these more serious postpartum disorders have been the presence of a previous personal or a strong family history of psychiatric illness, particularly of affective disorders.[4,12,16-19]

Our current knowledge of the incidence and prevalence of less serious emotional disturbances arising in pregnant and postpartum women is far less certain. Many of these disorders have received little investigative attention. Among those studies that have been undertaken, findings have been frequently contradictory or difficult and even impossible to compare. Samples have tended to be quite heterogeneous, the methods and timing of assessments have varied widely, and appropriate control groups have often been lacking. Findings from a number of more recent systematically conducted, prospective investigations do suggest, however, that the prevalence and severity of such states, particularly of depression occurring in the postpartum period, may well be quite extensive, affecting as many as 15% to 20% of all childbearing women.[16,20-24] Even more alarming are findings indicating that despite an increase in the number of health care contacts associated with the period of childbearing in women, the vast majority of these disorders goes virtually unrecognized and untreated.[25] The potential implications for adverse outcome among mothers and their infants as well as for society as a whole are only just beginning to be appreciated by psychiatry and obstetrics alike.

Review of Modern Literature

A comprehensive review of the existing literature is beyond the scope of this chapter. References cited here have been selected, based largely upon their representativeness with respect to available information on the disorders presented. For more extensive coverage of these areas, the interested reader is referred to Selected Readings (p. 46) which lists a number of excellent reviews and published monographs on the subject of mental and emotional disorders in pregnant and postpartum women.

We will begin by reviewing the various hypotheses that have been proposed to account for the excess of psychiatric disturbances in women during periods of childbearing and will also briefly highlight the normal reactions of women to pregnancy and motherhood.

Theories of Causation

Despite a large and growing body of evidence in support of a relationship between the period of childbearing and mental disturbances in women, causal mechanisms remain uncertain and controversial. Theories of hormonal or endocrine causation have understandably received considerable attention. The hormonal changes of pregnancy and parturition are unique, characterized by blood levels of both estrogen and progesterone gradually increasing to unparalleled highs during pregnancy, then falling dramatically and reversing to baseline within 2 to 5 days postpartum. Epidemiological patterns indicating low rates of illness in pregnancy followed by a sharp increase in impairment, particularly during the early weeks postpartum, have suggested that these changes might be etiological. To date, however, findings in these regards have been disappointing overall with few consistent or significant differences having been demonstrated between affected and nonaffected puerperal subjects and healthy nonpuerperal controls. The vast majority of this work, however, has been conducted among women with mild affective symptoms or the so called "maternity blues." These states are known to affect from 50% to 70% of women but are typically self-limited, resolving without any need for treatment, usually within 2 weeks postpartum. Although there is some support for hormonal causation in these states, there is virtually no information available on hormonal variables in women with more clinically significant levels of psychiatric impairment.[26,27]

Genetic and/or constitutional factors have received somewhat more support as causal factors, at least with respect to the more severe manifestations of these disorders. The presence of a past personal and/or family history of significant psychiatric illness, most notably of affective illnesses, has frequently been found in a large proportion of puerperally impaired women. Protheroe,[6] for example, found the morbid risk for nonpostpartum affective illness among first-degree relatives of affectively disordered puerperal patients to be 9% to 15%, which is higher than that for the general population. He also noted an increased morbid risk for schizophrenia in the relatives of his schizophrenic puerperal patients.

A number of investigators have reported increased rates of postpartum illness in women with manic-depressive disorder. For example, Whalley et al.,[28] in a sample of manic-depressive women, found the rate of postpartum illness to be 33 per 1000 births, far exceeding estimates for the general population that are 1–2 per 1000 births. Reich and Winokur and Kadrmas et al.[29,30] likewise noted an increase in the rate of postpartum episodes among bipolar women and further stated that the frequency of postpartum episodes was greater than that of nonpostpartum episodes in both the period of childbearing and the period of lifetime risk (15–80 years). Baker et al.[31] have reported that postpartum disorders may occur less frequently among women with unipolar as compared to bipolar illness. They found 40% of bipolar patients had had a postpartum episode as compared to 17% in the unipolar patients they examined and noted also that, among bipolar patients, 30% of pregnancies were followed by postpartum episodes as compared to only 7% in unipolar patients. Finally, a number of studies have demonstrated that among women who have experienced a prior postpartum episode, the risk of recurrence is quite high, ranging from 64% to 100%.[29,32–33] Garvey et al.[33] have suggested that this may represent a subset of affective disorder in which affected women are rendered particularly susceptible to factors associated with childbirth.

Psychological theories of causation have been proposed and are highlighted by the significant-event concept. Numerous factors, including ambivalence or negative attitude regarding a pregnancy, primary role conflict, lack of emotional and/or material support, and an increased number of life events have been reported to be differentially present among symptomatic as compared to nonsymptomatic women during pregnancy and the postpartum.[17,20,34–39] Although these factors have clearly been shown to contribute as risk factors in pregnant and postpartum woman, they have not as yet been demonstrated to be directly causal, particularly with respect to the more clinically significant psychiatric syndromes occurring in women at these times in their lives.

Prevailing views are perhaps best described as being reflective of a multifactorial or "stress summation" theory[40] in which all of these factors contribute. Empirically derived evidence in support of such a theory is, however, as yet not readily available.

Normal Psychological Reactions to Pregnancy and Motherhood

Pregnancy is one of a number of maturational crises in the female life cycle involving both physical and psychological changes, the implications of which are irreversible and lifelong. As is true for all developmental crises in the human life cycle, the event of pregnancy should be expected to elicit a variety of stressful and conflict-laden emotional responses. For any given women, the amount of disequilibrium experienced will depend not only upon the emotional environment within which a given pregnancy occurs but also on the degree to which previous psychological milestones have been achieved and earlier problems and conflicts resolved. Optimally, pregnancy, like other life crises, offers a unique opportunity for maturational growth through the resolution of both new and preexisting concerns. Issues commonly posed by the events of pregnancy and parenthood have been dealt with extensively in Chapter 5. Emotional responses to these adaptational tasks of pregnancy and parenthood can range from mild manifestations of ambivalence and anxiety to more extreme manifestations consistent with the onset of a clear-cut episode of psychiatric illness.

For the former, reassurance, support, and the provision of information relative to the concerns of pregnant women and new mothers will generally be the only intervention required. For the latter group of women, psychiatric consultation is clearly indicated and should be considered as well for women whose history suggests that they might be at high risk for the development of emotional difficulty. These historical risk factors include, among others, a past history of psychiatric illness, treatment, or hospitalization; previous difficulties with pregnancy, delivery, or postpartum psychiatric illness; a prior history of serious difficulty in adjustment at other maturational stages; marital discord or other family difficulties; unmarried status and/or poverty of resources for social support; previous history of miscarriage, premature birth, stillbirth, or the birth of a defective child and/or the possibility of such in the present pregnancy; and extremes of age (under 17 or over 40).[41-43]

Our overview of mental and emotional disturbances in pregnant and postpartum women has been arbitrarily divided into three categories: subclinical states and adjustment disorders, psychophysiologic conditions, and psychiatric disorders.

Subclinical States and Adjustment Disorders

As previously indicated, the periods of pregnancy and postpartum are inherently stressful and universally associated with characteristic disturbances in psychophysiological functioning. Ambivalence, anxiety, and lability of mood as well as disturbances in appetite, sleep, and sexual interest and activity are reported to be extremely common and "normal."[44] Maladjustment has been qualitatively described as being characterized by "excesses" in these responses, yet there are surprisingly few quantitative data available in these regards. The degree of social and occupational impairment in women with such adjustment problems is not known. Several more recent longitudinal studies aimed primarily at the identification of postpartum depression and using more standardized methods of assessment have reported the prevalence of "mild" or subclinical depression to range from 16% to 20% in pregnancy and postpartum.[45-49]

The condition for which the greatest amount of quantitative data is available is that of the so called "maternity or postpartum blues." This condition is estimated to affect from 50% to 70% of all women postpartum, rates that have been shown to be similar across cultures. Weeping is the hallmark of the blues. It generally begins between the third and the tenth postpartum days, peaking on day 5, and is frequently associated with other manifestations of emotional hypersensitivity and/or vulnerability. Other symptoms have included insomnia, irritability, forgetfulness, and headache. The blues typically last from 1 to 2 days to 2 weeks, are self-limited, generally requiring only reassurance and support, and have not been shown to be related to more severe forms of psychiatric impairment postpartum. Hormonal changes are suggested to be the basis of this condition.[24,49,50–54]

Psychophysiologic Conditions

Although a variety of psychophysiologic conditions such as asthma or migraine may be affected by pregnancy, the two conditions that are typically encountered in obstetrical practice and invariably require some psychiatric intervention are hyperemesis gravidarum and pseudocyesis.

Hyperemesis gravidarum is a severe form of intractable vomiting which occurs in pregnant women. The incidence of this disorder is quite low, having been estimated to occur in only approximately 1 per 1000 women in the United States and ranging from 0.5 to 10 per 1000 women cross-culturally.[55] Though the disorder was once considered merely a more severe form of the universally common "morning sickness" of early pregnancy, the two are currently viewed as being qualitatively different disorders. Morning sickness occurs in 50% to 75% of all pregnant women, does not seriously affect nutritional state or weight, and seems to have little psychological significance. It peaks at 8 to 12 weeks of gestation and generally disappears between weeks 12 and 16. In contrast, hyperemesis is much more severe, persists through the second trimester of pregnancy, may be life-threatening, and is often associated with psychological problems. We note here also, that although quite rare, anorexia nervosa may occur in pregnancy. It can usually be easily differentiated from hyperemesis, however, in its tendency to produce metabolic acidosis as opposed to the metabolic alkalosis more typically associated with the persistent vomiting of hyperemesis gravidarum.

Early psychoanalytic theory viewed hyperemesis gravidarum as a purely psychic disorder reflective of a symbolic rejection of the fetus.[56] Today, it is considered a psychophysiologic disorder being neither entirely organically nor psychologically based. Correlates of the disorder include a history of previously unsuccessful or unwanted pregnancy, multiple birth, below average IQ, unmarried status, poor social supports, and the preexistence of a number of psychiatric syndromes including histrionic personality disorder, borderline personality disorder, and somatization disorder. Treatment strategies include both medical intervention with hospitalization, intravenous fluid replacement and/or parenteral antiemetics, and supportive psychotherapy.

Pseudocyesis is one of the oldest known psychophysiologic disorders, having been described by Hippocrates many centuries ago, and presenting in this instance *as* pregnancy. It is marked by the absolute conviction of a nonpregnant woman that she is pregnant. Pregnancy signs and symptoms develop, and the disorder has been missed by more than a few excellent practitioners until the point of unproductive labor. The disorder typically occurs in older women but can present at any age, including prior to menarche and following menopause. The disorder has also been observed to occur in males. Pseudocyesis is an extremely rare disorder whose incidence seems to be decreasing,[57] perhaps owing to social change and the number of roles in addition to motherhood that are increasingly socially sanctioned.

Pseudocyesis must be differentiated from delusional disorders, pseudopregnancy resulting from tumor growth, and factitious disorder or simulated pregnancy in which the woman may *profess* to be pregnant but knows she is not.

Psychiatric Disorders

As earlier noted, epidemiological studies have reported rates of psychiatric contacts to be lower than for the general population during pregnancy but to rise sharply in the early postpartum period. Population-based rates for serious psychiatric illness arising in the postpartum period have remained surprisingly stable over time at approximately 1 to 2 per 1,000 births.[11–14,58–61] Rates of postpartum illness have been found to be significantly higher than this in populations of women with a history of affective illness, particularly among those with manic-depressive disorder.[28–30]

Examination of puerperally ill samples using established diagnostic criteria has shown from 50% to 75% of patients suffer from affective illnesses,[4,6,8,19,62–63] 10% to 20% from schizophrenic illnesses,[8,19,62,63] and only 2% to 12% from organic psychiatric disorders.[62,63] Anxiety disorders were found by Seager in 12% of his sample.[4]

In several more recent prospective studies among either selected or random samples of pregnant women, using DSM-III criteria for diagnosing illnesses, Cutrona et al.[21] reported a point prevalence for major depressive disorder of 3.5% in the third trimester of pregnancy and 8.1% for the first 2 months postpartum. O'Hara et al.[22] reported the prevalence of major and minor depressive disorders to be 9% in the second trimester of pregnancy and 12% in the first 6 months postpartum. Half of the postpartum episodes were noted to begin in the first month postpartum. At both assessment points, two-thirds of the depressed women met criteria for a major depressive disorder. Watson et al.[23] reported the following prevalence rates: at 16 weeks of gestation, 6.3% of their sample met criteria for psychiatric diagnoses, 62% with affective disorders, 25% with agoraphobia, and 12% with alcoholism; between 16 weeks of gestation and term, an additional 7% met criteria, 78% with affective disorders, 11% with agoraphobia, and 11% with obsessive neurosis; during the first 6 weeks postpartum, 16% of the sample met criteria, 75% with affective disorders, 15% with agoraphobia, 5% with alcoholism, and 5% with obsessive neurosis. In the only such study to compute incidence rates for disorders, Kumar and Robson[24] found in a sample of 119 first-time mothers, a 16% prevalence of clinical depression (13% were major, 73% minor, and 13% intermittent depressive disorder) at 12 weeks of gestation. Ten percent were actually new cases arising since the time of conception. Eighty-five percent of these cases had remitted by the time of delivery. In this sample of first-time mothers, 13% experienced a depressive disorder in the first 4 to 6 weeks postpartum.

Finally, McNeil et al.[38] examined the effect of pregnancy on the mental health of a sample of women with a past history of nonorganic psychoses, comparing them to demographically similar pregnant controls. Controls showed either no change or only a slight worsening of mental health during pregnancy, whereas index cases showed significant increases in rates of active mental disturbances. The most disturbed were those women with a history of schizophrenia. Only women with a history of affective illness did not differ from controls during pregnancy. It is interesting, however, that 27% of this group experienced a new episode of major depression within the first postpartum month. Despite the high rates of mental disturbances in these women, only one-third were in contact with a psychiatrist during their pregnancy.

Conclusion

Although the incidence of frank and severe psychiatric illness is relatively rare among pregnant and postpartum women, the incidence and prevalence of mild to moderately severe disorders is not fully known at present but is suggested to be higher than has previously been believed. There are also few data available on the degree of impairment among women as a result of the "normal" stresses of childbearing. As more women, particularly married women of childbearing age, are entering the workforce and more are delaying their childbearing until after beginning their careers, the economic consequences of even minor functional impairment could be quite serious. Clearly, more studies are needed not only to better define the extent of the problem but also to better understand ways in which we might facilitate the adaptational tasks of childbearing.

References

1. Jones WHS: *Hippocrates—With an English Translation,* vol 1. London, Heinemann, 1923.
2. Esquirol E: *Mental Maladies: A Treatise on Insanity* (translated by EK Hunt). Philadelphia, Lea & Blanchard, 1845.
3. Marcé LV: *Traité de la Folie des Femmes Encientes, de Nouvelles, Accouchées et de Nourrices.* Paris, Baillière, 1858.
4. Seager C P: A controlled study of post-partum mental illness. *J. Ment Sci* **106:**214–230, 1960.
5. Mora G: Historical and theoretical trends in psychiatry, Freedman AM, Kaplan HI, and Sadock BJ (eds): *Comprehensive Textbook of Psychiatry—II,* ed 2, Vol 1. Baltimore, Williams & Wilkins, 1975, pp 1–75.
6. Protheroe C: Puerperal psychoses: A long term study, 1927–1961. *Br J Psychiatry* **115:**9–30, 1969.
7. Garvey MJ, Tuason VB, Lumry AE, Hoffman NG: Occurrence of depression in the postpartum state. *J Affect Disorders* **5:**97–101, 1983.
8. Schopf J, Bryois C, Jonquiere M, Le PK: On the nosology of severe psychiatric post-partum disorders: Results of a catamnestic investigation. *Eur Arch Psychiat Neurol Sci* **234:**54–63, 1984.
9. American Psychiatric Association: *Diagnostic and Statistical Manual of Mental Disorders,* ed. 3. Washington, DC, Author, 1980.
10. Hamilton JA: The identity of postpartum psychosis, Brockington I F, Kumar R (eds): *Motherhood and Mental Illness.* London, Academic Press, 1982, pp 1–17.
11. Pugh TF, Jerath BK, Schmidt WM, Reed RB: Rates of mental disease related to childbearing. *N Engl J Med* **268:**1224–1228, 1963.
12. Paffenbarger RS: Epidemiological aspects of parapartum mental illness. *Brit J Prev Soc Med* **18:**189–195, 1964.
13. Kendell RE, Wainwright S, Hailey A, Shannon B: The influence of childbirth on psychiatric morbidity. *Psychol Med* **6:**297–302, 1976.

14. Kendell RE, Rennie D, Clarke JA, Dean C: The social and obstetric correlates of psychiatric admission in the puerperium. *Psychol Med* **11**:341–350, 1981.
15. Paykel ES: Contribution of life events to causation of psychiatric illness. *Psychol Med* **8**:245–253, 1978.
16. Pitt B: Depression and childbirth, in Paykel ES (ed): *Handbook of Affective Disorders*. New York, Guilford Press, 1982, pp 361–379.
17. Paykel ES, Emms EM, Fletcher J, Rassaby ES: Life events and social support in puerperal depression. *Br J Psychiatry* **136**:339–346, 1980.
18. O'Hare MW, Rehm LP, Campbell SB: Postpartum depression: A role for social network and life stress variables. *J Nerv Ment Dis* **171**:336–341, 1983.
19. Davidson J, Robertson E: A follow-up study of post-partum illness, 1946–1978. *Acta Psychiatr Scand* **71**:451–457, 1985.
20. Nilsson A, Almgren PE: Paranatal emotional adjustment: A prospective investigation of 165 women. Part II. The influence of background factors, psychiatric history, parental relations, and personality characteristics. *Acta Psychiatr Scand* **222**:65–141, 1970.
21. Cutrona CE: Causal attributions and perinatal depression. *J Abn Psychol* **92**:161–172, 1983.
22. O'Hara MW, Neunaber DJ, Zekoski EM: Prospective study of postpartum depression: Prevalence, course, and predictive factors. *J Abn Psychol* **93**:158–171, 1984.
23. Watson JP, Elliott SA, Rugg AJ, Brough DI: Psychiatric disorder in pregnancy and the first postnatal year. *Br J Psychiatry* **144**:453–462, 1984.
24. Kumar R, Robson KM: A prospective study of emotional disorders in childbearing women. *Br J Psychiatry* **144**:35–47, 1984.
25. Cox JL: *Postnatal Depression: A Guide for Health Professionals*. New York, Churchill Livingstone, 1986.
26. Gelder M: Hormones and post-partum depression, in Sandler M (ed): *Mental Illness in Pregnancy and the Puerperium*. Oxford, Oxford University Press, 1978, pp 80–90.
27. Campbell, JL, Winokur, G: Postpartum affective disorders: Selected biological aspects, in Inwood, DG (ed): *Recent Advances in Postpartum Psychiatric Disorders*. Washington, DC, American Psychiatric Press, Inc, 1985, pp 19–39.
28. Whalley, LJ, Roberts, DF, Wentzel, J, Wright, AF: Genetic factors in puerperal affective psychoses. *Acta Psychiatr Scand* **65**:180–193, 1982.
29. Reich, T, Winokur, G: Postpartum psychoses in patients with manic-depressive disease. *J. Nerv. Ment. Dis.* **151**:60–68, 1970.
30. Kadrmas, A, Winokur, G, Crowe, R: Postpartum manias. *Br J Psychiatry* **135**:551–554, 1979.
31. Baker M, Dorzab J, Winokur G, Cadoret R: Depressive disease: The effect of the postpartum state. *Biol Psychiat* **3**:357–365, 1971.
32. Bratfos, O, Haug, O: Puerperal mental disorders in manic-depressive females. *Acta Psychiatr Scand* **42**:285–294, 1966.
33. Garvey MJ, Tuason VB, Lumry AE, Hoffman HG: Occurrence of depression in the postpartum state. *J Affect Disord* **5**:97–101, 1983.
34. Bergler, E: Psychoprophylaxis of postpartum depression. *Postgrad Med* **25**:164–168, 1959.
35. Douglas G: Puerperal depression and excessive compliance with the mother. *Br J Med Psychol* **36**:271–278, 1963.
36. Frommer EA, O'Shea G: Antenatal identification of women liable to have problems in managing their infants. *Brit J Psychiat* **123**:149–156, 1973.
37. Brown GW, Bhrolchain NM, Harris T: Social class and psychiatric disturbance among women in an urban population. *Sociology* **9**:225–254, 1975.
38. McNeil TF, Kaij L, Malmquist-Larsson A: Women with nonorganic psychosis: Pregnancy's effect on mental health during pregnancy. *Acta Psychiatr Scand* **70**:140–148, 1984.
39. McNeil TF, Kaij L, Malmquist-Larsson A: Women with nonorganic psychosis: Factors associated with pregnancy's effect on mental health. *Acta Psychiatr Scand* **70**:209–219, 1984.
40. Herzog A, Detre T: Psychotic reactions associated with childbirth. *Dis Nerv Syst* **37**:229–235, 1976.
41. Gise LH: Psychiatric implications of pregnancy, in Cherry SH, Berkowitz RL, Kase NG (eds): *Rovinsky and Guttmacher's Medical, Surgical, and Gynecological Complications of Pregnancy*, ed. 3. Baltimore, Williams & Wilkins, 1985.
42. Helper MM, Cohen RL, Beitenman ET, Eaton LF: Life-events and acceptance of pregnancy. *J Psychosom Res* **12**:183–188, 1968.

43. Cohen RL: Maladaptation to pregnancy. *Seminars in Perinatology* **3(1):**15–24, 1979.
44. Nadelson CC: "Normal" and "special" aspects of pregnancy: A psychological approach, in Nadelson CC, Notman MT (eds): *The Woman Patient. Medical and Psychological Interfaces: Vol. 1. Sexual and Reproductive Aspects of Women's Health Care.* New York, Plenum Press, 1978, pp 73–86.
45. Hayworth J, Little BC, Carter SB, Raptopoulos P, Priest RG, Sandler, M: A predictive study of postpartum depression: Some predisposing characteristics. *Br J Med Psychol* **53:**161–167, 1980.
46. O'Hara MW, Rehm LP, Campbell SB: Predicting depressive symptomatology: Cognitive behavioral models and postpartum depression. *J Abn Psychol* **91(6):**457–461, 1982.
47. Bridge LR, Little BC, Hayworth J, Dewhurst J, Priest R G: Psychometric ante-natal predictors of post-natal depressed mood. *J Psychosom Res* **29(3):**325–331, 1985.
48. Saks BR, Frank JB, Lowe TL, Berman W, Naftolin F, Cohen DJ: Depressed mood during pregnancy and the puerperium: Clinical recognition and implications for clinical practice. *Am J Psychiatr* **142(6):**728–731, 1985.
49. Buesching DP, Glasser ML, Frate DA: Progression of depression in the prenatal and postpartum periods. *Women & Health* **11(2):**61–78, 1986.
50. Tobin SM: Emotional depression during pregnancy. *Obstetr and Gynecol* **10(6):**677–681, 1957.
51. Yalom ID, Lunde DT, Moos RH, Hamburg DA: "Postpartum blues" syndrome: A description and related variables. *Arch Gen Psychiatr* **18:**16–27, 1968.
52. Pitt B: "Atypical" depression following childbirth. *Br J Psychiatr* **114:**1325–1335, 1968.
53. Dalton K: Prospective study into puerperal depression. *Br J Psychiatry* **118:**689–692, 1971.
54. Harris B: "Maternity blues" in East African clinic attenders. *Arch Gen Psychiatry* **38:**1293–1295, 1981.
55. Fairweather DV: Nausea and vomiting of pregnancy. *Am J Obstet Gynecol* **102:**125–175, 1968.
56. Freud S, Breuer J: Studies on hysteria, in Freud S (ed): *Complete Psychological Works,* standard ed 2. London, Hogarth Press, 1955.
57. Murray JG, Abraham GE: Pseudocyesis: A review. *Obstet and Gynecol* **51:**627–631, 1978.
58. Jones R: Puerperal insanity. *Br Med J* **1:**579–585, 1902.
59. Boyd DA: Mental disorders associated with childbearing. *Am J Obstet Gynecol* **43:**148–163, 335–349, 1942.
60. Hemphill RE: Incidence and nature of puerperal psychiatric illness. *Br Med J* **2:**1232–1235, 1952.
61. Butts HF: Post-partum psychiatric problems: A review of the literature dealing with etiological theories. *J Nat Med Ass* **61:**136–139, 1969.
62. Brockington IF, Cernik KF, Schofield EM, Downing AR, Francis AF, Keelan C: Puerperal psychosis: Phenomena and diagnosis. *Arch Gen Psychiat* **38:**829–833, 1981.
63. Ifabumuyi OI, Akindele MO: Postpartum mental illness in northern Nigeria. *Acta Psychiatr Scand* **72:**63–68, 1985.

Selected Readings on Puerperal Mental Disturbances

1. Weissman MM, Paykel ES, Klerman GL: The depressed woman as mother. *Soc Psychiatry* **7:**98–108, 1972.
2. Pitt B: *Feelings about Childbirth.* London, Sheldon Press, 1978.
3. Sandler M (ed): *Mental Illness in Pregnancy and the Puerperium.* Oxford, Oxford University Press, 1978.
4. Dalton K: *Depression after Childbirth.* Oxford, Oxford University Press, 1980.
5. Welburn V: *Postnatal Depression.* London, Fontana Books, 1980.
6. Brockington IF, Kumar R (eds): *Motherhood and Mental Illness.* New York, Grune & Stratton, 1982.
7. Pitt B: Depression and childbirth, in Paykel ES (ed): *Handbook of Affective Disorders.* New York, Guilford Press, 1982, pp 361–379.
8. Stern G, Kurckman L: Multi-disciplinary perspectives on post-partum depression: An anthropological critique. *Soc Sci Med* **17:**1027–1041, 1983.

9. True-Sorderstrom BA, Buckwalter KC, Kerfoot KM: Post-partum depression. *Maternal–Child Nursing Journal* **12(2):**109–118, 1983.

10. Hopkins J, Marcus M, Campbell SB: Postpartum depression: A critical review. *Psychol Bull* **95(3):** 498–515, 1984.

11. Gise LH: Psychiatric implications of pregnancy, in Cherry SH, Berkowitz RL, Kase NG (eds): *Rovinsky and Guttmacher's Medical, Surgical, and Gynecological Complications of Pregnancy,* ed 3. Baltimore, Williams & Wilkins, 1985.

12. Inwood DG (ed): *Recent Advances in Postpartum Psychiatric Disorders.* Washington, DC, American Psychiatric Press, Inc., 1985.

13. Myles M: *Textbook for Midwives,* ed 10. Edinburgh, Churchill Livingstone, 1985.

14. Cox JL: *Postnatal Depression: A Guide for Health Professionals.* New York, Churchill Livingstone, 1986.

II

The Building Blocks

5

Developmental Tasks of Pregnancy and Transition to Parenthood

An Approach to Assessment

RICHARD L. COHEN

Introduction

This chapter embodies two closely related foci. The first involves a presentation of the developmental tasks of pregnancy (especially as they stand out during the first pregnancy). The second describes a conceptual framework and a clinical approach for using such developmental information in assessing the status of the pregnant woman's assets and liabilities and for developing an action-oriented approach to intervention where that is indicated. The learning of normal function and normal modes of adaptation must have practical application for the clinician and consultant or they will soon be forgotten. Retention of such knowledge is rapidly lost unless it is used on a daily basis in the helping process. It is for this reason that the two foci mentioned before are not presented consecutively in this chapter. Rather, an effort is made to interweave them so that the evolving developmental process of pregnancy is presented as a basis for organizing an interview process that integrates that developmental model. This is particularly important during pregnancy because the eliciting of isolated behavioral phenomena through unstructured interviewing or, conversely, highly structured rating scales may mislead the examiner into exaggerating the importance of an isolated episode. The context in which such behavior occurs during pregnancy is all important.

Intimate knowledge of pregnancy adaptational modes should be one of the crucial

Richard L. Cohen • Department of Psychiatry, Western Psychiatric Institute and Clinic, University of Pittsburgh, Pittsburgh, PA 15213.

data bases that the consultant brings to the evaluation process. It is, in fact, one of the three legs of the tripod on which an expert consultation is based. The other two will be discussed in subsequent chapters. They involve a knowledge of the prevalence and forms of major psychiatric disorders during pregnancy and a knowledge of the various settings in which childbirth care is given.

There is a temptation to skip this first leg of the tripod because most clinicians, by way of training and experience, are preoccupied with pathology and dysfunction. Yet no surgeon would dream of practicing without an intimate knowledge of anatomy and physiology; no metabolic specialist would dream of entering the office without first becoming intimately familiar with healthy metabolism; every cardiologist is an expert on normal cardiac function and must use this knowledge as his or her baseline data for understanding and intervening in pathologic states.

Unfortunately, it is the rare clinician who is taught or has learned the normal developmental process of pregnancy. Those who have experienced it directly through pregnancy and childbirth will certainly have more basic awareness than most. This is valuable and can be used but, in fact, the helping profession of medicine is still dominated by men whose knowledge of pregnancy is skimpy at best and by a significant number of nulliparous woman.

Reading this chapter and mastering this content may be initially helpful. However, this is not a substitute for investing time and energy in learning "normal" pregnancy development by observation and by interviewing large numbers of normal pregnant women at various stages of development.

A framework for conducting and recording such interviews is presented in this chapter. The same interview, in rather abbreviated form, can be used as a clinical instrument during consultations. The more expanded version should be used if one expects to grasp the significance of pregnancy in female development. Such interviews are more than "finger exercises." They should never become tedious or routine. When conducted well, they are stimulating and exciting journeys into the life course of a woman during what many judge is the most important developmental crisis that women experience.

There are several workable models that conceptualize the developmental course of pregnancy. One of these will be outlined in some detail as a basis for assessment, but others can be equally useful and are described in the literature.[1-16] Each has positive features and its own specific advantages and disadvantages. Unfortunately, there is no commonly accepted theory or approach, nor is there a framework for integrating the various models. Furthermore, although much is known about physiologic processes during pregnancy and the major changes that evolve in the pregnant woman's endocrine system,[17-22] there are no data that relate these changes on any kind of one-to-one basis to the personality, temperamental, and emotional developments that characterize the reproductive period. What is sorely needed is a unifying theory (supported by empirical data) that truly integrates what is known about physiologic changes with the psychological and interpersonal shifts that seem to be general themes for many women immediately before, during, and following pregnancy.

An excellent illustration of our inadequate understanding of the relationship between biochemical and behavioral changes during pregnancy has been discussed in a paper by Morgan and Hytten.[23] These investigators and others[24,25] reported that there is a large number of biochemical and hormonal shifts between the eighteenth and twenty-fifth week of pregnancy, yet many women describe this period of time as being the most tranquil, emotionally stable, and relaxed period of the entire pregnancy. Morgan and Hytten have reported a rising serum concentration of the enzyme polyamine oxidase around 20 weeks, whereas others have reported a marked increase in histaminase and diamine oxidase. Perusal of the literature suggests that there are many examples of important substances

Table 1. Laboratory Values in Pregnancy[a]

Value	Nonpregnant	Pregnant
Electrolytes and acid-base values		
Sodium (meq/liter)	135–145	132–140
Potassium (meq/liter)	3.5–5.0	3.5–4.5
Chloride (meq/liter)	100–106	90–105
Bicarbonate (meq/liter)	24–30	17–22
P_{CO_2} (mm Hg)	35–50	25–30
P_{O_2} (mm Hg)	98–100	101–104
Base excess (meq/liter)	0.7	3–4
Arterial pH	7.38–7.44	7.40–7.45
BUN (mg/dl)	10–18	4–12
Creatinine (mg/dl)	0.6–1.2	0.4–0.9
Creatinine clearance (ml/min)	3.5–5.0	2.0–3.7
Osmolality (mosm/kg)	275–295	275–285
Lipids and liver function tests		
Total bilirubin (mg/dl)	1.0	1.0
Direct bilirubin (mg/dl)	0.4	0.4
Alkaline phosphatase (IU/ml)	13–35	25–80
SGOT (IU/ml)	10–40	10–40
Total protein (g/dl)	6.0–8.4	5.5–7.5
Albumin (g/dl)	3.5–5.0	3.0–4.5
Globulin (g/dl)	2.3–3.5	3.0–4.0
Total lipids (mg/dl)	460–1000	1040
Total cholesterol (mg/dl)	120–220	250
Triglycerides (mg/dl)	45–150	230
Free fatty acid (μg/liter)	770	1226
Phospholipids (mg/dl)	256	350
Hematologic laboratory values		
Complete blood count		
Hematocrit (%)	37–48	32–42
Hemoglobin (g/dl)	12–16	10–14
Leukocyte (count/mm$_3$)	4,300–10,800	5,000–15,000
Polymorphonuclear cells (%)	54–62	60-85
Lymphocytes (%)	38–46	15–40
Fibrinogen	250–400	600
Platelets	150,000–350,000	Normal or slightly decreased
Serum iron (μg)	75–150	65–120
Iron binding capacity (μg)	250–410	300–500
Iron saturation (%)	30–40	15–30
Ferritin (ng/ml)	35	10–12
Erythrocyte sedimentation (mm/hr)	<20	30–90

[a]In Gleicher (ed): *Principles of Medical Therapy in Pregnancy.* Reprinted with permission. New York, Plenum Medical Book Company, 1985.

that reach their maximum or minimum serum levels between 18 and 25 weeks. Morgan and Hytten have suggested that some of these processes may be related to a delicate balance needed to ensure a firm implantation of the trophoblast on the endometrial wall while at the same time not causing myometrial damage or activating maternal immune systems. They have suggested that the consequences of failure of these delicately balanced systems may actually not become evident until later in the pregnancy and may have little or no effect on the woman's emotional state or adaptational modes.

Although few behavioral correlates to the many physiologic changes accompanying pregnancy have been clearly identified (and their clinical significance even less so), the aspiring consultant is urged to become familiar with the many shifts in body function that are common in the normal gravid woman. This understanding is helpful during the interviewing and assessment process in order to place changes in energy levels, sleep patterns, eating, elimination, and sexual behavior in proper context. The contribution of Elrad and Gleicher is particularly useful in this regard.[17]

In addition, it is unwise to prescribe psychotropic medications during pregnancy without a working familiarity with those physiologic functions that may be directly or indirectly influenced by those agents. An overview of the altered body states that are typical of pregnancy and the possible implications of these for the prescribing psychiatrist is provided in Chapter 12. Table 1 shows normal laboratory values in the pregnant female.

The importance of understanding the physiologic changes that occur during a normal pregnancy should not be underestimated. Except for their usefulness in understanding and monitoring the use of psychotropic agents, their direct clinical application to the consultation process is unclear at this time. Perhaps current studies that are examining behavioral correlates of neurohormonal processes will make it possible in the future to apply a truly psychobiologic model to the understanding and management of disorders of pregnancy.

Within the limits of our current understanding, it is important to maintain a consistent conceptual framework concerning the developmental stages of pregnancy because many clinical abnormalities are associated with failure to progress adequately from one stage to the next, regardless of which model a clinician employs.

For our purposes, a developmental crisis model has proven to be most useful. This construct draws heavily on the early work of Gerald Caplan,[26] John Rose,[27] and Grete Bibring.[28] Interviews with hundreds of normal pregnant women conducted by the author[29-32] over the past 25 years reinforce both the soundness and the utility of this model as will be illustrated in subsequent case material.

Developmental Model of Pregnancy

The model itself is a simple one and views the woman (and her immediate support figures) progressing through four easily identifiable periods. These are (1) acceptance of the pregnant state; (2) affiliation with the fetus; (3) preparatory (or nesting) behavior; and (4) development of a reality-based perception of the neonate.

Acceptance of the Pregnant State

On initial inspection, this step may seem so self-evident as to be trite. Yet we have seen several pregnant women who have actually never accepted the "condition" of pregnancy or have done so only partially even though the pregnancy has been far advanced. At the extreme, one may be confronted with a young woman at term who brings herself to a gynecology clinic because she has "a large tumor" in her abdomen and is seeking surgical intervention. Admittedly, this is rare, although I have seen five or six such cases over the years. What is more frequent is a partial acceptance of the pregnancy with ongoing ambivalence, denial, or conflict over becoming pregnant. This may manifest itself by continuing to engage in activities (e.g., horseback riding) or by dressing, eating, or drinking in a fashion wholly inappropriate to the pregnant woman while experiencing a kind of blithe indifference to one's health and appearance and to the welfare of the fetus.

During the first trimester, it is often difficult for a woman to conceptualize fully her pregnant condition. She has missed her usual menstrual periods, there may be some breast changes, she may experience some morning G.I. symptoms. These are all collateral to the state of pregnancy, however. Basically, she feels well, her appearance has not changed, she is not likely to experience energy depletion yet, and the whole idea of being pregnant is primarily a fantasy for several months. Accepting the pregnant state, in the truest sense of the word, is not as easy and simple as it may seem at first blush, particularly during the first trimester.

In the normal, healthy primagravida, it may sound something like this:

Mrs. K. is a 27-year-old primagravida who works as a senior laboratory technician in a large urban hospital. She is married and has recently been promoted to a more responsible position. At the time of this interview, she is reaching the end of her second trimester and has experienced a relatively uneventful obstetrical course.

DR. C.: Can you tell me a bit about the circumstances and the timing of your pregnancy?

MRS. K.: Well, we had been working at becoming pregnant for about 6 months and each month, it was, well it would be this month, and then when my period was late for about 8 days, it was well, this must be it! So I called my doctor and had a blood test done, and they knew within 2 days, and it was a little bit of a relief. I was beginning to worry that maybe we would have a problem getting pregnant. After 6 months you always assume that that's something you can do immediately. When you're 17 everyone seems to be able to do that immediately, so it was a relief about that and plus a lot of excitement and all of the things we saw coming after that . . . the baby . . . and we immediately started talking about names and thinking about those sorts of things.

DR. C.: What did you do when you found out you were pregnant?

MRS. K.: Well, I called my husband.

DR. C.: And then what happened, what did he say?

MRS. K.: Well, he was also very excited, but we had decided that we wouldn't really . . . we were going to keep the secret to ourselves for a little while; and waited until the doctor's appointment before we even told our families or anyone where we work . . . so it was like our little secret, and that was kind of fun for a few weeks, although it was hard not to tell.

DR. C.: The reason for keeping it a secret was what?

MRS. K.: Just till we had real verification that we really were pregnant, and no problems.

DR. C.: You wanted the doctor to examine you?

MRS. K.: Yes.

DR. C.: I see.

DR. C.:   So did you feel pregnant or not?

MRS. K.:   No, and that was hard especially, then, talking once other people knew. It seems that everyone is willing to . . . women talk to you about their . . . instantly you have something to talk to people about since they find out that you're pregnant. It really changes how other people look at you. People will start telling you, people that you hardly know, start telling you about their pregnancies and how they . . . problems they had and I by comparison, I had no morning sickness. I didn't really have any real symptomatology to go with this pregnancy so it didn't seem real at the time.

DR. C.:   What kinds of things were you hearing?

MRS. K.:   A friend of mine had been sick every day of her pregnancy. I wasn't at all disappointed that I wasn't sick, but I felt that I needed something real . . . some real symptomatology to go with it.

DR. C.:   Outside of the missed menstrual periods, what were the first signs that you were really pregnant?

MRS. K.:   I think the tenderness in my breasts and then emotionally I was a little . . . my husband said I was a little testy the first few months. I didn't think I was particularly testy! But other than that, no major changes, and then I had some low-back problems early, some changes there that I hadn't had before.

DR. C.:   But none of those things that you've mentioned are specific to pregnancy. Other things can cause those changes. We all have testy days, and we can all have low back pain. What was the first thing that happened to you that made you say to yourself, "Wow, I'm pregnant!"

MRS. K.:   I think it was the . . . when I went to the physician the first time, and she said how my uterus had grown and everything; and she said, "There's definitely a baby in there," and that was enough for me.

DR. C.:   So what happened to you then, did that change anything for you?

MRS. K.:   Well, from the very first I started taking better care of myself, making sure I got some rest, eating healthier than I probably ever have eaten in my life and trying to be this model pregnant person.

There is nothing dramatic about this particular interview segment. What it does illustrate is the search for reality anchors by a woman who has had no direct experience with pregnancy and is seeking to begin a transition to parenthood at a different level of responsibility. The need to maintain the pregnancy as a "secret" for a period of time is very common. It seems to be based simultaneously on a need to be "sure" while also reveling in this intimate and deeply personal experience with one's mate.

In order to evaluate the overall status of the pregnant woman's mate (a direct interview is best but often not feasible during a consultation). It is important to explore his changing role in the family, any shifts in the spousal relationship, and his participation in preparing for the new family member.[33-40]

Contrast Mrs. K.'s account of her early pregnancy experience with that of Mrs. A.:

Mrs. A. is a 25-year-old married paralegal who is also a primagravida now in the fifth month of her pregnancy. Earlier in the interview, she had indicated that the pregnancy was unplanned and that she had some partially formulated plans to attend law school during the coming year. She presents as a bright, articulate, energetic young woman.

DR. C.:   How have things been going so far for you?

MRS. A.:   [Several seconds of silence] . . . What do you mean?

DR. C.:	Well, to begin with, how have you been feeling?
MRS. A.:	Fine, fine.
DR. C.:	You are now 5 months into your first pregnancy. Has anything changed for you so far?
MRS. A.:	No, not really. I pretty much feel the same. I'm working very hard, but I don't see much that's different.
DR. C.:	Are you doing any other things differently from before?
MRS. A.:	[Several seconds of silence] . . . Like what?
DR. C.:	Just the normal routines of living. Eating. Sleeping. Recreational activities. Any area of your life?
MRS. A.:	Should I?
DR. C.:	I don't think there is any "should" about all of this. My purpose was simply to find out what the pregnancy has been like for you so far since it is a relatively new experience in your life.
MRS. A.:	My overall feeling about all of this is that too much fuss is made of being pregnant. Life goes on, you know. People have been pregnant for thousands of years. It's no big deal.
DR. C.:	Have your parents and your in-laws shown much interest in this coming grandchild?
MRS. A.:	You know, we don't have any family in this town. We both moved here from different parts of the country so that our families haven't been involved very much in this.
DR. C.:	Well, have they been writing and calling very much?
MRS. A.:	No one knows yet. We really haven't told anyone. I suppose we will have to face that pretty soon. I don't want people fussing all over me. I've been a very independent person all of my life. I've been working since I was 15 years old, and I plan to keep on working all of my life. It is very important for me to feel independent and on top of things.

Although Mrs. A. certainly presents as a young woman with considerable strength and resources, her current reaction to the pregnancy cognitively, affectively, and behaviorally suggests that she has not accepted the state of being pregnant. It is as if she plans to continue her life as if this were a minor illness such as a head cold or an inconvenience such as a faulty carburetor in her car.

To the casual (or not so casual) observer, Mrs. A. presents as a capable, well-adjusted, healthy young woman. It is not until one approaches her in the context of her adaptation to her pregnancy that any suggestion of potential difficulty emerges. One wonders especially whether her overriding need to be "independent" will allow her to use the kinship and marital support systems that might be available to her, and whether she will take care of herself appropriately (diet, nutritional supplementation, tobacco and alcohol abstinence, timely prenatal medical visits, etc.). These latter are often particularly important during the first pregnancy if the woman has had little contact with pregnant women in the past and little or no experience with infant care.

Affiliation with the Fetus

The process of attachment begins for the healthy parent long before birth. As the child becomes identified as an independent being growing and maturing within the uterus, it begins to be assigned various characteristics and identities by the parents. Daily conversations about the fetus give it the form and substance of a person, often with a name or nickname. Its activity is discussed, and its reaction to noise and movement and its presenting parts are explored and "identified." This process of affective involvement with the child may begin earlier in the pregnancy but is usually catalyzed by the onset of quickening. This is an appropriate point to have Mrs. K. continue to describe her experience.

Dr. C.:	Can you recall the first time you felt life?
Mrs. K.:	Yes, but it was sort of nebulous because I didn't . . . it was about four and a half months, and I felt something for a day or two just a little movement, but I thought maybe it was gas or something, and then when it became more consistent, then it was more exciting. I just didn't want . . . I wanted to be sure that's what it was before I got real excited about it. I tend to be a little tentative about excitement.
Dr. C.:	But when were you sure?
Mrs. K.:	Well, then I wanted someone else to be able to feel it, too, and my husband would get bored waiting for something to move.
Dr. C.:	And did he get to feel it?
Mrs. K.:	Well, eventually, but it wasn't till about 2 weeks later.
Dr. C.:	Did anything change for you after you began to really feel life in there? Did anything change in terms of your thinking about being pregnant or how you acted in any way?
Mrs. K.:	I think it made it much more real to me that we really are going to have this baby and that there is something in there that's moving around. I had thought for a while even though I wasn't having any symptoms there's just little about you that changes. It changes a little about everything about you . . . your skin, your hair, how much to go to the bathroom, your whole digestive system changes just a little bit, and you feel you really lost a little bit of control over your body, for one thing. Once I felt movement, it's well, I really have been taken over. It wasn't a complete sort of feeling about it, and it wasn't at all negative like I didn't feel totally taken over.
Dr. C.:	Did you say it was or wasn't positive?
Mrs. K.:	It was very positive.
Dr. C.:	Very positive feeling, but at the same time some sense of not being in total control of yourself.
Mrs. K.:	Right.
Dr. C.:	Because of this other person?
Mrs. K.:	Yes.
Dr. C.:	Moving around in there?
Mrs. K.:	Yes, and being responsible for that other person now. Totally dependent on what I eat, and the rest that I get.
Dr. C.:	What other kinds of things are going on? For instance, do you picture the baby or yourself with it?
Mrs. K.:	I can see myself bathing the baby or the three of us and the dog hiking or doing some of the things we enjoy doing now, but incorporating the baby into that. I've tried to pay attention to those fantasies and see if I can pick out what sex the baby is. I think, gee, I should be able to tell that or I should be able to see it in these fantasies but I can't.
Dr. C.:	Do you try to think of what's going on in there now and what it looks like?
Mrs. K.:	Yes.

DR. C.:   What do you see?

MRS. K.:   Well, at first I just saw this little . . .you see pictures, and they show all these
            pictures, this is how big your baby is now each month, and now I see this little
            person that was just sort of floating in there and I tried to pay attention to those
            and see if I could tell the baby's sex, but I can't!

In order to develop a relationship with another person, one must invest some energy
and "emotional work." Here one listens to a young mother struggling to identify the
characteristics of her child, to think about what it will be like, and most importantly, to
begin organizing herself at a higher level of integration in order to assume this increasing
responsibility. This drive to identify the baby as a new member of the family is usually
triggered by the increasing awareness of its ability to grow, to move, to rest, and to react
to stimuli in an independent manner.

Again, this does not happen in every instance or, more commonly, does not happen
in a way that leaves the interviewer comfortable that the growing fetus is being emotionally incorporated into the network of the family. The following interview excerpt is
illustrative: Mrs. P. is a 37-year-old para 2 gravida 0 who is married to a cardiologist. She
is not employed outside the home. They have been married for several years and have had
considerable difficulty in conceiving. Her first pregnancy was 2 years ago and ended in a
spontaneous abortion in the second trimester. We have reached a point in the interview
where I am attempting to learn something about her response to quickening in this, her
second pregnancy.

DR. C.:   Can you remember when you first felt life with this pregnancy?

MRS. P.:   Yes, I think so. It wasn't too definite. I have had a lot of abdominal discomfort with
            this pregnancy, and it really is kind of hard to be sure.

DR. C.:   Are you sure now?

MRS. P.:   Yes I am.

DR. C.:   Can you describe what it feels like?

MRS. P.:   It's just a kicking. Sometimes its rather hard, but you get used to it. I don't notice it
            too much anymore.

DR. C.:   Well now that you have felt life, has it changed in any way how you feel about this
            pregnancy or how you feel in general?

MRS. P.:   Well I really know that I'm pregnant. I don't think there is much other reaction to it.

DR. C.:   Do you think about what is going on in there or what the baby looks like?

MRS. P.:   No, I can't say that I do. Now that I recall, it seems to me I did a lot of that with my
            first pregnancy, but there isn't too much now. Maybe its just normal for the
            second pregnancy to feel this way.

DR. C.:   What way do you mean?

MRS. P.:   Well, that I don't think much about it. [Long pause.] You know, don't you, that my
            first pregnancy ended in a miscarriage. That's what I really think about especially
            at night when I am up. You can't imagine what that's like. One day you are
            pregnant and happy and thinking about the baby and getting ready. You are like a
            family. And the next day there is nothing. You have the nursery that you fixed up
            and the clothes you bought, and there is nothing. I could never stand to go
            through that a second time. I'm 37, and time is running out.

DR. C.:   Are you saying that you are so preoccupied about what happened to you the first time
            that you are a little bit afraid of getting too close to this baby?

MRS. P.:   I guess I never really thought of it that way, but that's exactly the point. I don't seem
             to be able to let myself go. You know, because I was 35 years old with the first
             pregnancy, we thought it would be a good idea to have an amniocentesis just to
             make sure the baby didn't have any genetic defects. A few days after the pro-
             cedure, I began to bleed and I lost the baby. It seems like you're damned if you
             do and you're damned if you don't. We tried to do the responsible thing and
             make sure the first baby was okay and we lost it. I would never do that again. But
             now I am uncertain about losing this one or whether there will be anything wrong
             with it because I am 37. I should be enjoying my pregnancy and I'm not. They
             say it is better to have loved and lost than never to have loved at all, but that has
             nothing to do with pregnancy. That's crazy. It's better not to love and lose when
             you're pregnant.

The contrast between Mrs. K. and Mrs. P. does not seem to require much highlighting. In the latter instance, we see a woman who is withholding emotional investment in
the pregnancy and in her fetus; she is still preoccupied with a previous fetal loss and
experiencing a kind of anticipatory grief reaction that blocks her affiliation with the
present child. Only if one actively searches for such phenomena are they likely to emerge
during the course of the assessment of a pregnancy. The information is most unlikely to be
volunteered, and yet it may prove to be crucial in designing appropriate management at a
later time.

Preparatory (or Nesting) Behavior

The reader may already perceive the early interplay of two contrapuntal themes
emerging in the interview excerpts so far. On the one hand, there are the strivings for
attachment and closeness with this emerging human being accompanied by the beginnings
of parental identity and behavior. On the other, there are the rumblings of discomfort at
the reshuffling of resources that will be necessitated by this newcomer and by the shift
both in internal identity in the woman and in family relationships that will be precipitated
by the new member. This latter theme repeats itself many times through parental feelings
of "loss of control" or a sense of not being able to manage one's life as efficiently and
autonomously as was the case before the pregnancy. In those pregnancies that are product
of a permanent relationship (usually institutionalized through marriage), both partners
have already yielded some sense of inner control and total autonomy to another individual. They now find themselves faced with yet another yielding of control and freedom
because the new member of the family is now not only a heavier responsibility, but for
some time, he or she is likely to be totally vulnerable and dependent.

There is a growing body of experimental work that highlights the importance of locus
of control issues[41-44] as they apply to health maintenance, to the acceptance of medical
care, and more specifically, to adapting to the demands required by transition to parenthood. Space does not permit a review of this literature here, but the reader is urged to
become familiar with it. For many new parents, particularly for young women emerging
into the expanded workforce, these issues assume particular importance as they impact on
the family's equilibrium during pregnancy and following childbirth.

The time clock of pregnancy is such that the approximate date when this new
responsibility must be assumed is known, and the process moves inexorably toward that

conclusion. In fact, pregnancy is probably the only developmental crisis that has so fixed a time clock attached (in contrast to adolescence, middle age, senescence, etc.).

It is as though biology has taken over and, even if the pregnancy is planned and wanted, conception has set in motion a series of developmental events that cannot be altered or arrested except by terminating the pregnancy itself.

The counterpoint of these two themes, the urgings to parent and to achieve intimacy with the child while at the same time struggling with loss of control and autonomy, represents one of the most important foci around which adult growth takes place.

As the need to parent and regain a sense of mastery over the situation becomes a possibility, most pregnant couples begin to display what is referred to as nesting behavior. They begin to act in a more adult fashion, to do less celebration about the pregnancy and more preparation for the baby-to-be. The preparation should be explored along multiple lines: in the fantasy life of the parents as they envision themselves in real-life situations with the new child; along cognitive lines as they plan how they will care for the child, what their child-rearing practices will be; and along behavioral lines, as they make space, prepare clothing, make arrangements for transportation and, perhaps most importantly, begin to shift in their behavior toward each other, becoming parental partners in addition to marital spouses. Again, it may be helpful to return to Mrs. K.:

DR. C.: As the baby became more real to you, did you begin to get ready for it in any different ways?

MRS. K.: Well we started going to general prenatal classes. That sort of thing. Like I said early, we talked a lot about names and that sort of took a backseat. We started more planning what would . . . where we were going to put the baby and making some plans but not really working on them. Just more in the planning stages. Where the baby would be and how much I was going to work and what arrangements we were going to make about that, child care and . . .

DR. C.: Well, can we go into that a little bit. What arrangements did you make?

MRS. K.: Really, we haven't made any arrangements. We've made some decisions that I probably, I will, go back to work full-time at least for a while because at about the third month I got this promotion, this new position at work. So I decided that I will go back full-time at least for a while and then decide. See how it goes. If I'm able to cope, and on the condition that the baby is well and not have special needs or anything like that.

During the past decade, there has been growing interest and a rapidly expanding literature on the advantages and disadvantages of continued work outside the home during pregnancy.[45-52] In the final analysis, the significance of gainful employment for each woman is a function of her perceptions of its rewards, demands, stresses and consequence with her long-term plans for herself.

DR. C.: You tell me you're fixing up a room in your home for the baby, right?

MRS. K.: Yes.

DR. C.: What about other things like clothing. Have you done anything with that?

MRS. K.: Some things but mostly through the grandmothers. They're knitting their fingers to the bone right now and making some preparations towards that. We've ordered a crib and some furniture, but we haven't gotten a lot of that; I think we're saving that for the last 2 months. We've just started to move on the room and getting the crib and we have a few things like blankets and T-shirts and whatever.

Dr. C.:   Will you need some assistance when you get home? Have you made preparations for that?

Mrs. K.:   I think both of our mothers will be coming to spend some time, and I think my husband will be taking off a few weeks of work so I think that will be . . . I think I'll have enough help. That was sort of assumed by the grandmothers, "We'll be there, whether you want us or not." [Laughs]

If the consultant is to evaluate the balance between stresses and supports, constant attention during the interview to the quality of not only the spousal relationship referred to previously but of the extended kinship, social, and professional support systems is essential.[53–57]

Dr. C.:   How would you compare your relationship with your husband now with, let's say, a year ago or how have things changed, if at all?

Mrs. K.:   In some ways I think we're closer because we have this new commitment . . . getting married is one commitment but now having this child and committing to the care of this child for 18 to 20 years is another commitment that I think we both see as a change in our relationship. So I think we're closer in some ways because of that. But in other ways this baby also came between us. Not between us but has taken over some parts of our life. Preparation for this baby. We spend all of our weekends now working on the baby's room, we spend time in preparation for the baby rather than time for us, and we've realized that it's going to be a big change in life-style for us.

Dr. C.:   So in some ways you're closer and in other ways you have a third partner in the business that dilutes some of that closeness?

Mrs. K.:   And some ways it takes over some of it.

Dr. C.:   That sounds like the issue of control you were talking about before only a slightly different context, right?

Mrs. K.:   Yes.

Dr. C.:   This little person who hasn't even come on the scene yet is controlling your lives to a certain degree?

Mrs. K.:   Right.

Dr. C.:   What's been your reaction to your change in appearance? When you get out of the shower and you stand in front of the bathroom mirror, what do you see?

Mrs. K.:   Well this blob! [laughs] I lost all shape . . . this part of me that is part of me but really isn't. I've lost control of my shape. I spent most of my life concerned about my weight and my appearance and everything, and all of a sudden there's not too much that you can do about your weight or your appearance. I can still see my toes if I make an effort!

Dr. C.:   What's been your husband's reaction to your change in appearance?

Mrs. K.:   Lately he laughs a lot, or he just chuckles, or he'll tap my belly and say, "Let's see it blossoming," or whatever.

Dr. C.:   He just laughs a lot?

Mrs. K.:   He laughs a lot, and that's not always the most supportive thing for him to do. I usually react rather well to it because . . . but sometimes I think he's being a little insensitive to my concerns of my loss of shape and also I'm concerned about how he looks at me. Physically I'm a different person than I was.

Dr. C.:   Do you talk about that?

MRS. K.: A little bit, but maybe not as much as we probably should talk about it . . . that I've changed so much.

DR. C.: This is part of what I was alluding to previously when I asked how things have changed between you, if at all. You are a different person?

MRS. K.: Yes.

DR. C.: In some ways?

MRS. K.: Yes, in a lot of ways I think it changes a little bit about everything about you and sometimes some things more than others.

DR. C.: Do you think he's pleased with that person?

MRS. K.: I think so, I think . . . I think he seems right now in his own sort of little euphoria about this, and I think he sees these changes in me as real positive and, well, it's getting closer but I don't know if I perceive as . . . I'm just not physically the same person.

Of course, there is nothing particularly eye-opening about the content of this interview. As with much that we have said so far, it may only be of real significance in the woman and family where these processes do not occur. For instance, let us consider this interview excerpt with Mrs. D.:

Mrs. D. is a 20-year-old primagravida who has moved to a new city with her young husband who is in the military service. She is now in her third trimester, reports that she has made few social contacts in her new city, and tends to see her husband sporadically because his duties require lengthy absences from the city. Her nearest relative is 500 miles distant.

DR. C.: It will not be very long now before you will be having a new baby. Do you feel ready to take that on now?

MRS. D.: I guess I feel pretty comfortable handling babies. I've done a lot of baby-sitting, and I had a younger sister. I took care of her a lot so it's not like I'm starting out cold.

The single best criterion for how a woman and her spouse will adapt to the pregnancy and to subsequent child rearing is their respective "track records." Their experience with success and failure in school, work, social relationships, avocations, and, in general, with stress coping deserves careful attention during the interview for this reason. People who are accustomed to mastery of novel challenges tend to persist in that mode.

DR. C.: Well that's helpful, isn't it. It's good to have some experience under your belt. It makes you more confident when you are facing a new responsibility. Have you and your husband done anything else to get ready for the baby?

MRS. D.: You mean like clothes and things?

DR. C.: Yes, that sort of thing. Also names for the baby and things like getting to the hospital, help, if you need it, when you come home with the baby and so on.

MRS. D.: I'm a little superstitious about those things. After all, what does a baby really need? We can do all those things if the baby comes and is all right. [Starts to cry.] I know it's wrong, but if there's anything wrong with the baby, if it's retarded or anything, I would have to put it in an institution. I just couldn't take that. That's terrible, isn't it?

DR. C.: I don't quite understand why you're bringing this up at this time? I was just asking about clothes and names for the baby. Is there something I don't know?

Mrs. D.:   My husband was on drugs, a lot of different ones. I haven't told anybody, but he was
             on drugs when I got pregnant. A lot of bad stuff that he picked up on the street.
             I've heard terrible stories about what can happen to the baby if you use a lot of
             drugs or alcohol.

Dr. C.:   Have you talked with anyone here in the clinic about this?

Mrs. D.:   No. No one knows. I haven't even talked with my husband about it. I'm just scared all
             the time. He wants to talk about names for the baby, but I won't do it. If the baby
             is okay, then we can worry about names, and he can go out and get some diapers
             and towels and that kind of stuff. After all, what does a baby really need?

In these two contrasting interview excerpts, one can already sense that the first couple is striving in several spheres for mastery and for learning new adaptive modes. In the second, one sees a relatively unsupported primagravida making little or no effort to prepare for this new task while tending to minimize the amount of reintegration it will mean for her and her husband.

Development of a Reality-Based Perception

In a very important sense, the final step in the process of pregnancy and the first "hands-on" step in the transition to parenthood occurs in the days following birth. This involves a clear demonstration on the part of the parents that they are now able to move from a fantasied image of the child that is being shaped by the real characteristics of the infant, both physical and behavioral. Immediately following a healthy, normal childbirth, both parents are usually on an emotional high, are quite tuned in to the new infant, and are able to incorporate an incredible amount of detail concerning its appearance and its behavior. The fatigue, drowsiness, and affective decline that often appears 12 to 36 hours following birth has not yet set in. The parents are in a considerable state of arousal (as may be the infant), particularly if neither mother nor child is heavily sedated.

In most instances, both parents are able to describe the child in exhaustive detail and, within a day or two, the mother is often able to distinguish the child's cry from that of others. As days progress, the normal physiological rhythms of the child begin to be perceived and reacted to by the parents, and its early temperamental characteristics (although these, of course, are not stabilized as a neonate) begin to be described. This "reality perception" of the child is one major factor that will determine the quality and responsiveness of the care it receives. The higher the level of accurate perception on the part of the parents, the less the perplexity concerning the child's cues and the less dependent the parents are likely to be on professionals to give advice concerning feeding, physical nurturance, and other aspects of early care. Mrs. M. is a 26-year-old married woman who was interviewed on a home visit 4 days following the birth of her first child, a girl. Her husband was also present during the interview and actively participated. The birth took place in an out-of-hospital alternative birthing center. Mrs. M. returned to her home 12 hours after Kathy's birth.

Dr. C.:   Now that the delivery is a few days behind you, how do you see things going with
             Kathy?

Mrs. M.:   Kathy was definitely ours from the very beginning. We held her for 2 hours before
             anyone else . . . she was with us the whole time . . . she never left us . . . no-

Mr. M.:	body interfered. We could really look at her and see all the little parts that you miss when you only see them for 15 or 20 minutes.
Mr. M.:	I think it was because she was with us so long when she was first born that she was really ours. There was no chance of sneaking anybody else's kid in there. We knew every little mark on her. They couldn't have brought us any one else's baby. We would have known.
Dr. C.:	You sound like you must have examined her from head to toe.
Mrs. M.:	I don't know if "examined" is the word, but we sure took her inside of us.
Dr. C.:	Well, I still haven't seen Kathy because she's asleep right now. Can you describe her for me?
Mrs. M.:	Have you got an hour? She's about this big [holds her hands a little less than two feet apart]. She has wide open, bright blue eyes and just a little brown peach fuzz on her head. She has that funny little bump in her nose just like Alvin does [Mr. M.] and she has two funny little freckles or birthmarks on the inside of her right leg. She has a funny little cry when she's hungry. I would know it anywhere anytime even if there were a hundred babies in the room. I think she has a couple of other cries too but I really don't know them yet. She sleeps like my husband too. Nothing wakes her. She's like a log.
Dr. C.:	[To Mr. M.] Anything else?
Mr. M.:	Yes, I think she's going to have my wife's disposition. You get the feeling of a friendly, cheerful, sort of up person. The only times she's in a bad mood is when she's sleepy or hungry. [Laughs] That's like my wife, too.

Although there is considerably more to this interview, the preceding excerpt should serve to reassure the interviewer that whatever fantasy life the M.'s may have had about their baby, these have been dispersed by the immediate impact of her real presence. There can be little doubt that they have accepted this person into the family as a separate and discrete individual with an identity of her own and that they will be observing her closely over time. Although the interview segment is not included here, one should always ask whether the baby was particularly different from what was expected and if so, in what ways. This may also elicit useful information about the parents' ability to differentiate the child as a separate individual.

Partial or complete inability to make that transitional step into in vivo parenthood may be revealed in the interviewing process in several ways. The two most common ways involve either (1) a tendency to fuse the baby's new identity with previously held fantasies about it that were developed during the pregnancy; or, (2) an inability to perceive the baby as a separate individual with distinguishing characteristics regardless of previous fantasies.

To illustrate, Mrs. L. felt that her baby was much too active during the pregnancy, often keeping her up at night with its kicking and movement. The fetus would respond, according to her report, to noises like slamming doors or music, and she predicted that it would be a very hard baby to take care of. When interviewed in the hospital only 24 hours postpartum, she reported that her fears had been confirmed. She explained that the baby was not only fussy but that there must be something wrong with him because he "snapped back" when she attempted to breast feed him. She could not accurately describe what she meant by this except that he was not compliant and that she felt he was going to be very oppositional to her because of his feeding behavior.

Mrs. Y., on the other hand, produced a postpartum interview that was either devoid of any specifics about the baby or revealed observations that could not have been based on any actual perceptions. She had great difficulty describing the baby physically (twice she commented that all babies look pretty much alike anyway), could not distinguish its cry, and revealed fantasies that were projected far into the future and had little or nothing to do with the baby's current infantile and dependent state. For instance, she pictured his first day of school and taking him to the schoolbus. She also pictured him playing football and pictured going to his wedding.

Although Mrs. L. and Mrs. Y. do not necessarily present pathological states at this point, they would appear to be headed for a difficult start with their babies because they have not taken the final transitional step of "connecting" or "locking in" with the baby as a person. The beginnings of what has been described as an attachment process do not seem to be taking place, and, although they may give perfectly adequate physical care to the baby and, in fact, may experience much tenderness and positive emotion for it, there may be a better than even chance that their care will be disruptive and jangling to the baby's normal rhythms because both mothers seem out of synchrony in the interactive process that begins immediately after birth.

Other Components of the Developmental Interview

Our emphasis, so far, has been the core of the developmental process in the assessment interview during pregnancy. However, several other collateral areas have been highlighted in passing. In order to reemphasize their importance, we will mention them once more.

1. *The parents' preparation for childbearing and child rearing.* This inquiry should not only explore their previous experience with children but the modeling that was provided for them by their own parents and by other significant adults, particularly for parenting behavior. In a broader but equally important sense, one should get an overview of their life experience and accomplishments, particularly in the educational, work, and social spheres. This is important because it tends to clarify whether the individual parents prepare adequately for novel experiences and what their "track record" has been with respect to success and failure in new and challenging experiences.

2. *Life apart from parenting.* An effort should be made to clarify the rewards and demands currently in their personal lives apart from childbearing and child rearing. This is particularly true for mothers who may become more socially isolated and more easily depleted as a result of the early experiences of parenting if they do not have other sources of gratification outside the home.

3. *Parental support systems.* An overall picture of parental support systems is useful. Of course, one explores quickly the marital support system but extended kinship, social, and professional supports are also crucial. It is helpful to know how the parents have related to professionals in the past, what their pattern of asking for help is like, and whether they can use help constructively when it is offered to them.

4. *Role and adaptive behavior of the father.* Finally, it is obvious from what has been described so far that much of the focus has been on the childbearing woman. There have been several references to the inclusion of her mate in the assessment process. The first

paternal experience with the mate's pregnancy and the early experiences of fathering are maturational catalysts for the man and important contributors to long-term outcome of the child's development. Much has been written[33–40] about the psychological crisis for men that accompanies the first pregnancy and early fathering, but very few empirical studies have been carried out in this area. It is unusual for the consultant to be used for services for the father but one should take a proactive stance in this regard. If the male partner is either deficient as a support or appears to be functionally decompensating himself, the consultant may be of considerable assistance in calling proper attention to this and suggesting a course of action in order to achieve access to appropriate counseling services.

Organizing and Formulating Information Gathered

The foregoing can be integrated into a summary that should highlight the strengths and deficits in the pregnant woman and her family. It should be action oriented and jargon free so that nonpsychiatric clinicians can "process" the data quickly and easily and collaborate with the consultant and the patient in the development of a plan of intervention if one is indicated. A sensible format that I have found useful and helpful to consultees follows:

History of Current Pregnancy

This section should include a review of the parents' current experience in this pregnancy with special emphasis on such areas as:

1. Circumstances surrounding conception.
2. The reaction of both parents to the pregnancy.
3. What changes, if any, the mother has made in her pattern of living as a result of becoming pregnant.

It is usually worthwhile to include some statement concerning the mother's reactions to her change in appearance (if this has occurred).

4. Reaction to quickening if this has occurred.
5. Mother's interaction with and use of supports indicated previously.
6. Any fantasies concerning the labor and delivery experience.
7. The nature of preparation for the baby including both fantasies about the fetus and the subsequent child, choice of name, physical preparations for transportation to the hospital, reception of the baby at home, and so forth.

Parents' Preparation for Child Rearing and Current Life Experience

Past History. The mother's preparation for the assumption of the roles of woman, wife, and mother. It is important to record information concerning her own views of her parents, how she was prepared to meet the developmental milestones of school, menarche, adolescent dating, vocational choice, choice of mate, and so forth. Where it is possible, it is valuable to collect like information from the father.

Current Support System. Describe the nature of supports available to the mother, including the potential role of husband and mate in the family as a resource for rearing the coming child and the nature of other supports, both social and kinship, available to the mother during this pregnancy.

Mother's Life Apart from Pregnancy and Child Rearing. This should include some picture of the degree to which interest in or conflict in these areas of life experience may be preempting the major portion of the mother's energy investment. Also, it should include some sense of whether the mother finds her current activities as a homemaker satisfying or as interfering with the accomplishment of other basic needs and ambitions. It would be important to include also in this area any information concerning such items as maternal reactions to her own illness currently (if any) and the degree to which disability in herself or others with whom she is closely associated may be depleting her resources.

Conclusions

The foregoing information should be integrated into a clear statement indicating the following:

1. Current status of developmental progression of the pregnancy with particular attention to the possibility of "arrest" or delay (see the second section of this chapter).
2. In connection with such arrest or delay, has there been appearance of serious and persistent maladaptive behaviors (e.g., denial of pregnancy, constant overreaction to minor physical complaints, failure to display nesting behavior, etc.)?
3. An evaluation of the severity and chronicity of current life stresses particularly as they are perceived by the pregnant woman.
4. On balance, what is the quality and nature of the marital, kinship, social, and professional support system, and how appropriate is the use of these when viewed in the context of current stresses?
5. One must take into account the adequacy of preparation for childbearing and child rearing with particular emphasis on past stress coping and mastery of novel experiences.
6. Finally, one must weigh strengths against deficiencies: To what degree can one predict further development of maladaptive behavior; what is the portent of this for favorable or unfavorable outcome of the pregnancy; and, if unfavorable, what is the nature of professional interventions that would be most likely to shift the balance of supports in a positive direction?

References

1. Osofsky HJ, Osofsky JD: Normal adaptation to pregnancy and new parenthood, in Taylor PM (ed): *Parent-Infant Relationships.* New York, Grune & Stratton, 1980, pp 25–48.
2. Shereshefsky PM, Plotsky H, Lockman RF: *Pregnancy Adaptation. Psychological Aspects of a First Pregnancy and Early Postnatal Adaptation.* New York, Raven Press, 1974, pp 67–102.

3. Chalmers B: A conceptualization of psycho-social obstetric research. *J Psychosom Obstet Gynaecol* **3**:17–26, May 1984.
4. Mercer RT, May KA, Ferketich S, et al: Theoretical models for studying the effect of antepartum stress on the family. *Nurs Res* **35**:339–346, November/December 1986.
5. Molfese VJ, Bricker MC, Manion L, et al: Stress in pregnancy: the influence of psychological and social mediators in perinatal experiences. *J Psychosom Obstet Gynaecol* **6**:33–42 February 1987.
6. Pohlman EW: Changes from rejection to acceptance of pregnancy. *Soc Sci Med* **2**:337–340, 1968.
7. Breen D: *Conflict and acceptance of pregnancy in the Birth of a First Child: Towards an understanding of femininity.* Tavistock Publications, pp 131–139, 1975.
8. Gloger-Tippelt G: A process model of the pregnancy course. *Human Development* **26**:134–148, 1983.
9. Flapan M: A paradigm for the analysis of childbearing motivations of married women prior to birth of the first child. *Am J Orthopsychiatry* **39**:402–416, April 1969.
10. Hofferth S: Childbearing decision making and family well-being: A dynamic, sequential model. *Am Sociol Rev* **48**:533–545, August, 1983.
11. Donaldson SM: Suddenly you've become somebody else: A study of pregnancy and the creative women. *Women's Studies Int Forum* **7**:227–235, 1984.
12. Jessner L, Weigert E, Foy JL: The development of parental attitudes during pregnancy, in Anthony EJ, Benedek T (eds): *The Psychobiologic Approach to Parenthood.* London, J & A Churchill, Ltd, 1970, pp 209–244.
13. Reading AE, Cox DN, Sledmere CM, et al: Psychological changes over the course of pregnancy: A study of attitudes toward the fetus/neonate. *Health Psychol* **33**:211–221, 1984.
14. Wideman M, Singer J: The role of psychological mechanisms in preparation for childbirth. *American Psychologist* **39**:1357–1371, December 1984.
15. Hern WM: The illness parameters of pregnancy. *Soc Sci Med* **9**:365–372, 1975.
16. Liley AW: The foetus as a personality. *Aust NZ J Psychiatry* **6**:99–105, 1972.
17. Elrad H, Gleicher N: Physiologic changes in normal pregnancy, in Gleicher N (ed): *Principles of Medical Therapy in Pregnancy.* New York, Plenum Medical Book Company, 1985, pp 33–56.
18. Bartl W, Riss P, Bieglmayer C, et al: Evaluation and correlation of hormone levels in normal and pathologic pregnancies. *Biol Res Pregnancy Perinatol* **5**:143–148, 1984.
19. Benedek T: The psychobiology of pregnancy, in Anthony EJ, Benedek T (eds): *The Psychobiologic Approach to Parenthood.* London, J & A Churchill, Ltd, 1970, pp 137–151.
20. De Flamingh JP, van der Merwe JV: A serum biochemical profile of normal pregnancy. *S Afr Med J* **65**:552–555, April 1984.
21. Challis JR, Patrick JE: Changes in the diurnal rhythms of plasma cortisol in women during the third trimester of pregnancy. *Gynecol Obstet Investment* **16**:27–32, 1983.
22. Liu J, Rebar RW, Yen SSC: Neuroendocrine control of the postpartum period. *Clin Perinatol* **10**:723–736 October 1983.
23. Morgan DML, Hytten FE: Midtrimester pregnancy: A time of tranquility or activity? *Br J Obstet Gynecol* **91**:532–537, 1984.
24. Detrick JM, Pearson, JW, Frederickson RC: Endophins and parturition. *Obstet Gynecol* **65**:647–651, May 1985.
25. Buster JE: Gestational changes in steroid hormone biosynthesis, secretion, metabolism and action. *Clin Perinatol* **10**:527–552, 1983.
26. Caplan G: Emotional implications of pregnancy and influences on family relationships, in Stuart HC, Prugh DG (eds): *The Healthy Child.* Cambridge, MA, Harvard University Press, 1966, pp 72–82.
27. Rose JA: Emotional growth and development of children, in Wallace HM (ed): *Health Services for Mothers and Children.* London, W. B. Saunders Company, 1962, pp 118–152.
28. Bibring GL: Some considerations of the psychological process in pregnancy, in Eissler RS, Freud A, Glover E, et al (eds): *The Psychoanalytic Study of the Child.* New York, International Universities Press, Inc. **14**:113–121, 1959.
29. Cohen RL: Pregnancy stress and maternal perceptions of infant endowment. *J Ment Subnormality* **22**:18–23, June 1966.
30. Helper MM, Cohen RL, Beitenman ET, Eaton LE: Life events and acceptance of pregnancy. *J Psychosom Res* **12**:183–188, 1968.

31. Cohen RL: Factors influencing maternal choice of childbirth alternatives. *J Am Acad Child Psychiatry* **20**:1–15, 1981.
32. Cohen RL: A comparative study of women choosing two different childbirth alternatives. *Birth* **9**:1–7, 1982.
33. Parke RD, Power TG, Tinsley BR, et al: The father's role in the family system, in Taylor P M (ed): *Parent-Infant Relationships*. New York, Grune & Stratton, 1980, pp 117–133.
34. May KA: Three phases of father involvement in pregnancy. *Nurs Res* **31**:337–342, November/December 1982.
35. Gerzi S, Berman E: Emotional reactions of expectant fathers to their wives' first pregnancy. *Br J Med Psychol* **54**:259–265, 1981.
36. Swartz MS, Cavenar JO: Countertransference in the expectant father. *Psychosomatics* **25**:566–568, July 1984.
37. Quill TE, Lipkin M, Lamb GS: Health-care seeking by men in their spouse's pregnancy. *Psychosom Med* **46**:277–283, May/June 1984.
38. Scott GH: Marital adaptation during pregnancy and after childbirth. *J Reprod Infant Psychol* **1**:18–28, May 1983.
39. Clinton JF: Expectant fathers at risk for couvade. *Nurs Res* **35**:290–295, September/October 1986.
40. Shapiro S, Nass J: Postpartum psychosis in the male. *Psychopathology* **19**:138–142, 1986.
41. Craig AR, Franklin JA, Andrews G: A scale to measure locus of control of behavior. *Br J Med Psychol* **57**:173–180, 1984.
42. Fisher S, Erlbaum S: The basis of personal control, in: *Stress and the Perception of Control*. Hillsdale, NJ, S. Fisher & L. Erlbaum Associates, Publishers pp 20–32, 1984.
43. Lefcourt HM, Martin RA, Saleh WE: Locus of control and social support: Interactive moderators of stress. *J Personality and Soc Psychol* **2**:378–389 1984.
44. Lieberman JJ: Locus of control as related to birth control knowledge, attitudes and practices. *Adolescence* **16**:1–10, 1981.
45. Saurel-Cubizolles MJ, Kaminski M: Work in pregnancy: Its evolving relationship with perinatal outcome. *Soc Sci Med* **22**:431–442, 1986.
46. Zuckerman BS, Frank DA, Hingson R, et al: Impact of maternal work outside the home during pregnancy on neonatal outcome. *Pediatr* **77**:459–464, April 1986.
47. Beral V, Grisso JA, Roman E: Is paid employment during pregnancy detrimental to the offspring? *Prog Clin Biol Res* **163B**:261–264, 1985.
48. Chamberlain G: Effect of work during pregnancy. *Obstet Gynecol* **65**:747–750, May 1985.
49. American College of Obstetricians and Gynecologists: Pregnancy, work, and disability. *Technical Bull* No. 58, May 1980.
50. Murphy JF, Dauncey M, Newcombe R, et al: Employment in pregnancy: Prevalence, maternal characteristics, perinatal outcome. *The Lancet,* **1,** 1163–1166, May 1984.
51. American Medical Association, Council on Scientific Affairs: Effects of pregnancy on work performance. *JAMA* **251**:1995–1997, April 1984.
52. Marbury MC, Linn S, Monson RR, et al: Work and pregnancy. *J Occup Med* **26**:415–421, June 1984.
53. Cronenwett LR: Network structure, social support, and psychological outcomes of pregnancy. *Nurs Res* **34**:93–99, March 1985.
54. Brown MA: Social support during pregnancy: A unidimensional or multidimensional construct? *Nurs Res* **35**:4–9, January/February 1986.
55. Brown MA: Social support, stress, and health: A comparison of expectant mothers and fathers. *Nurs Res* **34**:72–76, March/April 1986.
56. Parry G, Shapiro DA: Social support and life events in working class women. *Arch Gen Psychiatry* **43**:315–323, April 1986.
57. Perez R: Effects of stress, social support and coping style on adjustment to pregnancy among Hispanic women. *Hispanic J Behav Sci* **4**:141–161, June 1983.

6

Emotional Disorders and Mental Illness Associated with Pregnancy and the Postpartum Period

RICHARD L. COHEN

Introduction

It would be most desirable to have a precise and inclusive nosology of the emotional and mental disorders associated with pregnancy and the postpartum period. This is particularly true because of the far-reaching implications of pregnancy for the family and for the next generation. It inevitably has an impact on family dynamics and on the intrapsychic and interpersonal processes of the woman and her mate. Perhaps, most important of all, there is a need to conceptualize any disease process that occurs during this time in a way that takes into account another developing organism, both in terms of its possible significance for present (intrauterine) and future well-being. It is this fact more than any other that makes the assessment, diagnosis, prevention, and management of disorders during pregnancy unique.

Unfortunately, there is no commonly accepted nosology for the psychiatric disorders associated with pregnancy. Although many psychiatric illnesses occur during pregnancy, the typical DSM-III or ICD-9 types of classifications would not by themselves serve the pregnant population well. They could not encompass many of the problems to which the clinician is exposed on a frequent basis.

For instance, how would we label those problems that are at least in part related to

Richard L. Cohen • Department of Psychiatry, Western Psychiatric Institute and Clinic, University of Pittsburgh, Pittsburgh, PA 15213.

specific age groups such as young adolescents; or pregnancy occurring for the first time in a woman who is in her late 30s or early 40s? What about those problems associated with, or worsened, by drug or alcohol abuse? What about the specificity and management of the grief reactions associated with spontaneous abortion or stillbirth? How would one classify the emotional response to prolonged infertility, or the denial of pregnancy occurring in the third trimester?

In daily practice, these latter types of dysfunctions occur more frequently and are more often referred for consultation than those of the patient who warrants a major psychiatric diagnosis. It is, therefore, necessary to "jury-rig" a classification in order to approach comprehensiveness and in order to present a picture of emotional and mental disorders that is more relevant to the experience of practice. Admittedly, such a classification has not yet been subjected to the scientific rigors either of the epidemiologist or the medical taxonomist. It rests only on the weight of clinical observation. Its current use can only be justified because of the absence of an empirically documented nosology and the need for some bridging concepts that will be of assistance to the clinician for the immediate future.

Essentially, one must consider three types of "conditions":

1. Psychiatric disorders that can occur during pregnancy but are not necessarily associated with or characteristic of the pregnant state and that occur with equal or greater frequency in nonpregnant individuals.
2. Psychophysiologic disorders that may have some impact on the course of pregnancy, labor, or delivery.
3. Conditions or states of development that may interact adversely with pregnancy.

The essential ingredients, therefore, for such a classification are (1) comprehensiveness; (2) relevance to current consultative practice; and (3) wherever possible, an action-oriented approach.

What follows should be read for best understanding in conjunction with other companion chapters in this volume. Chapter 4 (Epidemiology) should be helpful in better understanding the importance of major psychiatric disorders during pregnancy. Chapters 3 (Prenatal Stress) and 5 (Developmental Tasks) bear important relationships with many of the psychophysiologic entities described later, whereas Chapter 5 itself cannot be separated from a discussion of maladaptive behavior. Chapter 9 (Direct Case Consultation) consists mainly of detailed case illustrations in which many of the disorders outlined here are described as they are encountered by the consultant in everyday practice. A thorough review of Chapter 13 concerning the problems of drug and alcohol use during pregnancy is essential because that area will be mentioned only in passing in this chapter. Finally, although little is known at this writing about the developmental and emotional outcome of the use of various new high-technology approaches to conception, we would be remiss if we did not include some mention of these in our nosology (what is known about the field is outlined in Chapter 15).

With these caveats in mind and in view of the need for some transitional system of "clinical cataloging" of the psychopathology of pregnancy and the postpartum period, the following classification is offered (see Table 1). A brief review of the disorders outlined in Table 1 may be useful.

Table 1. A Partial Classification of Emotional and Mental Disorders That Can Be Associated with Pregnancy and the Postpartum Period

I. Major psychiatric disorders (DSM-III Axis 1)
   A. Schizophrenia and schizophreniform disorders (Case 3)
   B. Affective disorders
      a. Endogenous (unipolar and bipolar) (Cases 8 & 9)
      b. Exogenous (e.g., reactive depression, mourning postabortion or stillbirth) (Case 10)
      c. Postpartum depression[a] (Case 7)
   C. Anxiety Disorders
      a. Acute and chronic anxiety disorders (Case 2)
   D. Adjustment disorders (maladaptive reaction to developmental tasks of pregnancy) (Cases 1 & 4). Exact form of maladaptive behavior depends on state of pregnancy (see Chapter 5).
   E. Organic and/or toxic syndromes
II. Conditions in which stress or emotional factors may contribute to the cause or pathogenesis of the disorder (Case 6)
   A. Pseudocyesis
   B. Couvade syndrome
   C. Hyperemesis gravidarum
   D. Pathological cravings and pica
   E. "Functional" sterility
   F. Prolonged and dystronic labor
III. Conditions or states that may interact adversely with pregnancy
   A. Pregnancy occurring in early adolescence (below age of 17) (see Chapter 9)
   B. First pregnancy occurring at advanced age (40 years or above) (in this chapter)
   C. Concomitant with drug and/or alcohol abuse (Chapter 13)
   D. Emotional disorders associated with alternative methods of conception (Chapter 15)

[a]There is some disagreement concerning whether postpartum depression or psychosis represent distinct clinical entities. For the purpose of this classification, it is helpful to consider them separately.

Major Psychiatric Disorders

Schizophrenia and Schizophreniform Disorders

On the whole, pregnancy does not alter the clinical picture of a schizophrenic episode.[1] Criteria for diagnosis remain the same. There are surprisingly few studies of the relationship between schizophrenia and pregnancy. Yarden and Eisenbach[2] described the course of schizophrenia in 30 pregnant women and followed them during the first postnatal year. They did not discern any long-term negative influence on the course of established schizophrenia but did find a significant "aggravating affect" during the first year postpartum. Thirteen of 30 patients were hospitalized within 6 months of delivery. The authors emphasize that of the 13 schizophrenic women requiring hospitalization, 21 reported spontaneous abortions in the past or present. The long-range effects on the infant's being cared for by a schizophrenic mother is a matter of greater significance[3-5] so that the implications for early intervention (see Chapter 10) are of critical importance. There is an impression among some clinicians that the incidence of schizophrenic episodes in established schizophrenics is actually decreased during pregnancy. This is not substantiated by any controlled studies, however. Psychopharmacologic management during pregnancy and the postpartum period is discussed in detail in Chapter 12.

Affective Disorders

In this category, there have been many more studies, and there is much more known. Nevertheless, extreme caution must be exercised in applying a clinical diagnosis of depression during pregnancy because of the marked lability of mood, the feeling on the part of some women that they are dependent, more needy, and more easily rejected during this period; and the tendency of family members to view normal placidity and introversion as depressed mood.

Conversely, there are several medical conditions that may masquerade as depression during their early stages and should always be considered in the differential diagnosis.[1] Among the most important of these are hypothyroidism, an adverse reaction to antihypertensive drugs that may have been used during pregnancy or Cushing's syndrome.

It is useful both in terms of prognosis and management to think of "depression" during this period as falling into one of four categories: that is, it may be major (reaching the proportions of a psychotic depression) or minor; it may occur during pregnancy or during the postpartum period. The epidemiology of depression during pregnancy itself is not as definitive as it is in the instance of postpartum syndromes (see Chapter 4). Most depression that occurs during pregnancy is self-limiting, responds to good psychosocial and professional support, and requires active intervention with psychotropic medication much less frequently. Suicidal attempts do occur during pregnancy, but there is little evidence that the incidence of either attempts or successful suicides varies significantly from those of nonpregnant females matched for age.[6,7] Most studies seem to support the contention that, in the absence of a history of major unipolar or bipolar affective disorder, depressions that occur during pregnancy tend to be more related to deficiencies in support systems.[8] An obvious exception to this occurs in the instance of pathological mourning following the loss of a fetus by spontaneous abortion or stillbirth. These situations may require more active intervention and more sustained care[9-20] (see also Chapters 9 and 11).

Although the literature on this subject is very large, perhaps the clearest explication of the process emerging from the paranatal loss of an infant was written from firsthand experience by a British resident in child and adolescent psychiatry. Oglethorpe,[21] in a paper that fills only one and one half journal pages, has described the process with exquisite accuracy; and what is just as important, she has indicated what proved to be helpful (or not) to her and her husband. The preparation and anticipation of the baby, the experience with hospital practices, the empty nest, the compulsive need to share the experience with others, the feelings of failure and uselessness, the search for causes and for help, and the eventual resolution of the mourning process are all described in unforgettable prose.

Postpartum depression is significantly more common and occurs in a variety of forms. Here, too, the literature is so large as to be barely encompassable, and it is not possible within the confines of this chapter to cover what is known about postpartum depression. Inwood[22] has edited an excellent monograph on the subject, and a representative sample of excellent publications can be found in the bibliography at the end of this chapter.[23-33]

1. *So-called "baby blues."* In some classifications, this would not be considered a "disorder" because it is so common as to be the rule rather than the exception. Up to 70%

of women experience episodes of sadness alternating with elation, crying, irritability, anxiety, headache, confusion, insomnia, forgetfulness, and negative feelings toward the baby. Usually, all of these do not occur in the same woman but may occur in almost any combination. Onset is usually on the third or fourth day after birth. Duration is sometimes only a matter of hours, although some women report that the episode may last for 2 or 3 days.

2. *Nonpsychotic postpartum depression.* This is the most common form of postpartum disorder and is variously reported to have an incidence of 10% to 15% in women following delivery. Severity of symptoms varies considerably. Onset is usually some time during the first 8 to 10 weeks after birth. There may be the presence of several premorbid risk factors, particularly a history of depression either in the patient or her family. The patient demonstrates frequent crying, physical agitation, various somatic symptoms of a nonspecific nature, extreme irritability, occasional panic attacks, anorexia, loss of interest in the family and usual activities, insomnia, and inability to carry out routine tasks. There is often expressed concern about loss of interest in the baby or inability to love it. Although the course of this disorder may be self-limiting, intervention is almost always indicated both in order to ensure proper care of the baby and in order to avoid self-destructive behavior on the part of the mother.

3. *Psychotic depression.* This is a very uncommon disorder probably occurring only about once in 1,000 deliveries. Onset is usually earlier than in the less serious depressions, often within 2 weeks of delivery. Onset may be rather sudden with marked irritability and insomnia progressing rapidly to a confusional state marked by disorganized cognitive functioning, bizarre behavior, mercurial mood swings, hallucinations, hyperkinesis, and in some instances, marked suspicion and distrust of family and professional caretakers. Obviously, prompt and thorough intervention is necessary in these disorders once a firm diagnosis has been made (see Chapters 9 and 12). Prolonged and unresolved grief reactions following spontaneous abortion or stillbirth are not uncommon.

Acute and Chronic Anxiety Disorders

Whether or not the incidence of anxiety states that meet DSM-III criteria vary with the state of pregnancy is not known. There are no controlled studies in this area. Again, a large part of the difficulty revolves around the degree to which transient states of ''nervousness,'' irritability, unusual fears, brief panic, or unusual degrees of dependency and ''helplessness'' are all typical of the normal pregnant state. Therefore, the reliable diagnosis of these relatively minor disorders is filled with diagnostic pitfalls. In any event, there is no reason to believe that their appearance during pregnancy takes on a different clinical picture.

My own observation is that the most commonly expressed fear which tends to be persistent in some pregnant women and is often intractable to counseling is the concern surrounding the intactness of the fetus as a result of some real or fantasied insult. The mythology surrounding pregnancy (see Chapter 1) is such that almost any maternal illness, putative toxic agent, or physical injury can cause an abiding fear in one or both parents that the child is irreparably damaged. In most instances, this will respond to careful and sensitive professional counseling. When it is persistent and refractory to intervention, long-term monitoring of the parent–child interaction long after birth is usually warranted[34,35] in order to avoid the so-called "vulnerable child syndrome" (see especially the discussion of screening procedures and interventive programs as described in Chapter 10).

Adjustment Disorders

It is particularly characteristic of pregnancy that the phenomenology of adjustment disorders will be tied to the developmental stage of pregnancy in which the patient finds herself.[36] A maladaptive reaction to stress can produce a kind of developmental arrest or distortion so that the clinical presentation may appear early in pregnancy, for instance, as an inability to accept the pregnant state; at midpregnancy as a failure to react to quickening; and in late pregnancy, as a failure to display appropriate nesting behavior. Generally, the clinician is able to identify a marked imbalance between the pregnant woman's perception of stress level and the strength of marital, kinship, social, and professional supports available to help in mediating that stress. (A review of the developmental tasks of pregnancy is outlined in Chapter 5, and a review of screening procedures for identifying women at risk of maladaptive behavior as described in Chapter 10 may be useful in gaining a better understanding of this area.)

Organic and/or Toxic Syndromes

In general, there is no reason to expect that these disorders will take on a different clinical picture during pregnancy.[37] The epidemiology of these syndromes has not been studied during the pregnant period. The one area in which severe confusional states or even a psychotic reaction may occur is in association with eclampsia. Whether this results from a severe metabolic and/or electrolyte imbalance or whether the etiology is basically that of cerebral ischemia is not clear. Such reactions do occur and the psychiatrist may be called upon to manage the pharmacotherapy of the patient.

Conditions in Which Stress and/or Emotional Factors May Contribute to the Disorder

In this category, the extensive mythology of pregnancy becomes extremely difficult to separate from what has been empirically demonstrated in the clinic or laboratory. A careful review of Chapter 3 that discusses much of what we know about the impact of stress on the developing fetus is indispensable to an understanding of this problem area.

The consultant may be invited to evaluate and make recommendations for a variety of disorders that have proven intractable to other forms of treatment and that are now considered to be "functional" by the attending physician.[38-43] In fact, in many instances, there is substantial literature to suggest that some form of psychological or psychiatric intervention may be helpful in some of these situations. Several fall into the category of "complications of pregnancy, labor, and delivery" (such as hyperemesis gravidarum,[44-48] pre-eclampsia,[49] or repeated premature births.[50]) Others are somewhat exotic in nature, such as pseudocyesis or the couvade syndrome. Both of the latter are quite rare, and it is unlikely that the consultant will see more than a few of these in a lifetime.

Pseudocyesis

Pseudocyesis[51-55] is the syndrome of false pregnancy. It may appear in delusional form, although some clinicians consider it to be a type of conversion hysteria. It is characterized by menstrual irregularity or amenorrhea, distension of the abdomen, breast enlargement, morning nausea, and sometimes, even softening of the cervix. The patient may report a sensation of fetal movement. The presence of these symptoms and signs in the absence of any objective corroborating evidence of pregnancy is diagnostic. Active intervention is always indicated and usually takes the form of dynamically oriented psychotherapy. Pseudocyesis is not unknown in males.[56]

Couvade Syndrome

The couvade syndrome[57-59] (in contrast to the ritual of couvade that in many cultures is a modal male adaptation to pregnancy and childbirth) is a psychogenic disorder in which expectant fathers are afflicted by symptoms that bear a resemblance to those which their wives experience during pregnancy and labor. Unlike ritual couvade, the syndrome is not a pretense. There is no deliberate acting out of the wife's pregnancy but rather a reaction to it by the acquisition of symptoms. In some instance, swelling of the abdomen occurs either through severe aerophagia or displacement of the abdominal viscera. Sympathetic labor pains are also quite frequent. The syndrome may occur at any time during the pregnancy. Again, the diagnosis is easily made, and the treatment usually involves psychodynamic intervention.

Hyperemesis gravidarum (see references 44–48 for more details)

Pathological cravings and pica (see references 38–43 for more details)

"Functional" Sterility

Over the ages, many writers have attributed a major component of functional sterility[60-63] to emotional factors. There is no incontrovertible evidence to this effect, though many obstetricians believe it to be so, and there is the oft-told tale of the couple who conceive after years of infertility shortly after they adopt a child.

Prolonged and Dystonic Labor

It is possible that emotional factors can be a contributory cause to prolonged or dystonic labor[37] but it is most unlikely that the psychiatric clinician will be consulted in such matters because these are usually dealt with at first pharmacologically and, if this modality is not successful, by cesarean section.

Conditions or States That May Interact Adversely with Pregnancy

Again, because of the unique nature of pregnancy and the various biological time clocks with which it is connected, when it occurs very early in the female's development or very late in her reproductive life span, there are often specific problems associated with the process.

Pregnancy Occurring in Early Adolescence

Hundreds of papers and scores of volumes have been written on the problems of teenage pregnancy.[64-79] Most agree that in Western cultures, the highest risk period is that between puberty and age 17. Not only does this occasion the greatest number of adaptational stresses for the young female, but it is also associated with the highest incidence of pregnancy complications and reproductive casualties. Although no specific syndrome can be described here, the essential concepts revolve around the fact that the young adolescent (and her mate) are engaged in a complex and difficult developmental step themselves; to have the demands of pregnancy, childbirth, and parenting superimposed on this process can be catastrophic for some young people. Extreme conflict over keeping the baby or placing it for adoption can create both major intrapsychic turmoil and serious dissension within the family. Major interferences with the female's current and future heterosexual contacts, her career and educational goals, and her self-image and self-esteem emerge as frequent themes. The mental health consultant can be most helpful not only in dealing with the adolescent and her family but in assisting the hospital in program planning and development for this growing population of child parents and their offspring. (For a more detailed description of the types of problems presented by the young, pregnant adolescent and their management, see Cases 11 and 12, Chapter 9.)

First Pregnancy Occurring at Advanced Age

At the opposite end of the reproductive cycle, a woman who becomes pregnant for the first time may also experience significant stress and her own development may seem compromised at least for the time being.[80,81] She may not only be experiencing the pregnancy as an intercurrent stress in her own personal and professional advancement, but she may be beset by concerns that she is bearing a child who is at much higher risk for mental or physical abnormality. A recent review of the literature by Mansfield[82] uncovers little convincing evidence to support such fears. Again, there is no specific syndrome connected with this period, but the woman may report panic attacks, depression, irritability, persistent fears about the intactness of the fetus, marital discord, decreasing work productivity, and sleep disorders.

Concomitant with Drug and/or Alcohol Abuse

The problems and risks attendant to substance abuse during pregnancy are outlined in detail in Chapter 13.

Emotional Disorders Associated with Alternative Methods of Conception

Although we are only at the dawn of understanding problems that may be associated with the advanced technologies for improving fertility, inducing conception, and for surrogate parenting, we can anticipate the emergence of significant problems in these areas. Our current knowledge about such circumstances is described in Chapter 15.

An Alternate Conceptualization

Having imposed upon the reader this tedious but necessary cataloging of disorders that may be associated with childbearing and with childbirth, I would like to add that this nomenclature has considerable shortcomings. Although it is necessary to have such a format because it assists in "labeling" for statistical and for reimbursement purposes, it is not likely to be the one used in everyday practice.

The most important reason for this is that it is not the way in which problems present

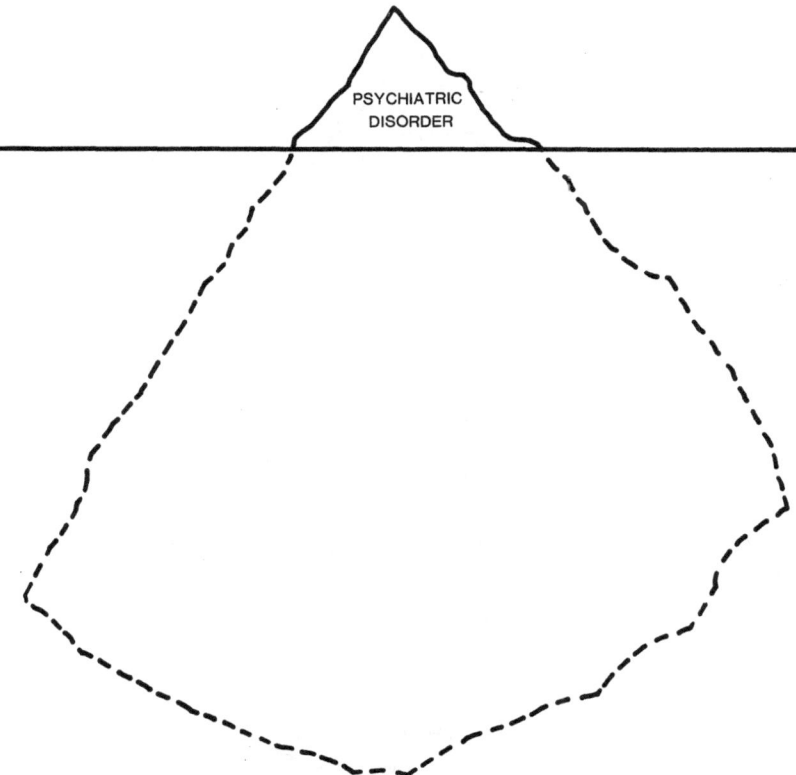

Figure 1. Schematic model of emotional disturbance and psychiatric disorder in a university prenatal clinic: The "tip of the iceberg."

themself generally, and it is not "action-oriented." That is, these labels with some exceptions, do not suggest a course of action.

It is deceptive to suggest that what the consultant is most confronted with in daily practice is a spectrum of frank psychiatric disorders. Actually, if one carefully screens and evaluates a randomly selected population of pregnant women, those who need some form of mental health intervention do not fall into any conventional diagnostic category (for more detail, see Chapter 10). Those with psychiatric disorders are actually the tip of an iceberg (see Figure 1).

Programs that have more systematically evaluated the nature of problems being presented by a population of pregnant women have the ability to look at the entire iceberg (see Figure 2).

Of course, each clinician or investigator would describe this population differently because it does not always present in the same way and because there is no formal classification to which to refer. In my own experience, by far the largest number of problems revolve around inadequate or distorted preparation for pregnancy, labor, and delivery; acute or chronic problems associated with deficiencies in support systems; persistent fears about the welfare of the fetus that have proved intractable to authoritative

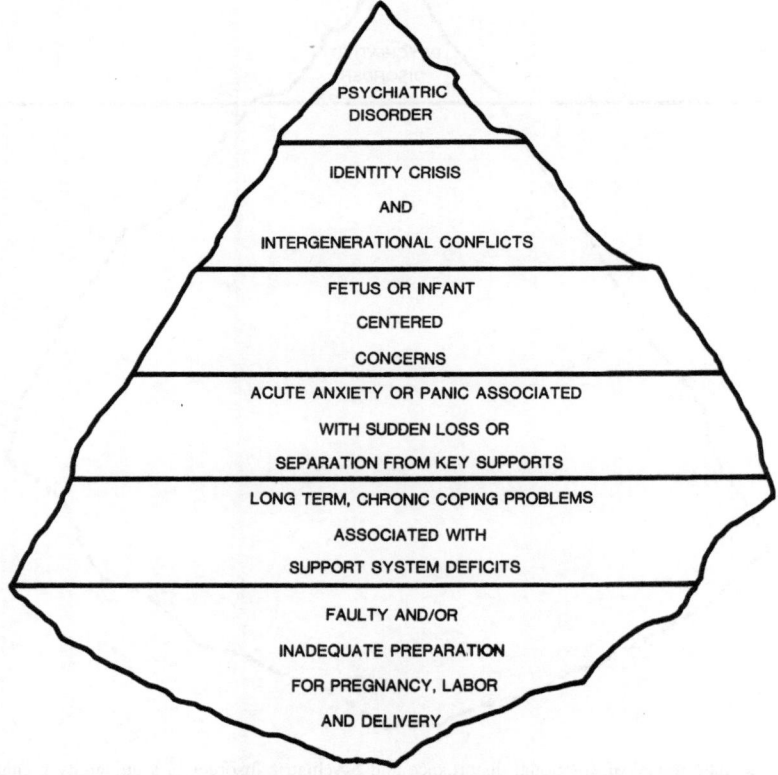

Figure 2. Schematic model of emotional disturbance and psychiatric disorder in a university prenatal clinic: The "iceberg."

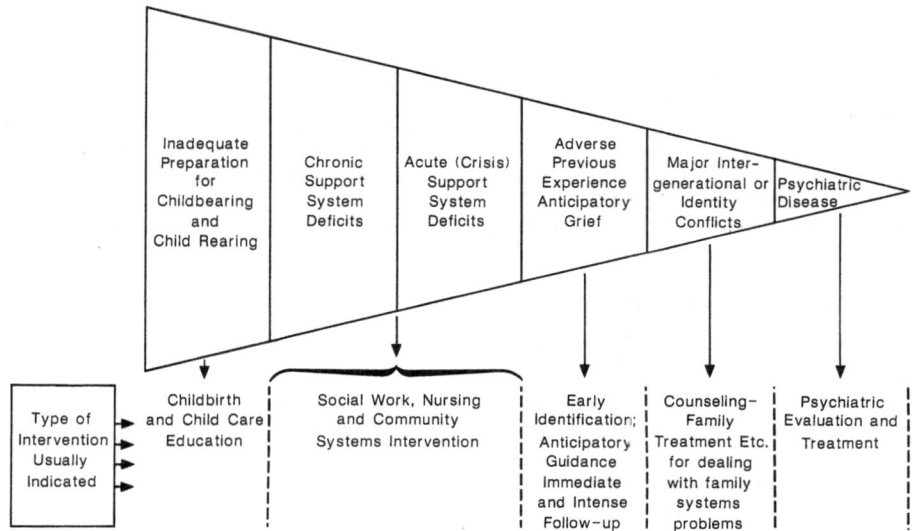

Figure 3. Schematic representation of types of problems identified by psychosocial screening.

medical counseling; and identity crises or intergenerational conflicts associated with the woman's comfort with her gender identity, her assumption of a parenting role, and her readiness to shift her relationships with her spouse and parents.

Looking at the problem complex in this format has been more useful and more adaptable to teaching and liaison activities within the hospital.

In fact, the iceberg can be also schematized as a wedge or triangle set on its side, and, in this form, it becomes easier to represent the various modalities of intervention that most commonly are employed for each of these clinical presentations (see Figure 3).

However one conceptualizes the disorders associated with reproduction, it is important to remember that one is dealing with a condition ordinarily identified as a healthy physiologic process and that most parents enter this experience expecting a pleasant, happy, and rewarding outcome. Stresses and intercurrent events that complicate the developmental process can produce cognitive, affective, and behavioral deviations that may give the appearance of conforming to the conventional psychiatric disorders described in the literature. Designing long-term management of these, however, requires a shift in thinking on the part of the consultant/clinician because there is always a "hidden patient" involved in this interaction—the fetus and the baby-to-be.

References

1. Kane FJ: Postpartum disorders, in Kaplan HI, Sadock BJ (eds): *Comprehensive Textbook of Psychiatry*/IV. Baltimore, Williams & Wilkins, 1985.
2. Yarden PE, Max DM, Eisenbach Z: The effect of childbirth on the prognosis of married schizophrenic women. *Br. J. Psychiatry* **112**:491–499, 1966.
3. Anthony EJ: A risk-vulnerability intervention model for children of psychotic parents, in Anthony EJ,

Koupernik C (eds): *The Child in His Family: Children at Psychiatric Risk*. London, Wiley, 1974, pp 99–121.

4. Anthony EJ: The influence of maternal psychosis on children—folie à deux, in Anthony EJ, Benedek T (eds): *Parenthood: Its Psychology and Psychopathology*. London, J & A Churchill, 1970, pp 571–595.

5. Lidz T, Cornelison AR, Terry D, et al: The transmission of irrationality, in Lidz T, Fleck S, Cornelison AR (eds): *Schizophrenia and the Family*. New York, International Universities Press, 1965, pp 171–187.

6. Gabrielson IW, Klerman LV, Currie JB, et al: Suicide attempts in a population pregnant as teen-agers. *Am J Public Health* **60:**2289–2301, 1970.

7. Whitlock FA, Edwards JE: Pregnancy and attempted suicide. *Compr Psychiatry* **9:**1–12, 1968.

8. O'Hara MW: Social support, life events, and depression during pregnancy and the puerperium. *Arch Gen Psychiatry* **43:**569–573, June 1986.

9. Peppers LG, Knapp RJ: Maternal reactions to involuntary fetal/infant death. *Psychiatry* **43:**155–159, May 1980.

10. Kirkley-Best E, Kellner KR: Grief at stillbirth: An annotated bibliography. *Birth and the Family Journal* **8:**91–99, 1981.

11. Stack JM: The psychodynamics of spontaneous abortion. *Am J Orthopsychiatry* **54:**162–167, 1984.

12. Lovell A: Some questions of identity: Late miscarriage, stillbirth and perinatal loss. *Soc Sci Med* **17:**755–761, 1983.

13. LaRoche C, Lalinec-Michaud M, Engelsmann F, et al: Grief reactions to perinatal death—A follow-up study. *Can J Psychiatry* **29:**14–19, 1984.

14. Bourne S, Lewis E: Pregnancy after stillbirth or neonatal death. *The Lancet*, July 7, 1984, pp 31–33.

15. Kellner KR, Donnelly WH, Gould SD: Prenatal behavior after perinatal death: Lack of predictive demographic and obstetric variables. *Obstet Gynecol* **63:**809–814, 1984.

16. Herz E: Psychological repercussions of pregnancy loss. *Psychiatric Ann* **14:**454–457, 1984.

17. Benderly BL: The aftermath, in: *Thinking about Abortion: An Essential Handbook for the Woman Who Wants to Come to Terms with What Abortion Means in Her Life*. New York, Dial Press, 1984, pp 127–155.

18. American College of Obstetricians and Gynecologists: Grief related to perinatal death. ACOG Technical Bulletin No. 86, April 1985.

19. Leon IG: Psychodynamics of perinatal loss. *Psychiatry* **49:**312–324, 1986.

20. Leon IG: The invisible loss: The impact of perinatal death on siblings. *J Psychosom Obstet Gynaecol* **5:**1–14, March 1986.

21. Ogelthorpe RJL: Stillbirth: A personal experience. *Br Med J* **287:**1186–1199, October 1983.

22. Inwood DG: *Recent Advances in Postpartum Psychiatric Disorders*. Washington, DC, American Psychiatric Press, 1985.

23. Dalton K: Prospective study into puerperal depression. *Br J Psychiatry* **118:**689–692, 1971.

24. Dalton K: *Depression after Childbirth*. Oxford, Oxford University Press, 1980.

25. Oakley A, Chamberlain G: Medical and social factors in postpartum depression. *J Obstet Gynecol* **1:**182–187, 1981.

26. Little BC: Psychophysiological ante-natal predictors of post-natal depressed mood. *J Psychosom Res* **26:**419–428, 1982.

27. Schreuder-Hoekstra JCE: Post-natal(-partum) depression illness or disease? *J Psychosom Obstet Gynaecol* **2:**56–58, 1983.

28. Atkinson AK, Richel AU: Postpartum depression in primiparous parents. *J Abn Psychol* **93:**115–119, 1984.

29. Davidson J, Robertson E: A follow-up study of post partum illness, 1946–1978. *Acta Psychiatr Scand* **71:**451–457, 1985.

30. Bagedahl-Strindlund M: Parapartum mental illness: Timing of illness onset and its relation to symptoms and sociodemographic characteristics. *Acta Psychiatr Scand* **74:**490–496, 1986.

31. Gard PR, Handley SL, Parsons AD, et al: A multivariate investigation of postpartum mood disturbance. *Br J Psychiatry* **148:**567–575, 1986.

32. Chalmers BE, Chalmers BM: Post-partum depression: A revised perspective. *J Psychosom Obstet Gynaecol* **5:**93–105, 1986.

33. Rose JA: The prevention of mothering breakdown associated with physical abnormalities of the infant, in Caplan G (ed): *Prevention of Mental Disorders in Children*. New York, Basic Books, 1961, pp 265–282.

34. Cohen RL: Pregnancy stress and maternal perceptions of infant endowment. *J Ment Subnormality* **22:**18–23, June 1966.

35. Cohen RL: Maladaptation to pregnancy, in Taylor PM (ed): *Parent-Infant Relationships*. New York, Grune & Stratton, 1980, pp 49–67.
36. Guise LH: Psychiatric implications of pregnancy, in Cherry SH, Berkowitz RL, Kase NG (eds): *Rovinsky and Guttmacher's Medical, Surgical and Gynecologic Complications of Pregnancy*. Baltimore, Williams & Wilkins, 1985, p 645.
37. McDonald RL: The role of emotional factors in obstetric complications: A review. *Psychosom Med* **30:**221–237, 1968.
38. Crandon AJ: Maternal anxiety and neonatal wellbeing. *J Psychosom Res* **23:**113–115, 1979.
39. Chalmers B: Psychosocial factors and obstetric complications. *Psychol Med* **13:**333–339, 1983.
40. Georgas J, Giakoumaki E, Georgoulias N, et al: Psychosocial stress and its relation to obstetrical complications. *Psychother Psychosom* **41:**200–206, 1984.
41. Rizzardo R, Magni G, Andreoli C, et al: Psychosocial aspects during pregnancy and obstetrical complications. *Psychosom Obstet Gynaecol* **4:**11–22, 1985.
42. Istvan J: Stress, anxiety, and birth outcomes: A critical review of the evidence. *Psychol Bull* **100:**331–348, 1986.
43. Majerus PW, Guze SB, Delong WB, et al: Psychologic factors and psychiatric disease in hyperemesis gravidarum: A follow-up study of 69 vomiters and 66 controls. *Am J Psychiatry*, November 1960, pp 421–428.
44. Farkas G, Farkas G, Jr: The psychogenic etiology of the hyperemesis gravidarum, in Morris N (ed): *Med Obstet Gynaecol* (Third International Congress). London, Karger, Basel, 1971, pp 175–177.
45. Fitzgerald C: Nausea and vomiting in pregnancy. *Br J Med Psychiatry* **57:**159–165, 1984.
46. Katon WJ, Ries RK, Bokan JA, et al: Hyperemesis gravidarum: A biopsychosocial perspective. *Int J Psychiatry Med* **10:**151–162, 1980–81.
47. Gise LH: Psychiatric implications of pregnancy, in Cherry SH, Berkowitz RL, Kase NG (eds): *Rovinsky and Guttmacher's Medical, Surgical, and Gynecologic Complications of Pregnancy*. Baltimore, Williams & Wilkins, 1985, pp 635–637.
48. Cardenas-Escovar A: The place of psychosomatic factors in toxaemia of pregnancy and allied syndromes, in: Morris N *P Medicine in Obstetrics and Gynaecology* (Third International Congress). London, Karger and Basel, 1971, pp 180–182.
49. Newton RW, Webster PAC, Binu PS, et al: Psychosocial stress in pregnancy and its relation to the onset of premature labour. *Br Med J* **2:**441–413, 1979.
50. Gise LH: Psychiatric implications of pregnancy, in Cherry SH, Berkowitz RL, Kase NG (eds): *Rovinsky and Guttmacher's Medical, Surgical, and Gynecologic Complications of Pregnancy*. Baltimore, Williams & Wilkins, 1985, pp 637–639.
51. Fried PH, Rakoff AE, Schopbach RR, et al: Pseudocyesis: A psychosomatic study in gynecology. *JAMA* **145:**1329–1335, 1951.
52. Lapido OA: Pseudocyesis in infertile patients. *Int J Gynecol Obstet* **16:**427–429, 1979.
53. Guzinski GM, Conrad SH: Pseudocyesis and sonography. *Am J Obstet Gynecol* **138:**230–232, 1980.
54. Starkman MN, Marshall JC, Ferla JL, et al: Pseudocyesis: Psychologic and neuroendocrine interrelationships. *Psychosom Med* **47:**46–57, 1985.
55. Barglow P: Pseudocyesis: To be and not to be pregnant: A psychosomatic question, in Howells JG (ed): *Modern Perspectives in Psycho-Obstetrics*. New York, Brunner/Mazel, 1972.
56. Clinton JF: Expectant fathers at risk for couvade. *Nurs Res* **35:**290–295, 1986.
57. Lipkin M, Lamb GS: The couvade syndrome: An epidemiologic study. *Ann Int Med* **96:**509–511, 1982.
58. Reid KE: Fatherhood and emotional stress: The couvade syndrome. *J Social Welfare* **2:**13–14, 1975.
59. Trethowan WH, Conlon MF: The couvade syndrome. *Br J Psychiatry* **111:**57–66, 1965.
60. Rosenfeld DL, Mitchell T: Treating the emotional aspects of infertility: Counseling services in an infertility clinic. *Am J Obstet Gynecol* **135:**177–180, 1979.
61. Kraft AD, Palombo J, Mitchell DE, et al: The psychological dimensions of infertility. *Am J Obstet Gynecol* **50:**618–628, 1980.
62. Lalos A, Lalos O, Jacobsson L, et al: Depression, guilt and isolation among infertile women and their partners. *J Psychosom Obstet Gynaecol* **5:**197–206, 1986.
63. Edelmann RJ, Connolly KJ: Psychological aspects of infertility. *Br J Med Psychol* **59:**209–219, 1986.
64. Centers for Disease Control (Atlanta): Teenage pregnancy and fertility trends–United States 1974 and 1980. *JAMA* **253:**3064–3065, June 1985.

65. Jones EF: *Teenage Pregnancy in Industrialized Countries*. New Haven, Yale University Press, 1986.
66. McAnarney E, Thiede HA: Adolescent pregnancy and childbearing: What we have learned in a decade and what remains to be learned. *Sem Perinat* 5:91–103, 1981.
67. Phipps-Yonas S: Teenage pregnancy and motherhood: A review of the literature. *Am J Orthopsychiatry* 50:403–431, 1980.
68. Elster AB, Panzarine S: Teenage fathers. Stresses during gestation and early parenthood. *Clin Pediatr* 22:700–703, 1983.
69. Leynes C: Keep or adopt: A study of factors influencing pregnancy adolescents' plans for their babies. *Child Psychiatry Hum Dev* 11:105–112, 1980.
70. Freeman E, Sondheimer SJ, Rickels K: Influence of maternal attitudes on urban, black teens' decisions about abortion vs delivery. *J Reprod Med* 30:731–735, 1985.
71. Morin-Gonthier M, Lortie G: The significance of pregnancy among adolescents choosing abortion as compared to those continuing pregnancy. *J Reprod Med* 29:255–259, 1984.
72. Landy S: Teenage pregnancy: Family syndrome? *Adolescence* 18:679–694, 1983.
73. Leppert PC: The effect of pregnancy on adolescent growth and development. *Women Health* 9:65–79, 1984.
74. Vernon M: Teenage pregnancy: A prospective study of self-esteem and other sociodemographic factors. *Pediatr* 72:632–636, 1983.
75. Zabin LS, Hardy JB, Streett R, et al: A school—a hospital—and university-based adolescent pregnancy prevention program. A cooperative design for service and research. *J Reprod Med* 29:421–426, 1984.
76. Black C, DeBlassie RR: Adolescent pregnancy: Contributing factors, consequences, treatment, and plausible solutions. *Adolescence* 20:281–290, 1985.
77. Copeland AD: The impact of pregnancy on adolescent psychosocial development. *Adolescent Psychiatry* 9:244–253, 1981.
78. Simkins L: Consequences of teenage pregnancy and motherhood. *Adolescence* 19:39–54, 1984.
79. Group for the Advancement of Psychiatry: *Crises of Adolescent Teenage Pregnancy: Impact on Adolescent Development,* Report No. 118. New York, Brunner/Mazel, 1986.
80. Eichholz A, Offerman-Zuckerberg J: Later pregnancy, in Blum BL (ed): *Psychological Aspects of Pregnancy, Birthing and Bonding*. New York, Human Sciences Press, 1980, pp 94–102.
81. Kirz DS, Dorchester W, Freeman RK: Advanced maternal age: The mature gravida. *Am J Obstet Gynecol* 152:7–12, May 1985.
82. Mansfield PK: Re-evaluating the medical risks of late childbearing. *Women Health* 11:37–60, 1986.

7

Current Childbirth Options and Parental Decision Making

RICHARD L. COHEN

Introduction

It is essential that the mental health consultant have a working understanding of the spectrum of childbirth care options now available (at least in many large metropolitan areas) together with a grasp on the intellectual and emotional factors that influence the decision-making process for parents choosing a particular option. Because of the nature of pregnancy and childbirth, such choices are inextricably bound up with attitudes about becoming a parent in the first place, with attitudes toward the medical and allied health professions, and with value systems related to child care. These issues become much more complicated than choosing a surgeon or a hospital in which to have one's gallbladder removed.

In this chapter, I will focus primarily on two surveys that describe the spectrum of current childbirth options, that explore some of the factors impacting on choice of care, and that compare two populations of women electing widely different options.

The interested reader may also wish to consult a variety of other surveys[1-6] that examine various aspects of parental decision making with respect to childbirth care. Space does not permit a comprehensive review of the large literature on this subject. My own work is fairly representative of much of the work already conducted and, for the most part, the general findings and conclusions are in agreement.

In Chapter 16 of this book we will describe in much more detail the conflicting forces operating in the strident controversy about childbirth care. There is no need to reiterate those here except to say that this professional- and consumer-generated controversy tends

---

Richard L. Cohen • Department of Psychiatry, Western Psychiatric Institute and Clinic, University of Pittsburgh, Pittsburgh, PA 15213.

to heighten rather than resolve the tension experienced by many young parents in choosing the kind of care that may be best for them.

Factors Influencing Maternal Choice of Childbirth Alternatives*

During the mid-1970s, the New York District Branch of the American College of Obstetricians and Gynecologists (ACOG) issued a position paper on out-of-hospital maternity care.[7] This document extolled the advances of modern obstetrics with particular emphasis on the increasing ability of that speciality to predict which mothers and babies were at risk and to intervene in those situations, thereby preventing morbidity and mortality.

The statement gave recognition to the fact that hospital costs were skyrocketing as a result of tertiary care and that, unfortunately, high-technology settings have sometimes "not adequately met the individual, personal, emotional, and family needs increasingly felt and properly expressed by the public." Further, the ACOG indicated its continued efforts to make improvements both in cost-containment and in individualizing maternity care. The document was clearly a reflection of the growing concern of organized obstetrics about the enormous proliferation of out-of-hospital (in some instances, home-based) maternity programs during the past decade.

In April of that same year, the International Childbirth Education Association responded to the ACOG statement with a long list of problems and issues that its membership insisted were virtually being ignored.[8] In summary, the ICEA accused organized obstetrics of (1) ignoring the fact that neither the individual nor the professional is responsible for her own health and for her choice of care; (2) contravening the individual's right to define health or illness in terms different from those of the professional; (3) operating a health care delivery system that was not trustworthy and that often produced unnecessary physical and/or psychological trauma and interference; (4) disregarding the value systems of consumers and failing to give them a voice in the planning and operation of programs; (5) failing to acknowledge that childbirth is actually a normal physiological process, not a pathological one; and (6) taking full credit for improvement in maternity mortality and morbidity statistics when much of this may have been due to many other factors, "such as improved living standards, hygiene, nutrition, antibiotics, and educational level of the populace" (p. 3).

These opposing statements have been paraphrased in some detail because they characterize the polarity that has emerged in the field of childbirth care during the past 10 years. At one extreme, one finds proponents of health care who maintain that the only place to give birth is within the safe and secure confines of a modern, high-technology, university-affiliated hospital.[9-11] At the other extreme, there is a growing body of parents and caregivers who insist that, barring certain clearly understood at-risk medical conditions, a woman and her mate have a much better chance of providing their baby with a good start in life within the confines of their own home.[12,13]

A whole range of choices has appeared between these extremes. The value and

---

*The second section of this chapter was originally published under the same title by this author in the *Journal of the American Academy of Child Psychiatry* **20**:1–15, 1981. Reprinted with permission.

efficacy of these choices are documented by the bewildering barrage of lay and scientific publications.[14-20] Much of the data presented in these publications emphasizes the importance of making options available to pregnant women and their mates and assisting them, where possible, in making appropriate choices. The broad spectrum of childbirth services available in the United States today is outlined in Table 1. All may not be available within a given urban area, but an increasing number of them tend to be.

The major innovation involves the development of a variety of childbirth or maternity centers in which the desired outcome is to combine some of the safety and security of the hospital with the naturalistic, family-centered environment of the home.

Family-Centered Hospital Care (Birthing Room)

Many obstetric hospitals and services now have sequestered one or more rooms adjacent to or within labor suites where special procedures apply. Family members, especially the father of the baby, may be in constant attendance. Labor, delivery, and the postpartum recovery all take place in one setting and in one bed that may be especially designed for the purpose. Efforts are made to decorate the room so that it will have a more homelike atmosphere. High-technology equipment and procedures are kept to a minimum, and the length of stay during the postpartum period, barring complications, is a matter of family choice and is often considerably shorter than a conventional hospitalization for childbirth. The patient's physician is in attendance as well as trained nurses or nurse-midwives, and all of the specialized back-up staff and equipment of a modern hospital are within easy reach if unforeseen fetal or maternal complications arise.

Out-of-Hospital Birthing Center

Many variations of this particular type of facility are developing. Some are operated by trained obstetricians and are physically within the group practice. Others are operated primarily by nurse-midwives with obstetric consultants available. Most of these require medical certification of low-risk pregnancy and have a back-up hospital available in the event of labor and delivery difficulties. Both types of facilities are characterized by an even greater informality than the birthing rooms of hospitals. Families often prepare their own meals, and any number of family members may be in attendance. Patients are given

Table 1. Current Options in Childbirth Care

1. High technology (tertiary) OB hospital*
2. Conventional OB hospital service
3. Family-centered hospital care (birthing room)*
4. Out-of-hospital birthing center
   a. M.D. type*
   b. R.N.–midwife type*
5. Home birth
   a. With professional attendants
   b. Lay or family attendants

*Options involved in this study

practically total freedom to establish the ground rules under which they will labor and deliver the baby. Invariably, prerequisites are attendance by both partners at natural childbirth classes during the pregnancy and the availability of one or more support persons during labor and delivery. Often, older siblings are permitted to attend the birth. The length of stay for most women is about 8 to 12 hours postpartum, even shorter on average than in hospital birthing rooms. Emergency equipment is available and episiotomies can be performed, but general or regional anesthesia usually is unavailable.

The overall purpose of this study was to learn something about the factors that are leading women and their mates to choose one method of childbirth over another. This information may be important in understanding some of the precursors of parenting attitudes and practices and may also throw some light on the way in which parents get started with their new offspring.

It is pertinent to offer some justification for the involvement of several child psychiatrists and other similar mental health professionals in this area of scientific interest. There are at least three basic reasons: (1) There is a growing body of literature that at least suggests that the manner in which parents and a new baby get started in their interactional life together is one important variable in the long-range developmental outcome for the child.[21,22] (2) Scientific study of prenatal and childbirth care is uncovering additional developmental data with which professionals who are interested in the mental health of children should be familiar.[23,24] (3) It is possible that techniques for psychological and other interventions during pregnancy will become an important clinical area because there is a small but convincing body of information that pre- and perinatal stress may have a direct physiological impact on the growth of the fetus and the functioning of its central nervous system.[25-28]

These reasons seem compelling and should, over the coming years, direct the attention of child mental health professionals to the pregnancy period and to the professional boundary areas between child psychiatry and obstetrics—a neglected area of consultation and collaboration.

Method

The data for this study were collected over a 6-month period during which 14 different obstetric and childbirth centers were visited in the United States. Prenatal questionnaires, previously administered by nursing personnel at most sites, were aimed at identifying the presence of prenatal stresses and accompanying supports. The information derived from those questionnaires is reported later and elsewhere.[29,30] The findings reported here are derived from 125 postnatal interviews conducted in six programs (two university hospitals, two out-of-hospital birth centers, and two in-hospital birthing rooms). The distribution of this sample is indicated in Table 2.

Although it was not feasible to achieve a one-to-one match for demographic and obstetric variables, a comparison of the samples reveals surprisingly similar profiles. The typical woman in this study was between 24 and 29 years of age, Caucasian, married, had at least a high-school education, and was lower-middle class or middle class in socioeconomic status. About two-thirds of each group were having their first babies, and slightly less than one-third their second. In most instances, mates were present and participating in the postnatal interviews.

Table 2. Site of Childbirth Care of Population Studied

Population studied		N
University-based obstetric hospitals		34
Hospital-based birthing rooms		34
Out-of-hospital birth centers		57
a. M.D. type	27	
b. R.N.-midwife type	30	
TOTAL		125

The sample was selected simply by interviewing all mothers giving birth consecutively in the particular program during the period of the site visit who gave informed consent to be interviewed. When possible, interviews were conducted within 24 hours postpartum. However, some were conducted as much as 7 days postpartum during home visits. Only those women whose choice of hospital-based birth was elective (without obstetric or medical complication) are included in this sample.

The interview was semistructured and included the following questions, although both parents were encouraged to expand upon these in any way they deemed appropriate to the subject: (1) How did you prepare for having this baby? (2) What programs or services did you explore? (3) How did you choose the doctor (or midwife) who took care of you? (4) What were the most important things you wanted during your childbirth experience? (5) How did the actual experience compare with what you expected? (6) How would you rate the quality of care you received? (7) Did your experience seem to have any effect on how you reacted to the baby? Or how your husband reacted to the baby? (8) Would you use this service again?

Where possible, all interviews were tape recorded for future analysis. Detailed health, obstetric, and work history and other data were collected. This information will form the basis of other reports soon to be published. In about one-third of the cases, the father was present at the interview, and his comments were recorded separately. Because of the difficulty in achieving closely matched samples, these data cannot be treated statistically. The findings will therefore be reported in descriptive fashion.

Findings

Factors influencing the choice of childbirth option fall along four major axes that are both attitudinal and experiential. In addition, there is a group of other decision-influencing factors that do not lend themselves to simple categorization and must be discussed separately. All of these factors are reflected in Table 3.

Attitudes Reflecting Individual Responsibility

For Self. The women who chose out-of-hospital birthing centers expressed strong needs to be in a decision-making position concerning the care they received, including when and how they would receive analgesia (if at all). There was a strong interest in the continuity of care—these women preferred to have only a few well-known and well-

Table 3. Responses Influencing Choice of Childbirth Service

	University hospital (N=34)			Hospital birthing room (N=34)			Out-of-hospital center (N=57)		
	N	% of group	% of total	N	% of group	% of total	N	% of group	% of total
Related to responsibility for self									
Overall control of birth process	0	0	0	18	52.9	5.2	48	84.2	9.3
Risk-taking reduced	27	79.4	17.1	20	58.0	5.8	2	3.5	0.1
Pain management	28	82.3	17.7	12	35.2	3.5	4	7.0	0.1
Prenatal classes									
Lamaze type	3	8.8	1.8	34	100.0	9.9	57	100.0	11.0
Conventional	26	76.4	16.4	12	35.2	3.5	0	0	0
Distrust for medical profession	2	5.8	1.2	8	23.5	2.3	26	45.6	5.0
Related to responsibility for baby									
Overall control of baby care	0	0	0	28	82.3	8.1	51	89.4	9.9
Risk-taking reduced	30	88.2	18.9	27	79.4	7.8	4	7.0	0.1
Family attitudes									
Childbirth a family event	2	5.8	1.2	30	8.2	8.7	57	100.0	11.0
Constant attendance by mate	4	11.7	2.5	34	100.0	9.9	57	100.0	11.0
No separation from baby	4	11.7	2.5	31	91.1	9.0	57	100.0	11.0
Related to hospital environment									
Discomfort with routines	5	14.7	3.1	22	64.7	6.4	30	68.4	7.6
Continuity of care	4	11.7	2.5	25	73.5	7.3	40	70.1	7.8
Extended length of stay	23	67.6	16.4	25	73.5	7.3	43	75.4	8.3
Other	0	0	0	16	47.0	4.6	31	54.3	6.0
TOTAL	158			342			516		

trusted caregivers rather than a large complex of specialists prepared to deal with any medical or obstetrical emergency. Most did not claim that there were no risks in out-of-hospital childbirth but believed the risks were worth taking in return for what they perceived to be greater freedom of choice and a more relaxed and natural beginning with the new infant.

Virtually all of the 57 women had made special preparation by taking Lamaze or other similar natural childbirth classes, reading extensively, questioning relatives and friends, and visiting the birthing center and exploring its program in detail.

Many expressed open distrust of the medical profession (and often the nursing profession) and cited past experiences that they had found unsatisfactory. Several claimed that health professionals tended to treat them as if they were stupid or unthinking, failing to convey a sense of trust in the mother's ability to cope. Many mothers emphasized the importance of being totally conscious and alert during the childbirth process so that they could fully participate in it and accept immediate responsibility for their children upon delivery.

This brief excerpt from an interview with a young mother in San Diego may serve to illustrate the major points:

> I just wasn't satisfied with my obstetrician, and he "discharged" me. He felt my requests were above and beyond the call of duty. He felt it wouldn't be worth it to him for what he would have to go through with me. I wanted to know everything I could and I questioned everything. I

wanted my husband to stay with me before the baby was born and after. He thought that was a little severe. I wanted to know about the silver nitrate drops. I wanted to know legally why they were necessary . . . if you knew, you didn't have venereal disease. It wasn't like I was trying to be fanatical, but maybe that's the way I came off to him. Eventually I decided silver nitrate was a good thing because they can pick up infections that aren't venereal. It's just that he wasn't open and responsive to me. He said, "I'm not going to be strait-jacketed by a patient." I wasn't trying to do that. I just wanted somebody to talk to. I waited 30 years to have a baby. If somebody says "do this," I'm not going to say "yes" without questioning it.

In a similar vein, a young mother in New York City said:

I wasn't going to be told what I was going to get. I knew what I wanted . . . something more relaxed and a doctor who would take into consideration what you wanted, not a doctor who told you he was on the golf course and would be there in 2 hours when he finished his game. This American syndrome of "the doctor's convenience" is not what I want. I just don't want to be pushed around. My mother had her babies in Europe, and she told me to stay away from U.S. doctors and to look for a midwife.

In contrast, mothers who actively chose a more conventional hospital setting in which to have their babies conveyed a much higher sense of trust in the medical and nursing professionals, tended to be less concerned about personal decision making, and were more likely to take traditional prenatal classes rather than natural childbirth classes. They expressed more directly a sense of dependency on their caregivers; they were more concerned about risks and wanted an environment that they perceived as modern, medically safe, and scientifically up to date. Many others wanted to be cared for and stated freely that they had had previous experiences when they returned home from giving birth too early, tiring quickly in the first days and weeks of infant care. Almost universally, they were concerned about excessive pain and wanted reassurance that their physicians would quickly and expertly provide significant relief when it was necessary.

For Baby. The expressed spectrum of attitudes about responsibility for self was mirrored in a similar set of attitudes concerning the baby.

Mothers who elected out-of-hospital care strongly connected their own decision-making abilities with being responsible parents, with knowing their babies immediately, and with being identified as the primary caretakers from the first minutes of life. Each seemed almost resentful of intrusive professionals who "took over" the baby and wanted to perform medical or nursing care procedures upon him or her. Separation from their babies, even for brief moments, left them with a sense of discomfort and distrust.

Again, it may be useful to have a mother speak for herself. This 25-year-old mother of two children living in a large urban area on the East Coast had this to say about her new baby daughter:

I believe it made a difference [even allowing for being more experienced now and less afraid] . . . because she [the baby] was with us every single minute. She never really left us. We really saw what she was like . . . every single action. I was trying to think back with my son. When we went home with him we didn't know him. I didn't know what he was like the first couple of days. I just feel much more comfortable with our daughter. I just know her.

It would not be accurate to state that mothers who chose a more conventional hospital experience in which to have their babies did not want to feel close to or responsible for the new infants. Their interviews seem to indicate that they experienced less pressure and less of a sense of urgency about this. The prime concern was for the safety and health of the baby, and the first minutes and hours of the baby's life did not seem to hold such paramount importance for interactional purposes. They, too, felt that they were being responsible and involved parents by providing the best possible obstetric care. Their reading, however, was less focused on attachment and bonding than on the perils of perinatal asphyxia, respiratory distress syndrome, and other major problems of the perinatal period.

Family Life Attitudes and Values

All of the women who chose out-of-hospital birth experiences clearly communicated their attitudes about childbirth by portraying it as a major experience in the life of a family. They were turned off by discussions that implied that there were illness parameters to pregnancy and childbirth and tended to place much greater value on being attended by loved and trusted family members than by highly trained professionals. The latter were viewed as potentially or actually intrusive and as wanting "to take the experience away from us." As one mother said, "If you go to a hospital I just know from previous experience that having a baby is a medical event. I wanted my experience this time to be a family event."

The concept of childbirth as a period of celebration and a time of expanding one's kinship system seemed important to every one of these mothers. It was not important that large numbers of people be present: Most did not want this, but, rather, a small gathering of a few selected individuals (often including older siblings) with whom the event could indeed be celebrated.

Conversely, mothers who chose hospital care, although each may have had a sense of well-being and happiness at having a new baby, did not think of the event as a family experience. They tended to value the relative privacy and social isolation of the hospital for a few days and were quite comfortable with the sterile procedures and the restrictions concerning visiting.

It is important to add, however, that in each of the 57 instances of out-of-hospital care, there were available supportive individuals, including the woman's mate, who would participate with her in the childbirth-experience.

For 11 of the 34 hospital patients no genuinely supportive person was available, and in several of the remaining instances, the woman's mate was seen as ambivalent or somewhat distanced from the childbirth experience.

Attitudes Concerning Hospital Environment

The next group of attitudes is expressly related to perceptions of hospitals as caretaking environments. Of the 57 women who chose out-of-hospital care, 39 expressed moderately to highly negative attitudes about hospitals (as distinguished from doctors and nurses). There were frequent comments, such as "in hospitals, they don't tell you anything"; "you have to keep on guessing what's going on"; and "they don't like to communicate with you." Hospitals were also seen as places where even the most sympathetic professionals would be subordinated to fixed procedures and would be unable to provide individualized or personalized care. Continuity was also seen as a problem in hospitals because of the constant changing of shifts, the strong possibility that a woman's own doctor might not deliver her, and the constant intrusions from curious students and house officers. One woman summed it up like this: "In some hospitals, you have the feeling that you are really in the way—that if they could have the baby without you, they would." Another mother, who had to be transferred from her birthing center to a hospital because of failure of progress, described it as follows:

> I didn't like it. The doctor cut the cord right away. He gave the baby to the pediatrician before he gave it to me. I was under the hospital regulations. I felt that they were taking over my baby. They took him away. I couldn't keep him with me when I wanted to. They were in control. If they wanted to do something, they just did it. It just didn't seem like it was my baby any more. It was pretty much the way I was afraid it was going to be.

On the other hand, another mother who had used a birthing room in her local hospital for her first delivery decided against such an experience when it was time to return. She stated her reasons as follows:

> I felt I was not prepared physically or mentally. The birth of my first son went so beautifully. I just figured I had to stay 3 days this time. Last time I misjudged and went home very early after one day . . . I was a wreck at home. This time I'm going to feel a lot better. The care at the hospital was really super. They really did a wonderful job.

It is clear from this latter statement (and from many others in this sample) that there is a large group of women who still perceive the hospital as a protective and supportive environment and who accept what may sometimes be impersonal, discontinuous, and routinized care while they relax and prepare themselves for the vicissitudes of the first weeks and months at home.

Other Factors

As might be expected, there is a large group of factors that defy categorization but that seem to play an important part in the decision making for some women and their mates.

Finances. Many families chose an alternative birth center because it was cheaper; yet others reported that their third-party health insurers would not cover care at an alternative birth center but would cover conventional obstetric care, so that it was really less expensive to go to the hospital.

Specific Procedures. For some women, a crucial factor in using a particular setting, often an out-of-hospital birth center, was the belief that a particular childbirth method was possible within that setting. Some wanted to be free to move about physically during labor and to have their babies in a position they chose. Others wanted a nurse-midwife rather than a physician to attend them. Still others (4 of 57) felt that the most important thing was to go home as soon as possible after delivery and believed that such an attitude would meet less resistance from a birthing center than from a hospital. For some women, it was important to settle down within a specific nest and to be able to go through labor, delivery, and the immediate postpartum period in one room and in one bed without being moved to different physical environments and to different caregivers. This group was all multiparous women who had been unhappy with the constant shifting of locale that they had experienced during their previous deliveries in hospital settings. They would have gone to a hospital if this option had been available, but they chose the environment with regard to this particular factor.

Compromise with Mate. Of the 57 women who had their babies in birthing centers, 6 indicated that this had been a compromise choice. In each of these instances, the mother had wanted to have the baby at home, whereas the father insisted on the hospital. The birthing center was simply a convenient compromise that each could accept.

Note on Birthing Rooms Located within the Hospital

Finally, little has been said so far about the women who chose to have their babies in a birthing room within a hospital. Although space does not permit a detailed reporting of this population, the findings do suggest a compromise between the attitudes of women selecting conventional hospital care and those selecting out-of-hospital programs. Essentially, this middle group viewed the birthing room as offering proximity to technology and specialized hospital personnel and an environment where the care seemed more personalized, more family-centered, and more focused on the needs of the parents to affiliate early with the neonate.

Discussion

On initial inspection, there appears to be a wide disparity between what different groups of women with their mates are seeking as a childbirth experience. The differences, however, may not be as great as they appear on the surface. Although approaches for achieved desired goals during childbirth vary as much as individuals do, the actual choice of setting depends on previous life experience, current kinship and social support systems available, the woman's perception of her own health needs, and the perceived needs of her infant.

Common denominators emerge in the decision-making processes of all of these parents. What they appear to want is a childbirth experience that they perceive as (1) safe and secure; (2) providing mastery over the body of information and skills they need to parent the new child with confidence; and (3) promising positive outcome of the child's development. It is most unlikely that any single type of experience could provide this for the millions of individuals who have babies every year. Therefore, a broad variety of options is necessary and a careful prepregnancy and prenatal educational experience is required in order for parents to do some intelligent decision making.

One nurse-midwife with whom I spoke recently scoffed at the idea that women are attempting to rebel against medical authority or to usurp the position of nurses and physicians during childbirth. She said:

> When women say they want control, I don't think they're saying "I want to do my own thing." They're saying "I want to know what I'm getting into so that when I let down and become totally vulnerable, I can really let go without losing my self-respect or my dignity. I want to be able to relax and really give my baby a good welcome."

This nurse-midwife is saying most eloquently that some women need to know that everything in the environment is set up so as to make them feel safe, secure, confident, and well-attended, so that they can yield to their needs to be totally dependent and trustful of those who are looking after them during the childbirth experience.

As the claims that certain kinds of childbirth care are best for mothers and babies become more strident, it is extremely important for those of us who have some opportunity to remain focused on long-range developmental needs of children to become involved in the process by which these various options are investigated and their results documented. There are indeed few, if any, long-range studies that support any claims at all.

The second study referred to in the introduction of this chapter was prompted by the fact that there is not only a dearth of long-range developmental observations of children delivered in different settings, but also there is comparatively little known about possible differences in groups of women choosing different settings.

A Comparative Study of Women Choosing Two Different Childbirth Alternatives*

Because it appears that no single childbirth option provides the same sense of safety, security, and personal autonomy for all parents, we decided to compare two groups of women who had selected widely divergent childbirth options in the hope of learning more about the characteristics of these groups and more about their decision-making process. In addition, there is the possibility that such data might suggest important precursors of long-range parental attitudes and behavior that might be significant in influencing subsequent child development. Such information could be useful for the rendering of care both within the hospital and during the early weeks and months of the baby's life.

Method

For this study, we selected two groups of 30 women each who delivered their babies consecutively in two different childbirth settings, both in large urban centers. The first group delivered in a major university medical center known for its advanced technology, the research expertise of its faculty, and the immediate availability of the most modern perinatal and neonatal support systems. The second group of mothers delivered their babies in an out-of-hospital alternative birth center operated by certified nurse-midwives in a residential neighborhood of a large city, without a physician in attendance (although a consulting obstetrician was on call). This service is known for its emphasis on family-centered childbirth care, active participation of family members in the childbirth process (including siblings, if desired), and early discharge to home (usually within 12 hours). Because an effort was made to compare the two populations both clinically and demographically, it was not appropriate to match the populations for race, age, parity, and

*The third section of this chapter was originally published under the same title by this author in *BIRTH* 9:13–19, 1982. Reprinted by permission.

other similar features because one or more of these criteria might have proved to be differentiating characteristics between the two populations. Rather, they were accepted into the study on the basis of being delivered in succession in each center within a short period. Women who required admission to the university hospital on the basis of medical or obstetric complications (who, therefore, could not be considered to have actively elected that setting) were eliminated from the sample. Only those parents who chose the high technology setting with awareness that other out-of-hospital alternatives were available are included in the university hospital sample.

Both populations were administered a structured interview during the third trimester of their pregnancies. In addition to the usual demographic data and relevant obstetric information, each woman was questioned concerning (1) previous experience with childbirth and child rearing; (2) the nature of her childhood and adolescent preparation for pregnancy, labor, and delivery; (3) the quality and extent of her current marital, kinship, and social support systems; and (4) concerns about her own health during pregnancy and postnatal.

Each woman was also rated for the level of appropriate adaptive behavior during pregnancy (e.g., nesting behavior following quickening, denial of the pregnancy, overreaction to minor physical complaints, etc.), and their knowledge of out-of-hospital birth services was ascertained.

Results: Demographic Comparison

A comparison of the two populations along demographic lines (Table 4) revealed that the only difference unlikely to have occurred by chance was that of age distribution. This pattern, in which one-half of the women in the university hospital group were between 18 and 25 years, while 76.7 percent of the alternative birth center women were between 26 and 34 years, represents a difference that is significant ($\chi^2 = 6.05$, $p = .014$). More of the university hospital group of women were unmarried, less educated, and pregnant for the first time. Except for age distribution, these differences were not statistically significant and thus could be due to change. Because both the out-of-hospital birth center services and the tertiary center services are reimbursed by Medicaid and medical insurance companies, the choice of care was not dictated by ability to pay.

Women in both samples were likely to be married, Caucasian, in their 20s, reasonably well-educated, and having their first or second child. Considering that both samples came from a large urban area, the relatively low incidence of separation and divorce is surprising and probably would not be representative of a larger sample.

An analysis of the structured prenatal interviews conducted with each of these women during her third trimester suggests more noteworthy differences between the populations, however. In each category, we will report both numbers of responses we considered ominous for the family ("at-risk" responses) and also comment on any qualitative differences in the content.

Previous Experience with Childbearing or Child Rearing

Experience in other settings[31-33] has led to the prediction that women who have had previous adverse experiences with childbearing or child-rearing report higher levels of

Table 4. Comparison of University Hospital and Alternative Birth Center Groups by Demographic Characteristics

	University hospital (N=30)		Alternative birth center (N=30)		
	N	%	N	%	p
Age					
17 and under	1	3.3	0	0	N.S.
18–25	15	50.0	6	20.0	
26–34	14	46.7	23	76.7	p=.014[a]
35 and over	0	0	0	0	N.S.
Race					
Caucasian	26	86.7	26	86.7	N.S.
Black	4	13.3	4	13.3	N.S.
Marital Status					
Married	23	76.7	28	93.3	N.S.
Single	6	20.0	2	6.7	N.S.
Separated/Divorced	1	3.3	0	0	N.S.
Years Education					
Less than high school	3	10.0	1	3.3	N.S.
12	17	56.7	13	43.3	N.S.
13–16	9	30.0	13	43.3	N.S.
More than 16	1	3.3	3	10.0	N.S.
Parity					
0	14	46.7	10	33.3	N.S.
1–2	10	33.3	17	56.7	N.S.
3 or more	6	20.0	3	10.0	N.S.

[a] $\chi^2=6.05$

concern about the welfare of the present pregnancy and, therefore, might also be expected to elect a high technology setting for childbirth. Although there was a slightly higher incidence of concern about the fetus in the university hospital population, this was not significant (Table 5). Nineteen of the 30 university hospital patients (63.3%) expressed concern about the fetus, whereas fifteen (50%) of the alternative birth center patients did. There were no qualitative differences between their concerns. For example, typical responses of the university hospital group to the question, "Have you had any past difficulties that would give you concern about your baby?", included:

- "I had a miscarriage at about 6 months. The baby was dead for 2 months. That was very hard for me."
- "I thought I was going to have a miscarriage because my mother-in-law hit me in the stomach."
- "I didn't go to a doctor for the first 6 months and didn't take my vitamins like I was supposed to."
- "I have epilepsy. It scared me—whether the baby would be all right. I take Dilantin, and they told me the baby might have a cleft palate because of this."
- "I hemorrhaged in September, and I've been worried ever since then."

Table 5. Comparisons of Incidence of At-Risk Responses in University Hospital and Alternative Birth Center

		University Hospital (N=30)		Alternative birth center (N=30)		
		N	%	N	%	p
A. Adverse previous experience	Pts.*	19	63.3	15	50.0	N.S.
with childbearing	Resp.**	25	—	21	—	
B. Preparation for childbearing	Pts.	18	60.0	16	53.3	N.S.
and child rearing	Resp.	22	— .	18	—	
C. Maternal health concerns	Pts.	6	20.0	7	23.3	N.S.
	Resp.	6	—	7	—	
D. Marital support system	Pts.	19	63.3	10	33.3	p=.020***
	Resp.	32	—	11	—	

*Indicates number of patients with codable responses.
**Indicates total number of responses in this category.
***$\chi^2=5.41$.

Some typical responses to the same questions from the alternative birth center patients included:

- "I've been taking headache medication. I'm worried about this medication going through my body for the last 2 years."
- "I had a strange miscarriage before."
- "There's a lot of Down's syndrome in my family."
- "I got an electric shock from my iron during my pregnancy."

There is nothing unusual about these responses; many would be elicited from any randomly selected prenatal population. In terms of concerns about the fetus, the two populations are remarkably similar.

Early Preparations for Childbearing and Child Rearing

Another area that was explored in the structured interview was the woman's view of her preparation for childbearing and child rearing and whether she planned to rear her child differently from the way she was raised. It is interesting that there was no significant quantitative difference in the responses. Eighteen of the 30 women in the university hospital group (60%) indicated some dissatisfaction with the way in which they were prepared for childbearing by their families and their intent to handle things differently with their own children, whereas 16 in the alternative birth center group (53.3%) gave similar responses to these questions. An examination of the content of these responses indicates a noteworthy difference. Typical responses from the university hospital group to the question, "Do you plan to raise your child any differently from the way you were raised?" included:

- "I'll share more with my children. Not like I was. I guess she did the best she could. She worked for the government and wasn't home much."

- "My parents are divorced. I lived with my grandmother, my aunts, uncles. I was shifted around a lot."
- "I had a little brother who was 10 years younger than I. I was like his mother. I'll never do that to my kids."
- "I'm going to be around more. My mother wasn't around. She was working all the time."
- "My dad was too strict. I wouldn't be pregnant now if he hadn't tried to keep me from seeing my boyfriend. I'll talk to my kids more. My mom didn't talk to me that much."
- "I only plan to have one child. I like to think I'll have a more personal relationship if it's an only child."
- "I was with baby-sitters too much. That's something I'll never do. I really didn't get to know my parents very well."

In contrast, typical alternative birth center patient responses included:

- "I'll be less strict and freer with them."
- "How many pages do you want me to write in answer to that question? I'll place much less emphasis on material things and more on emotional matters. I'll try to give the baby more self-respect and self-confidence."
- "I'll try to teach them to be less conservative and give them more freedom and more experiences."
- "There will be more co-parenting in our house—and real nonsexist education with no set rules for parents of each sex."
- "I'll let them be more flexible—explore more and not feel so guilty about things."
- "I'll give them more emotional support and try to respect their individuality more."
- "I'll allow my children to be more active. I was told to be quiet and listen all the time."

Although the differences between these responses may lend themselves to several interpretations, it seems reasonable to suggest that the university hospital group placed much more emphasis on their own sense of emotional deprivation during childhood and a strong intent to avoid duplicating this situation with their own offspring. The alternative birth center group appeared to place much more emphasis on supporting the child in developing as an individual with autonomy and independence.

Concerns about Maternal Health

Another important area explored in the interview had to do with the woman's concern about her own health and how the pregnancy might affect it. Again, previous experience might have suggested that the university hospital women would have greater health concerns and would have selected a tertiary care facility for this reason. In fact, it was in this area that there was the least difference between the two groups. Six university hospital patients had expressed health concerns, whereas seven of the alternative birth center group did so. In most instances, these were of a minor nature and had to do with illnesses that had occurred during adolescence or were related to manifestations of fatigue, tension headaches, or mild anemias. The two groups were indistinguishable, both quantitatively and qualitatively, regarding maternal health concerns.

Perceived Deficits in Marital Supports

An exploration of the support systems of these patients revealed the most remarkable differences between the two groups. Nineteen of the university hospital group (63.3%) indicated significant deficits in either their marital or kinship support systems, whereas only 10 (33.3%) of the alternative birth center group did ($p = .020$). Again, there were also qualitative differences in these responses that may be even more significant. For instance, typical responses to questions exploring the nature of the supportive relationship with the spouse during pregnancy in the university hospital group included:

- "He helps me as much as he can, I guess. He fishes a lot. Sometimes he's gone for as much as 9 days at a time."
- "I hardly ever see him at all."
- "I guess he helps if he can. He's so nervous. I had a very hard first labor."
- "My God, what a big mess! He was real good until I started getting big and then it scared him. He doesn't like responsibility."
- "He's in Louisiana. I guess I never really see him at all very much."
- "He's determined that I'll go back to him after the baby is born. If he stops hitting me, I'll go back. I figure it's safer with the baby. I figure he won't beat me with the baby."

Contrast the preceding comments with these typical responses from the alternative birth center group:

- "He helps sometimes but not as much as I like him to."
- "Yes, he helps most of the time."
- "I guess I'll take the fifth amendment on that one."
- "Sometimes he's a big help, but sometimes he's a big pain."

It should be emphasized that we considered the latter responses at-risk ones. Most responses from the alternative birth center group that explored the marital relationship were highly positive and indicated a view of the spouse that was very supportive and involved. The university hospital women's responses appear much more ominous in nature and indicate frequent separation and/or underinvolvement of the spouse in the pregnancy and in the childbirth process.

Response to Pregnant State and Nesting Behavior

Finally, the structured interview explored responses of the pregnant woman to various changes in her body during the pregnancy and to her preparation for the coming delivery and new offspring. In the first category of reactions to the pregnancy, one again sees a noteworthy difference between the two groups. On the whole, the university hospital group tended to react with more extremes—to be more reactive to the events of conception and to the pregnant state—or conversely, displayed more tendency to deny the changes. The alternative birth center group displayed a fair number of negative reactions to the pregnancy, but these seemed more reality-based with less tendency to deny or overreact. Specially, some typical responses to the question, "What was your reaction when you learned you were pregnant?", included:

From the university hospital group:

- "I was very upset. I didn't want any more babies."
- "I'm a lot fatter. I had to quit my job that I had worked at since I was 15 years old so I'm very bored."
- "I feel the same. I don't even feel pregnant."

This interview was conducted in the third trimester of pregnancy:

- "I don't feel any different."
- "I was horrified." [laughing]
- "God! It never stops moving."
- "I feel worse. Very depressed all the time. I feel trapped."
- "I don't know. I feel bad. I'm depressed all the time."
- "Wow! I think he's going to kick my ribs out."

From the alternative birth center group:

- "When I found out I was pregnant, I was both afraid and happy."
- "When I learned I was pregnant, I realized it was going to mean an awful lot of changes for me."
- "There's no comparison. I'm really very uncomfortable when I'm pregnant."
- "I'm anxious about how things are going to turn out for me now."

A useful indicator concerning adaptive behavior during pregnancy is so-called "nesting" behavior. The women's responses to the experience of quickening, particularly as expressed in preparation for labor, delivery, and the care of the new baby, have proved to be important indicators of her coping style[34,35] (see Table 6). In this category, there are wide disparities between the two groups. Fifteen (50%) of the university hospital group

Table 6. Behavior Suggesting Maladaptation to Pregnancy Reported in Third Trimester

		University Hospital (N=30)		Alternative birth center (N=30)		
		N	%	N	%	p
A. Denial of, or overreaction to pregnant state	Pts.[a]	16	53.3	12	40.0	
	Resp.[b]	30	—	13	—	
B. Absence of "nesting" behavior	Pts.	15	50.0	1	3.3	p=.001[c]
	Resp.	17	—	1	—	

[a]Indicates number of patients with codable responses.
[b]Indicates total number of responses in this category.
[c]$\chi^2=16.71$.

gave responses that suggested inadequate or inappropriate preparation for childbirth and child care, whereas only one (3.3%) of the alternative birth center group gave such a response ($p = .001$). Illustrations from the former group include:

- "We haven't done anything to get ready for the baby. We wait until the baby comes. If something happens, I don't want to come home to that."
- "I haven't picked any names. My husband usually picks the names."
- "No, I haven't done anything. I don't have any money. I haven't bought anything. I don't see how I can get ready for this baby."

The one rather maladaptive response out of 30 in the alternative birth center group came from a nurse who was working long hours on a Pediatric Intensive Care Service:

- "I've been trying to redo the apartment. I'm exhausted from that and going to classes and I can't really get ready for the baby."

Discussion

Our communication with obstetricians suggests that their image of women who select out-of-hospital birth centers may involve a stereotype: typically a superadequate, highly educated, very independent, feminist-oriented, and sometimes antiestablishment woman. Our interviews of this small population do not support this image. Although the alternative birth center group is moderately older, this difference does not explain the choice of childbirth setting.

On the other hand, themes of autonomy, independence, and an emphasis on coping did emerge in one form or another. Although our data do not reveal specifically how the early preparation for and child rearing of these two groups vary, what does seem consistent is that the university hospital group wishes more closeness, more intimacy, and more involvement with their children than they themselves experienced during their own childhoods. In contrast, the alternative birth center group repeatedly placed a high priority on fostering independence and self-reliance in their children and giving them space to grow and develop on their own. There seems to be less emphasis on intimacy and more on individuation for these mothers.

When we review the ways in which the two groups perceive the support and involvement of their spouses in the pregnancy and birth, themes of deprivation, neglect, and isolation emerged more from the university hospital group. With very few exceptions, the women who selected an alternative birth center perceived their marriages as strong, at least in the area of the mutual responsibility for parenting. One is left with the question: Because certain women feel more supported in their marriages, do they feel freer to select the option to have their babies outside of hospitals? Or is there something more fundamental about the mate selection process for these women that also operates in their choice of childbirth experience? These are chicken-or-egg questions that probably cannot be answered by available data. Our data suggest that women who perceive their closest relationships as more involved and more supportive of the childbirth experience are also the ones who tend to have their babies in settings that are family-centered and in which the staff is more oriented toward the psychosocial aspects of childbirth care.

Our data concerning maternal responses to changes during pregnancy and maternal nesting behavior also suggest that the university hsopital population adapted less adequately, or at least more slowly, to the changes imposed or required by pregnancy than did the women who selected an out-of-hospital birth center. This also may be a signal of a woman's need for greater involvement and support of caregivers in tertiary settings.

This represents an unfortunate paradox. High-technology hospitals are not renowned for their emphasis on providing strong emotional support to patients. Yet our study seems to indicate that it is this very population that may require the most individualized attention. It is especially true of those women who are having their first child that the need for constant support and sensitive responses to expressed fears and concerns may be more crucial to the conduct of labor and delivery than the administration of the most highly technical and advanced medical procedures.

This suggests important considerations, particularly for obstetricians, house officers, and nursing personnel in hospitals. It is a truism that patients in labor need support. It may be less obvious that women who find themselves in tertiary medical settings may actually need more support than others and, by the very nature of the technological priorities established in large hospital units, may actually get less support during childbearing.

Conclusions

As this volume goes to press, we are confronted with many uncertainties about the future of out-of-hospital birthing facilities. It is almost impossible to summarize their status accurately because the states (and, of course, other countries) each have 50 sets of different laws and regulations governing the delivery of health care and the licensing of nurse-midwives. The overall third-party reimbursement situation has made it easier in some areas and more difficult in others for birthing centers and nurse-midwives to deliver care in a climate that is fiscally secure. And last, the national crisis in liability litigation with its subsequent malpractice insurance cancellations has forced some nurse-midwives to terminate their practices or to seek positions in hospital settings where they can enjoy liability coverage. All of these factors are under active discussion and negotiation. The decisions that eventually will emerge from these interactions will have a major impact on the form and diversity of childbirth services in every locale.

References

1. Wertz R, Wertz D: *Lying In: A History of Childbirth in America.* New York, Free Press, 1977, pp 132–177, 178–200.
2. Riley E: What do women want? The question of choice in the conduct of labor, in Chard T, Richards M (eds): *Benefits and Hazards of the New Obstetrics.* London, William Heinemann Medical Books, 1977, pp 62–71.
3. McClain C: Women's choice of home or hospital birth. *J Fam Pract* **12**:1033–1038, 1981.
4. McClain C: Perceived risk and choice of childbirth. Soc Sci Med **17**:1857–1865, 1983.
5. Adamson GD, Gare DJ: Home or hospital births? *JAMA* **243**:1732–1736, 1980.
6. Schiff M, LaFerla JJ: Childbirth at home or in the hospital: A prospective study of decision-making. *J Psychosom Obstet Gynecol* **4**:41–50, 1985.
7. American College of Obstetricians and Gynecologists: Position paper on out-of-hospital maternity care. Adopted January 1976 (District 2).

8. International Childbirth Education Association: *ICEA News* **15**:1, 1976.
9. Pearse WH: Home birth. *JAMA* **241**:1039–1040, 1979.
10. Renou P, Chang A, Anderson I, et al: Controlled trial of fetal intensive care. *Am J Obstet Gynecol* **126**:470–476, 1976.
11. Shamsi HH, Petri RH, Steer EM: Changing obstetric practices and amelioration of perinatal outcome in a university hospital. *Am J Obstet Gynecol* **133**:855–858, 1979.
12. Mehal LE, Peterson GH, Whitt M, et al: Outcomes of elective home births. *J Reprod Med* **19**:281–290, 1977.
13. Stewart D, Stewart L: *Safe Alternatives in Childbirth.* Chapel Hill, NC, Association of Parents and Professionals for Safe Alternatives in Childbirth, 1976.
14. Baum D, Macfarlane A, Tizard P: The benefits and hazards of neonatology, in Chard T, Richards M (eds): *Benefits and Hazards of the New Obstetrics.* Philadelphia, Lippincott, 1977, pp 126–138.
15. Blankfield A: Conflicts created by childbirth methodologies, in: *Psychosomatic Medicine in Obstetrics and Gynecology.* Proceedings, Third International Congress. Basel, Karger, 1972, pp 87–89.
16. Cox CA, Fox JS, Zinkin PM, et al: Critical appraisal of domiciliary obstetric and neonatal practice. *Br Med J* **1**:84–86, 1976.
17. Freeman R: Where will your patient deliver—at home? in a hospital? in an alternative birth center? *Contemp Obstet Gynecol* **12**:104–130, 1978.
18. International Childbirth Education Association: The Pregnant Parent's Bill of Rights and the Pregnant Patient's Responsibility, New York, 1977.
19. Lubic RW: The impact of technology on health care—The childbearing center. *J Nurse-Midwifery* **24**:6–10, 1979.
20. Lubic RW, Ernest, EKM: The childbearing center. *Nurs Outlook* **26**:754–760, 1978.
21. Broussard ER: Neonatal prediction and outcome at 10/11 years. *Child Psychiatry Hum Dev* **7**:85–93, 1976.
22. Klaus MH, Kennell JH: *Maternal–Infant Bonding.* St. Louis, C.V. Mosby, 1976.
23. Korner AF, Grobstein R: Individual differences at birth, in Rexford EN, Sander SW, Shapiro T (eds): *Infant Psychiatry.* New Haven, Yale University Press, pp 68–78, 1976.
24. Stone LJ, Smith HT, Murphy LB: *The Competent Infant.* New York, Basic Books, 1973.
25. Crandon AJ: Maternal anxiety and neonatal wellbeing. *J Psychosom Res* **23**:113–115, 1979.
26. Morishima HO, Pederson H, Finster M: The influence of maternal psychological stress on the fetus. *Am J Obstet Gynecol* **131**:286–290, 1978.
27. Ward IL: Exogenous androgen activates female behavior in noncopulating, prenatally stressed male rats. *J Comp Physiol Psychol* **91**:465–471, 1977.
28. Zax M, Sameroff AJ, Babigian HM: Birth outcomes in the offspring of mentally disordered women. *Am J Orthopsychiatry* **47**:218–229, 1977.
29. Cohen RL: Parental experiences in out-of-hospital birthing centers, in Taylor PM (ed): *Parent-Infant Interaction.* New York, Grune & Stratton, 1980, pp 189–209.
30. Cohen RL: Modern Science, High Technology and the childbirth process. Paper presented to Joint Meeting of Pittsburgh Pediatric Society & Pittsburgh Society of Obstetricians and Gynecologists, December 1980.
31. Cohen RL: Maladaptation to pregnancy. *Sem Perinat* **3**:15–25, 1979.
32. McDonald RL: The role of emotional factors in obstetric complications. A Review. *Psychsom Med* **30**:222–237, 1968.
33. Rose JA: The prevention of mothering breakdown associated with physical abnormalities of the infant, in Caplan G (ed): *Prevention of Mental Disorders in Children.* New York: Basic Books, 1961, pp 265–282.
34. Doering SG, Entwisle DR: Preparation during pregnancy and ability to cope during labor and delivery. *Am J Orthopsychiatry* **45**:825–837, 1975.
35. Beck N, Siegel LJ, Davidson NP et al: The prediction of pregnancy outcome: Maternal preparation, anxiety and attitudinal sets. *J Psychosom Res* **24**:343–351, 1980.

III

Consultation Practice

8

Models of Consultation and Liaison
General Principles

RICHARD L. COHEN

Introduction

As indicated in several previous chapters, mental health consultation to childbirth services bears many similarities to conventional consultation and liaison services in a general hospital but with several significant adaptations. In Chapter 1 (Introduction), there is reference to the long history of development of the fields of psychosomatic medicine and consultation and liaison and the manner in which these paths have bifurcated to some degree over recent years. It is important to remember that the basic tenets of consultation and liaison in general medical and surgical hospitals have many applications to the field of obstetrics and childbirth, and it must be assumed that the reader enjoys a working knowledge of this data base.

In the same chapter, we also reviewed the reasons for considering consultation and liaison services to obstetrics as unique in many ways and as requiring an additional data base and level of sophistication for the consultant.

The most important data base that should be factored into the assessment process in a consultation is contained in Chapter 5. The detailed knowledge of the developmental process of pregnancy (using whatever philosophical approach is acceptable) combined with the interviewing skills necessary to elicit the relevant current and historical information represents the core of the consultant's expertise.

A very pointed and powerful rationale for the development of mental health interventions long before the intrapartum period is documented in the chapter concerned with the

Richard L. Cohen • Department of Psychiatry, Western Psychiatric Institute and Clinic, University of Pittsburgh, Pittsburgh, PA 15213.

impact of prenatal stress on the fetus and infant (Chapter 3). This growing body of knowledge should be made available to clinical administrators and to academic leaders in the field of obstetrics as a cogent argument for the identification of at-risk populations and the development of sensible, cost-effective programs to reduce morbidity both in mother and infant.

In Chapters 4 and 6, we have attempted to provide an overview of the epidemiology of mental disorders during pregnancy and the postpartum period together with a nosology that takes into consideration not only the frank psychiatric disorders but the developmental delays of pregnancy and the characteristics of at-risk populations.

We also considered the impact of ever-changing forces and the financing of liability coverage on emerging alternative models of childbirth care and the potential significance of these forces for mental health programs.

In the final chapter, we will also review some of the information that is available concerning what is known about the cost/benefit ratios both of consultation and liaison programs, their impact on hospital length of stay, and on overall expenditure for medical care.

All of this background represents a necessary foundation for considering a variety of consultation and liaison models that, if implemented with both expertise and sensitivity, should result in a high level of benefit to families, to infants, and to the stressed and often overstressed staffs of childbirth units.

Entrée into the System

It is a truism that the manner in which the consultant first becomes engaged with a new consultee (whether an individual or an organization) is a crucial determinant in how the interaction proceeds from that point. Sensitivity to the needs of the service, its priorities, its attitudes about mental health professionals and, last, about mental illness per se are all matters about which the consultant needs to be informed from the onset. The social-political-economic environment in which the childbirth services are being delivered should have a major influence on how the consultant conceptualizes his or her work and how he or she decides on the best form in which to offer his or her own services.

It is important before becoming active even as a single case consultant to understand fully the resources for psychosocial, environmental, and crisis intervention that already exist in the obstetric unit or hospital. Almost all services have medical/obstetrical social workers assigned. These professionals usually have excellent backgrounds in counseling, in understanding and using community resources, and in providing appropriate family supports within the limits of the resources available. It is natural and predictable that a social work staff will look upon many forms of mental health consultations with jaundiced eyes. Many may feel they can provide equivalent or even better service because they are constantly available and know the patients better. It is vital to "connect" with these staff members, in order to learn what they already know about the patient and to establish a collaborative relationship that recognizes their expertise in the hospital and that includes them as a part of any team that may plan crisis or ongoing interventions. Failure to handle this process sensitively and promptly may result in behind-the-scenes deprecation of the mental health consultant or, worse yet, sabotage of the consultant's efforts. There may be other professionals whose skills include supportive counseling and the use of referral services. These may be called clinical nurse specialists or obstetrical nurse practitioners. In any event, they represent experienced and respected members of the nursing hierarchy of the hospital. The same caveats apply to them as to the social work staff.

The traditional manner in which a mental health consultant progresses through a human service system has been from single-case-centered consultation over a period of time (during which he or she demonstrates his or her expertise and usefulness), to a more consultee-centered focus in which he or she becomes a part of the support system of the staff in a liaison relationship, and to, finally, a program consultant in which he or she advises around ways in which to improve existing delivery systems and generates ideas for planning and implementing new programs that incorporate preventive and public health concepts. This all may later lead to collaborative training and research projects.

In most situations, this may still be the most logical and feasible order of events, but one should not assume this without exploring the ground carefully. Indeed, the interests and priorities of a highly organized and academically centered department of obstetrics may not be congruent with this kind of agenda. There are occasions when a more sensible approach is first to engage senior faculty in the department of obstetrics to collaborate in a joint investigation around which a grant proposal can be developed and external funding can be generated. There are now many areas of mutual interest to obstetricians and mental health professionals such as risk factors in teenage pregnancy, the impact of alcohol or drug abuse on pregnancy outcome and child development, the diagnosis and management of depressive disorders during and following pregnancy, and the reliability of current high-technology methods for assessing the long-range effects of perinatal hypoxia, to name just a few.

The development of strong and mutually respectful working relationships that can occur in a well-designed and well-run research project can easily blossom into much broader programs of consultation and intervention that are well received in the obstetric unit because they have the support of the academic leadership.

Conversely, there are many programs in which the consultant must first gain credibility and visibility through making important contributions to the understanding and care of difficult patients. This usually leads to other kinds of working relationships and the generation of programs that have broader goals than the management of an individual patient.

The essential point is that the consultant is unlikely to progress very much in any direction without a careful look at the priorities of the organization. This should not be misinterpreted to mean that one needs to engage in "the soft sell" or any manipulation of one's colleagues. It means only that a consultant who is not genuinely responsive to perceived need within a program or service is likely to be discounted summarily.

Perhaps the most informative (because it is so personal) and detailed account of one experience that was both successful for the psychiatrist and productive for the obstetrical service is that of Pasnau.[1] This report of a 5-year experience in consultation and liaison with obstetrics has many lessons to teach. Pasnau himself makes the point, often emphasized by Lipkowski,[2-4] that one should be extremely careful about generalizing from one experience. Nevertheless, some of Pasmau's successes and failures do have generic implications for this work and deserve careful review.

I would like to paraphrase a few of the highlights here before proceeding further with specific recommendations and case material of my own. Pasnau makes the following major points that warrant special attention:

1. Enormous emotional demands are made on the obstetrician/gynecologist. He or she must learn to function in the widely varying settings of the labor suite and maternity ward, the gynecology ICU, the prenatal clinic or private office, the surgical amphitheater, and so on. These shifts in function and role may be more characteristic of the practice of obstetrics and gynecology than any other specialty and require major shifts in role, approach, and relationship with patients and families, often over the space of a few hours. In addition, these roles involve relating to many different kinds of support personnel in these settings and many different types of subspecialists. All of this must be carried out within the context of frequent sleep deprivation and chronic fatigue.

2. Physicians in this specialty are often faced with life and death situations both in mother and in infant for which their training has provided them little preparation by way of both personal coping styles and by way of appropriate counseling for parents. So much emphasis has been placed on the acquisition of technical skills that proper time and energy have not gone into other kinds of preparations for interpersonal skills.

3. Obstetricians and gynecologists are essentially surgeons who thrive on great attention to detail and on specific, concrete approaches to treatment and diagnosis. They are accustomed to acting and doing rather than more contemplative approaches.

4. The support staffs of obstetric programs, primarily nursing personnel, tend to be overstressed and easy victims to burnout both because of the emotional and physical nature of the work. This may be further complicated by the fact that they must often act quickly and in the absence of the physician at crucial points.

5. As with any specialty, obstetricians and gynecologists tend to have more respect and more trust in consultants who know something about their own specialty. It is important for the psychiatrist or other mental health professional to become knowledge-able, at least at a minimal level, about the nature of the obstetric complications and the latest diagnostic treatment methods being employed so that he or she will have some understanding of what the patient is experiencing and what the obstetrician is attempting to accomplish.

Pasnau makes many other important points but the previously mentioned ones seem to me to be ones that would apply to all programs and that the consultant must keep in the back of his or her mind at all times. With reference to the last point, for instance, I can recall how gratifying it was when the obstetric personnel with whom I was working learned that I had taken a postgraduate course in electronic fetal monitoring; that as a result of some of the writing I was doing, I had been elected an associate fellow of the American College of Obstetricians and Gynecologists, and that I was collaborating with a perinatologist in studying the long-range effects of hypoxia in the offspring of patients with failure to progress in labor. I rather suddenly became someone who understood and appreciated their problems and the vicissitudes of their practices and someone with whom they could discuss patients without having to explain everything.

Another, perhaps obvious, but enormously significant point deserves further empha-sis. Because the medical profession is still largely populated by males who have only indirect knowledge of pregnancy and childbirth, the psychiatric consultant (if indeed he is a man) must constantly find ways not only to increase his intimate knowledge of the pregnant state and the vicissitudes of the labor room, he must also make every effort to use available female support personnel to assist him in understanding the specific nature of the patient's problem he is confronting and in designing recommendations that are appropriate. How, for instance, is a young, male, unmarried psychiatrist able to establish credibility with a 35-year-old, multiparous woman who is now rejecting her pregnancy, who is depressed and unwilling to continue with mothering her children or with life in general? The first rule is to establish a clear and unmistakable posture of listening. Mental health personnel are trained to do this well, but in the rush of everyday hospital business, there is a tendency to cut people short, to look for quick answers, to hand people rating scales and questionnaires and to seek yes-or-no answers to questions that cannot be answered in that fashion. This is the best way to cut off communication with the pregnant woman and to reduce the reliability of information collected to a point where it is almost useless.

There are always knowledgeable and experienced professional women in the environment. If one is very fortunate, one has a consultation team for collaboration purposes. This may contain a female psychiatric social worker or clinical nurse practitioner who is not only a woman but a mother and can therefore be extremely helpful in communicating with the patient and in establishing clear directions for future intervention, if appropriate. If such personnel are not available, it is important to identify empathic females on the obstetrical staff (e.g., an obstetric nurse practitioner or hospital social worker). Collaboration and planning with these individuals not only helps to establish attachments within the hospital (so that the consultant is not a ''foreign body'') but is also likely to maximize the level of intervention because these latter individuals already enjoy credibility with the medical staff and are consistent figures in the patient's daily environment.

Last, in subtle and unobtrusive ways, the consultant must communicate to the patient his or her understanding of the developmental processes of normal pregnancy and his or her ability to enter empathically into the process at its current phase. This can only come from increasing mastery of the concepts that have been outlined in Chapter 5 and the large body of the literature that has been developed on this subject. Simply demonstrating a knowledge of what it is like to manage one's sleeping position or bladder during the latter stages of pregnancy (let alone the more complex intrapsychic and interpersonal issues) immediately establishes the consultant as someone who has talked with many pregnant women, has listened to them, and knows something about the experience.

Overview of Models

This chapter will outline three broad categories of consultation and liaison that can be related to childbirth services. These are as follows:

Direct Case Consultation

The most common examples of this category include:

1. Patients displaying gross psychiatric symptomatology (nonemergencies).
2. Patients displaying gross psychiatric symptomatology (emergencies, e.g., suicide risk).

3. Patient-initiated requests for psychiatric consultation.
4. Persistent preoccupation with fetal damage in the absence of medical documentation.
5. Some "psychophysiologic" disorders of pregnancy such as hyperemesis gravidarum.
6. Grief reactions following abortions or stillbirth.
7. Need to assess competency to care for an infant:
8. Postpartum depression or psychosis.
9. Pregnancy or childbirth as a precipitant to psychiatric disorder in the mate.
10. Serious emotional disturbances involving a pregnant adolescent.
11. No gross psychiatric symptomatology but professional concerns about an at-risk mother or family (e.g. severe marital crisis occurring during pregnancy).

Obviously, this list could be extended significantly but the preceding illustrations do cover the most common categories of direct consultation requests. In Chapter 9, we will describe in modest detail several such referrals, the kind of information gathering that is essential to understand them, and the interactive process with childbirth professionals that follows such assessment. With the understanding that no list of case illustrations can be all inclusive, I believe it is a fair statement that a working familiarity with the previously mentioned types of situations will place the consultant in a position where he or she is unlikely to encounter severe "culture shock" while doing direct case consultations in a childbirth environment.

Consultation and Education Activities with Medical, Nursing, Social Work Staff, and Others

Under this rubric is included a wide variety of efforts from the informal hallway consultation with house officers and others (during which teaching is an inevitable by-product) to the more formal structure of case conferences, seminars, lectures, grand rounds, and other activities. The purposes of the latter are to heighten awareness of the following:

1. The significance of stress factors during pregnancy; normal versus abnormal developmental processes in pregnancy.
2. The way in which psychiatric disorders appear differently during pregnant states.
3. The risks and benefits in using medication during pregnancy.
4. Other similar topics that may be useful in daily practice (e.g., how best to make a psychiatric referral, management of delayed grief reactions, and recognition of the "vulnerable child syndrome").

It is important to remember that a large part of the "message is in the medium." Mental health personnel are particularly prone to use jargon with which other professionals are unfamiliar and to use allusions having to do with intrapsychic constructs that have meaning only to "insiders." There is no easier way to turn off the listening apparatus of an obstetric resident or perinatologist than to resort to such language. Just as it is important to establish credibility with the pregnant woman by demonstrating one's working knowledge of the process of pregnancy, it is equally important to establish with childbirth personnel at least a superficial knowledge of current childbirth care practices, their risks, and benefits. The consultant who attempts to teach primary care mental health interventions that are totally inapplicable in a high-technology environment in the 1980s is wasting everyone's time. In Chapter 10, we will describe some specific types of educational and liaison activities that may be gratifying to the consultant and quite useful to the childbirth care givers.

Program Consultation and Participation

These activities, if they occur at all, result from an institutional commitment to use mental health expertise to do the following:

1. Help design new programs for screening at-risk pregnant women.
2. For early identification of psychiatric disorders.
3. For the development of innovative techniques based on newer information about the developmental processes of pregnancy.
4. Heightening staff sophistication about productive use of high technology interventions.
5. Other related programs.

Although all of the previously mentioned activities are important, in the final analysis, the consultant has reached the peak of his or her productivity and usefulness when he or she is in a position to influence the planning and development of institutionwide programs that serve to identify women and their families who may require some form of attention earlier in the pregnancy process than is likely to occur through the direct case consultation mode. The large numbers of women who can be reached through such efforts and the overall cost-benefit ratio that can be demonstrated through such approaches can have major impact on how the obstetrical environment operates. They may also have a positive impact on the incidence and prevalence of childbirth complications and on the overall outcome of the caregiving activities. In Chapter 10, we will also describe how such programs may be conceptualized and implemented.

References

1. Pasnau RO: Psychiatry and obstetrics-gynecology: Report of a five-year experience in psychiatric liaison, in: *Consultation Liaison Psychiatry*. New York, Grune & Stratton, 1975, pp 135–147.
2. Lipowski ZJ: Review of consultation psychiatry and psychosomatic medicine, I. General principles. *Psychosom Med* 29:153–171, 1967.
3. Lipowski ZJ: Review of consultation psychiatry and psychosomatic medicine, II. Clinical aspects. *Psychosom Med* 29:201–224, 1967.
4. Lipowski ZJ: Review of consultation psychiatry and psychosomatic medicine, III. Theoretical issues. *Psychosom Med* 30:395–422, 1968.

9

Direct Case Consultation

RICHARD L. COHEN AND KATHERINE L. WISNER

Introduction

Because this aspect of practice tends to be the most straightforward and best understood, let us begin with a discussion (together with some specific case illustrations) of one model for carrying out direct case consultations in an obstetric setting. Space will not permit a description and an illustration of all possible situations in which the consultant may become involved, but the following conceptual points and illustrative cases may serve as a basis for developing a deeper understanding.

It is vital to remember that most obstetric patients come into the hospital not expecting to be ill, not seeking psychiatric assistance, and certainly not connecting any physical symptoms they may have with any mental health problems.

To the degree possible, the consultant should "force" the resident or staff member to be specific concerning the need for consultation. The simple written request that may say "rule out psychiatric disorder" is almost worthless in these situations (or perhaps in any situation!). A telephone contact with the referring clinician during which there is some opportunity to exchange ideas, to ask questions, and to help the referring source be explicit about the reasons for seeking help are important. It is also essential to clarify that the patient has had the need for consultation explained and that either the patient (or if appropriate) the family have agreed to it. The game of charades should not be played during consultation.

The usual conferences with involved house staff and, especially, the patient's primary nurse are indispensable. Prior chart review is a given. Obviously, this takes time. It is important to explain to all concerned that psychiatric consultations cannot be performed in 15 minutes and that there is no magic bag of tricks or mind-reading act that the consultant can perform to come up with easy answers or quick fixes.

Richard L. Cohen and Katherine L. Wisner • Department of Psychiatry, Western Psychiatric Institute and Clinic, University of Pittsburgh, Pittsburgh, PA 15213.

Often patients are in semiprivate rooms or in rooms with as many as four to six patients. It should be made clear in advance that a private setting is necessary in which to interview the patient. This does not mean curtains drawn around the bed. It means an office or an empty room if the patient does not have her own private room. Patience and forbearance will be necessary until the working style of the consultant becomes more familiar and until there is better timing for consultations than is typical in many settings. It is not appropriate for the consultant to express irritation or anger at being called at the last moment when all other specialists have not been successful in "coming up with an answer." It may be appropriate to experience such irritation, but the open expression of it is more likely to be alienating and to be seen as critical. The realities of everyday medical practice are such that, particularly among surgical specialists, the use of psychiatric consultation as an early intervention is simply not a part of the mind set.

In conceptualizing the approach to the consultation, having reviewed the chart and having become familiar with the setting in which pregnancy and childbirth care are being delivered is to constantly recall the triad of factors that must be included in the assessment process:

1. The specific nature of the presenting clinical problem.
2. The developmental stage of pregnancy (not simply the gestational stage but the developmental stage).
3. The setting in which clinical care is being delivered.

If one considers only the first point, one is at risk of making erroneous conclusions and, therefore, recommendations. At the extremes, consider two patients being referred because of persistent fears of labor and delivery that are interfering with the use of prenatal care. The first patient is a 17-year-old unmarried woman in her second trimester being cared for in a high-technology university hospital; she is alienated from the father of the child, not caring for herself appropriately during the pregnancy, and she has not reacted to quickening with any preparatory behavior with respect to future care of the infant. Compare her with a 35-year-old primigravida who is in her last trimester and who is a partner in a two-career professional marriage, having spent much of the last several months preparing a nursery in her home, purchasing baby clothes and furniture, and arranging for substitute care for the baby so that she can return to work a few weeks following delivery. Also, she does not wish to be cared for in a hospital and has sought care in an out-of-hospital alternative birthing center run by nurse-midwives.

The presenting complaint of both of these patients is precisely the same, yet any attempt to deal with these based on the nature of the complaint alone is doomed. The developmental stage in question is not only that of the women themselves but of their pregnancies. The physical and professional resources available to participate as a part of the intervention team are so different that the consultant must be compelled to factor these into the equation prior to drawing any conclusions or making any specific recommendations.

Although many other influences, both positive and negative, must be factored into the assessment process, it is the three clinical "building blocks" described in Chapters 5, 6, and 7 that are likely to be most helpful in understanding the needs of the pregnant woman and in planning an intervention, if one is needed. The cognitive model I have

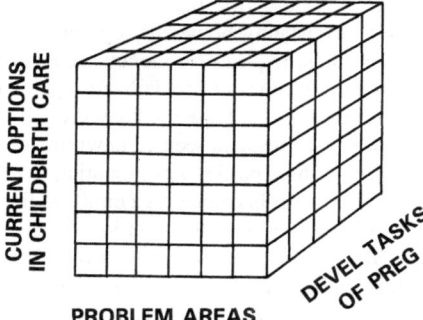

Figure 1. "Building blocks" of consultation model.

found most useful is to conceptualize all referrals as lying at some point in a three-dimensional matrix (see Figure 1).

The particular nature of the presenting problem, the developmental status of the pregnant woman, and the characteristics of the setting in which care is being delivered are all important and must be related to each other in order to fully grasp the implications of the referral.

How do these concepts appear in practice? Perhaps a review of a dozen or so cases may serve to illustrate some of the answers to that question.

The following consultations are not presented because there is any illusion that it is possible to cover this subject in exhaustive detail but to display the variety of situations to which the consultant may be exposed and to demonstrate how much flexibility and creativity may be necessary in order to tailor an approach in each of these.

Case Histories

Case 1

Type of referral. No current disorder identified. Staff concern about impending dysfunction. This case illustrates the function of psychiatric consultation in a situation where there is currently no gross psychiatric disorder but in which the obstetrician and nursing staff suspect impending problems and are seeking assistance in averting a major disorder.

Consultation request. Mrs. J. is a 19-year-old white, married primigravida who was referred because she complained of increasing nervousness and "grouchiness" toward everyone around her, especially her husband. She is in her seventh month, and the obstetric course of her pregnancy has been within normal limits. The clinic staff has become concerned about Mrs. J.'s fears that her marriage may be disintegrating and that she may be increasingly negative toward the pregnancy.

Data collection. Mrs. J. reluctantly accepted the consultation suggestion but did follow through. She was visibly irritable and abrupt. An abbreviated developmental review of her pregnancy revealed that, except for occasional back pain and lower abdominal discomfort, the pregnancy had gone smoothly from a physical standpoint. She has been married for 1 year to a man 12 years her senior whose first marriage ended in a very stormy and conflicted divorce. Now she found herself "constantly bothered" by her husband's former wife who lived only a few miles away, made constant requests for money and attention upon her husband, and, not infrequently, called the patient at odd times of the day and night. The latest telephone call ended with her husband's first wife screaming, "I hope the baby dies!"

Mrs. J.'s husband seemed unwilling or unable to cope with these disturbances, and the tension between all three parties was mounting to fever pitch. The patient was now wondering whether she should have ever become pregnant in the first place, whether her husband really cared enough about her, and whether he was regretting the dissolution of his first marriage.

Mrs. J. showed only a low level of interest in her pregnancy and her baby, was preoccupied with the mounting dissension, and feared she might be "stuck" with a new baby at the age of 19 and with inadequate supports.

Prenatal care was being delivered in a university hospital prenatal clinic. In addition to the usual attendants, there were two social workers and a mature obstetric nurse practitioner assigned to the team.

Because Mrs. J. now lived several hundred miles away from her family of origin, there were no family supports available, and she had had little opportunity to make new social relationships since marrying and moving to a new city.

Recommendations and disposition. The staff was reassured that Mrs. J.'s symptoms were largely situation-specific and that she appeared to be basically a healthy, well-adjusted young woman. The team social worker was encouraged to hold a series of counseling interviews with Mr. and Mrs. J. during which Mr. J. was assisted in recognizing the significance of his wife's reaction to his lack of involvement and support in resolving the disturbance being caused by his previous wife. He began to look at the long-range implications of this for his current marriage and for his ability to maintain a stable home for his new child. Although apprehensive about intervening, he was "rehearsed" through a series of contacts with his first wife during which he was able to take a firm position with her and to establish both a separation from her and a sense of permanency and commitment to his second marriage. During this process, follow-up reports from the social worker indicated that Mrs. J.'s mood began to lift, that she became much less irritable, and that she began to plan actively for the coming baby in a very realistic fashion.

Case 2

Type of referral. No current disorder identified. Staff concern about impending dysfunction. This case also illustrates the function of psychiatric consultation in a situation where there is currently no gross psychiatric disorder but in which the obstetrician and nursing staff suspect impending problems and are seeking assistance in averting a major disorder.

Consultation request. Mrs. B. is a 23-year-old white, married primigravida who works as a grade-school teacher. She is now in her sixth month of pregnancy and is referred for psychiatric consultation because of growing marital tension associated with her refusal to have any further physical contact with her husband and because she is beginning to decompensate on the job for reasons she cannot explain.

Data collection. Mrs. B. presented as a thin, pale, tense young woman. Early in the consultation, she made it clear that she was rather uncomfortable because the consultant was a male and that she would have preferred to speak to a woman. However, she did make every effort to participate in the interview. She stated that she felt guilty that ever since she had become aware of her pregnancy at about 8 or 10 weeks following conception, she had refused sexual contact with her husband. She went on to describe that this extended even to casual physical contact like touching and kissing. She said, "I hate to have him touch me now." She was not only guilty but puzzled by this. She maintained that she had always liked children, that this was a planned pregnancy, and that she very much looked forward to becoming a mother. It was the intimacy of heterosexual contact that she now found disturbing, even alarming. Although she did not describe their relationship as "passionate," she indicated that prior to the pregnancy, she and her husband had had a close and affectionate physical relationship. Apparently the state of pregnancy had precipitated a crisis related to some unresolved anxiety about heterosexual relationships.

Reluctantly and with much agitation, she was finally able to describe two or three incestuous experiences with a young maternal uncle when she was about 9 or 10 years of age. There had been no contact since, and she had never mentioned this to anyone, even her husband. She had hoped that this episode was behind her, but clearly it was not. She described her husband as hurt, rejected, and "destroyed" by her behavior, and this only heightened her guilt.

Although there were the beginnings of some "mechanical" preparations for the baby such as space and clothing, there seemed to be little fantasy about, or emotional attachment to, the pregnancy at this time.

This patient was being seen in the private office practice of a full-time faculty obstetrician at a university hospital. Aside from a secretary and nurse assistant, no other staff was available to work with Mrs. B. and her husband.

Recommendations and disposition. Although this patient did not warrant a psychiatric diagnosis, it seemed apparent that the pregnancy had precipitated a crisis related to wholly unacceptable incestuous behavior during late childhood.

Within the limits of Mrs. B.'s constraints on confidentiality (the consultant was limited to generalities by way of sharing information with the obstetrician), the general nature of the crisis was explained to the referring obstetrician, and a recommendation for referral for individual psychotherapy with a female therapist was made and accepted. Mrs. B. also gratefully accepted the referral. Follow-up information indicates that she participated well in the psychotherapeutic process and is making excellent progress in her new role as a mother.

Comment. The preceding two cases illustrate several points worth remembering. First of all, they remind us how gratifying the work of a consultant can be in situations where so modest an investment can have such far-reaching results. It is important for the consultant to remember and for him or her to be constantly reminding his or her obstetrical colleagues that these kinds of complaints should be taken seriously and not dismissed, that they may be the harbingers of more serious problems to come, and that they may, by their very nature, interfere with the developmental progress of pregnancy.

We may be reminded once more that it is often the private patient who may have the least professional resources available. These cases illustrate clearly how important it may be to have a diverse team of professionals available for intervention purposes. Often this team is available for "service" patients but not necessarily in the private sector. Indeed, it may take more improvisation to deal with these at-risk patients in private practice than in the clinic. By the same token, these are also the most valuable cases for heightening awareness among health professionals about such matters as developmental delays during pregnancy, the vulnerable child syndrome, and the impossibility of separating the entire process of pregnancy from the dynamics of the family in which it takes place.

Most of all, they remind us that intervention is not only possible and effective but does not have to be carried out directly by the mental health consultant provided he or she is aware of available resources and approaches for activating them.

Case 3

Type of referral. Suicidal risk.

Consultation request. The patient is reported as expressing serious suicidal intentions and also homicidal wishes toward her common-law husband. The consultation request was submitted 48 hours after delivery. By the time the consultant arrived on the unit, Mrs. D. had signed herself out against medical advice. The baby remains in the hospital. On discharge, Mrs. D. had been given a follow-up appointment at a community mental health clinic in the neighborhood where she lives. The appointment is 4 weeks from the date of her discharge from the hospital.

Data collection. Mrs. D. is a 22-year-old black woman who is a gravida three para one. Her common-law marriage extends over the past 4 years, and her first two pregnancies have ended in early spontaneous abortions. The present birth has just ended with the delivery of a 880-gm premature male infant with a ventricular septal defect. Delivery was by C-section. Chart review revealed that there is a strong family history of schizophrenia on the mother's side with several hospitalizations in public institutions for close family members. During some of her prenatal visits, Mrs. D. was noted to have made bizarre comments (e.g., "this god-damned baby better be good, or I'll stick it on a pole outside the hospital"). Mrs. D. was viewed by the staff as being "different and a little weird," but no staff member entertained a diagnosis of psychosis or impending psychosis, and no genuine suicidal or homicidal ideation was elicited during her prenatal visits. The congenital defect in the fetus had not been identified by sonography or any other diagnostic technique. Mrs. D. is believed not to have any knowledge of it. There had been no opportunity to inform her of the defect during the postpartum period because she had seemed to be too agitated to deal with such information.

Recommendations and disposition. Because direct patient contact was not possible, a brief meeting of the involved staff members was held with the consultant to discuss options. The consultant made a conscious effort to avoid finger pointing or blaming either at the prenatal staff or at the resident who was involved in the AMA ("Against Medical Advice") discharge. In fact, there is the distinct possibility that Mrs. D. met the criteria for involuntary commitment in view of her suicidal and homicidal threats. This might have been a choice had the consultant been involved earlier in the process.

Nevertheless, it was agreed that the staff and consultant had some ongoing responsibility in this situation and that a concerted effort should be made to recontact Mrs. D., especially in view of the extremely vulnerable state of her baby. The consultation/staff meeting resulted in agreement of the following points:

1. Continued effort should be made by phone and mail to bring Mrs. D. back to the obstetric unit and to reinvolve the psychiatric consultant if this is at all possible.

2. In any event, she should be encouraged to return for visits to her infant and to work with the staff around long-term disposition for this child assuming the infant's viability.

3. There was an ethical and legal obligation to contact Mr. D. in view of the open homicidal threats being made by his wife, particularly because no demands for confidentiality or secrecy had been claimed on her part. There was much debate on this last point. Consultation with the hospital's legal counsel supported the recommendation that Mr. D. be alerted to the threats on his life.

4. Because it seemed unlikely that Mrs. D. would be able to meet the baby's needs (especially in view of the level of its impairment), a series of contingency plans was to be developed by the neonatal and social work staffs that would allow for a stepwise system of interim care for the infant upon discharge from the hospital, using both kinship supports and child welfare service facilities in the community.

5. In the event that Mrs. D. could not be persuaded to return to the hospital, contact was to be made with the community mental health clinic where she had been referred to underscore the urgency of the situation and the inappropriate nature of a 4-week delay in clinical contact. They were to be urged to contact Mrs. D. directly and to invite her in for an immediate appointment. The possibility of a home visit by one of the mental health workers was to be discussed, and cooperation on the part of the consultant in assisting with certification for involuntary commitment was assured if this was indicated.

Comment. This type of consultation, unfortunately not an infrequent one, places the consultant in a difficult position. Because a referral for mental health assistance has been made and because the patient had signed out AMA, the course of least resistance would be to say that the consultant has little or nothing more to offer. The consultant is not fulfilling his responsibility if he ''steps aside'' at this stage of developments. First of all, one cannot assume that nonmental health professionals are in a position to evaluate lethality issues. In fact, they tend to either overreact or underreact to them, often not being clear either on the practical steps that may be taken to protect the patient and relevant others or acknowledge their own liability as professionals in these situations. They need an experienced consultant on whom to lean, and it is much better to have a clinician on whom to depend than to turn to the hospital's attorney for legal assistance and advice. That all too often happens in such dilemmas, and although the attorney may act in the best interest of the hospital and its staff, he or she cannot be expected to apply mature clinical judgment and to develop an intervention plan.

The obstetrical staff should not have accepted an appointment 4 weeks away for this patient at a mental health facility but should have insisted on earlier contact. They also need the advice of a consultant on how best to develop a long-term plan for this infant that involves more than expert neonatal care but takes into consideration the developmental issues that may be paramount for this child if it survives the early weeks or months of extrauterine life.

Case 4

Type of referral. Patient initiated request for psychiatric consultation.

Consultation request. Mrs. W. is a 38-year-old black woman who is a gravida five para four. She is married for the second time. Her three older children (ages 16, 13, and 12 are from her first marriage; her youngest child, age 4, is from the second marriage). Mrs. W. has reacted ''violently'' to the news of her fifth pregnancy and cannot understand how she became pregnant because she is using birth control pills. Finally, when seen by her obstetrician (because she delayed seeking prenatal care for many months), she admitted to being extremely upset and requested psychiatric consultation in so many words. The obstetrician concurred and made the referral.

Data collection. Mrs. W. presented as a well-groomed, articulate, intelligent woman who stated that when she learned she was pregnant several months ago ''went haywire.'' Although the possibility of seeking an abortion crossed her mind, she never pursued it, making, instead, every effort to ''calm myself down.'' She described herself as never feeling well during her pregnancies, always seeming to have a cold or some upper respiratory infection that drained her. At first she did not believe that she was pregnant and took castor oil and quinine tablets to bring on her menstrual period; now she is wondering that perhaps she damaged the baby. She believes she is ''too small'' for so advanced a time in her pregnancy. (The obstetrician reports all findings are normal from his point of view.)

Mrs. W. was obviously a mature and experienced mother, had been through several normal pregnancies, and described her children as doing well and being basically happy and well-adjusted youngsters. She simply could not contemplate going through the experience of another pregnancy, birth, and the stress of rearing a young child again at what she considered to be such an advanced age and with so many other children to care for. She described her nerves as being "very bad" and that matters were not helped at all by what she considered to be her husband's nonchalance about the whole matter. She described herself as being torn between wishes to end the pregnancy (now manifestly impossible) and her strivings to accept the situation, make the best of it, and get on with her life. She stated that she was "stuck" and so "crazy" about the overall situation that she could think of nothing else, was neglecting her family and her usually well-cared for home.

Recommendations and disposition. Because there was no staff member in the obstetrician's office to work in an ongoing role with Mrs. W. and because it appeared that a brief, time-limited intervention (in view of her track record) was likely to be effective, the consultant offered a "contract" for three or four sessions to include Mrs. W. and relevant family members. This was promptly accepted. What emerged very quickly was the picture of an overfunctioning wife and mother who often rejected help when it was offered to her and who was so compulsive about meeting the needs of her family and her home that other family members despaired of ever meeting her standards. What also emerged was Mrs. W.'s fear that she would "never have anything for myself," like a career or activities outside the home. Within a few sessions, the oldest offspring, a daughter of 16, was making it clear that she would welcome the opportunity to learn how to care for a baby and to be of help to her mother. Mr. W. was making it clear that supplementary child care help from others was available and that he would be happy to pay for this and to assist his wife in continuing with her advanced education in addition to participating himself much more actively in the care of the younger children.

The treatment goals were easily accomplished within three sessions with rapid restoration of emotional stability for Mrs. W. The obstetrician called a few weeks later to express his gratitude for the intervention and to inquire in some detail concerning how it had been accomplished.

Comment. There are situations in which brief, direct intervention by the consultant may be the best course of action. This, of course, can only be done with the full approval of the referring obstetrician and of the patient. This can be carried out in less severe cases where there are good family resources and where the clinical issues seem to be largely exogenous or situational. Also, if there is no mental health team available for direct intervention, this is an added reason for the consultant to become more active. These cases lend themselves to a time-limited contract. In the preceding case, a relatively simple shift in the family system and its way of operating around child care that involved both the husband and the siblings worked "magic."

Case 5

Type of referral. Fixed ideas concerning fetal damage in the absence of factual documentation. This type of situation may be a precursor of the so-called "vulnerable child syndrome." In one or both parents, there is a conviction that the fetus is damaged as a result of some intercurrent experience during pregnancy. These ideas tend to persist despite a plethora of medical tests and repeated reassurance by the obstetrician that all signs both with the mother and baby are now within normal limits.

Consultation request. Mrs. I. is a 26-year-old white, married, gravida two para one. She is now almost at term. During her seventh month, she had a brief episode of acute pyelonephritis that responded well to chemotherapy but did require a brief hospitalization. She has read that serious infections and/or medications may have an adverse effect on the fetus and is now terrified that she will give birth to a retarded baby or one with a serious congenital defect. Both her obstetrician and pediatrician have assured her that these events occurred much too late in her pregnancy to represent any serious risk to the baby who, by all signs including sonography, is growing and developing normally. In fact, all laboratory and other findings are well within normal limits. Mrs. I. has a 3-year-old son who was the product of a normal pregnancy and is now doing very well developmentally.

No amount of reassurance or answering her questions has had the effect of reducing her anxiety or alleviating her premonition that the outcome of this pregnancy will be a negative one.

The telephone referral from the obstetrician conveyed a mixed note of perplexity and irritation at Mrs. I. because of her refusal to accept his "word" that everything was all right. The obstetrician was convinced that Mrs. I. was "slipping her ratchet" and that this clinical presentation might be the beginning of a serious postpartum illness. Consultaton was being requested both in an effort to identify new approaches to reassuring Mrs. I. but also for an estimation of the risk level for postpartum illness.

Data collection. Mrs. I. appeared to be about her stated age and was clearly in the last trimester of her pregnancy. Both her obstetrician and pediatrician felt that she would be very resistant toward psychiatric consultation, and she stated that at first she had been but then began to wonder, "Maybe I'm going crazy." She went on to describe how different this pregnancy had been from her first one that had been such a happy and healthy experience for her and her husband. She talked at some length about how she and her husband "doted" on their 3-year-old, Timmy. She described in overinclusive detail her relatively mild bout of pyelonephritis and how different it might be with this coming child. She admitted that both her obstetrician and pediatrician whom she had trusted implicitly seemed impotent in the face of her overriding concern that she now carried a damaged fetus. She knew that she was so preoccupied with this that there was something "abnormal" about it; hence the fear that she might be going crazy and her final willingness to accept psychiatric consultation.

A developmental review of her pregnancy up until the seventh month revealed entirely modal patterns. And an exploration of her kinship and social support systems revealed a most involved and supportive husband who was equally puzzled by Mrs. I.'s inability to move beyond her intractable fears about the baby and several close female peers, all of whom were experiencing the early years of motherhood. Almost in passing, Mrs. I mentioned that a close friend had recently suffered a stillbirth. Further exploration of this uncovered the fact that her friend had become depressed during the pregnancy and had been treated with what Mrs. I. believed to be lithium.

The experience had been deeply shocking for the small group of women who served as mutual supports for each other and especially for Mrs. I. who was then about 5 months pregnant. It was not long after this that she began to experience the symptoms involving her renal system, and now she felt convinced that her fate would be similar to that of her friend. She revealed nighttime fantasies of delivering a dead baby and felt for fetal movement scores of times during the day, often not being sure whether the movement was adequate.

She further stated that even if the baby were born "normal," this would not mean anything. It might have some hidden defect, and then she would not know for years.

Recommendations and disposition. No direct reassurance was given to Mrs. I. that her baby was fine and that there was no cause for concern. In the face of the failure of two trusted physicians to alleviate her fear previously, this would have been folly.

She was told by the consultant that among his areas of interest was considerable expertise in infant and child development and that he would meet both with her obstetrician and pediatrician to discuss future management. The consultant urged both physicians to "back off" until the actual status of the newborn could be determined. Assuming that it was a normal baby (in fact, this was the case), Mrs. I. was to be encouraged on frequent visits with the pediatrician to report in detail on the infant's changes from visit to visit. She was instructed to keep a daily log and to bring in pictures showing how the baby had changed over time.

This in fact was a consultation that lasted for several months, although there was only one direct contact with the patient. Considerable liaison with the pediatrician was indicated in order to help Mrs. I. get locked in on the baby as a healthy, developing young person. No further efforts were made to give reassurance, but the emphasis was placed on holding Mrs. I. to carefully observing the baby's changes, to recording them, and to reporting on them constantly to the pediatrician.

Within a period of 4 or 5 months, her fears appeared to have dissipated, and she has come to experience her second child as a healthy, constantly changing infant, quite different from her older son but equally rewarding and exciting to care for.

Comment. Although this case also represents an illustration of the so-called "at-risk" family, it is included here because the model of intervention is one that deserves closer attention. Although there was only a single contact with the patient herself, it was clear that ongoing liaison with both obstetrician and pediatrician was essential for the proper resolution of this dilemma. This type of fixed ideation about potential damage to the fetus that has not responded to repeated expert reassurance is the kind that is least likely to respond to one intervention on the part of the consultant. The mother (or both parents, if appropriate) need to discover for themselves with constant support and guidance that the emerging development of the child has positive dimensions, that caring for the child can be rewarding and exciting, and that daily preoccupation with the child's growth and development soon supersedes fantasies about possible hidden defects. The constant emphasis on assets rather than pathology focuses the parents on the pleasures of being "connected" to a growing child that is, after all, the essence of parenthood.

Case 6

Type of referral. Request for opinion for use of psychotropic medication with hyperemesis gravidarum. Note the specificity of this consultation request. The case represents an excellent illustration that a focused consultation request does not always make for a productive use of the consultant. Perhaps even to a greater extent, this case is a lesson in humility for any consultant who begins to experience even a slight twinge of omnipotence. We have all had the experience of doing the right things for the wrong reasons. This is an instance in which all of the wrong things were done for the right reasons.

Consultation request. Mrs. McA. was referred for consultation because of intractable vomiting that did not respond either to the use of compazine, continuous bed rest, or counseling by the obstetrical staff. She is a 23-year-old married, white, primigravida who is at 33 weeks gestation. The consultation request is now made at Mrs. McA.'s fourth hospitalization during the past several weeks because of concerns about her vomiting. She is reported to experience severe vomiting daily, sometimes as many as six or eight times. She now suffers from esophagitis and has reported occasional hematemasis probably on a traumatic basis.

She is an insulin-dependent diabetic, has gained 20 lb, and is also reported to have a history of being anorectic and bulimic during her late adolescence.

In desperation, her obstetrician is now requesting an opinion concerning shifting her from compazine to amitriptyline in the hope of reducing her vomiting and avoiding serious problems with electrolyte balance and possible serious pregnancy complications.

At the time of referral, all physical laboratory and findings are reported within normal limits.

External fetal monitoring and ultrasonography revealed a fetus of normal size for gestational age, normal activity patterns, and the absence of any discernible physical abnormality.

Data collection. The usual conference with the nursing staff that should proceed any direct contact with the patient failed to reveal the specific reason for the need for an opinion concerning the use of amitriptyline. In view of the multiple variables in the past medical history and in the current situation, this seemed to be a rather unusual request and, if anything, too focused. It originated from an obstetrician whose occasional requests for consultation in the past tended to be quite diffuse and coming at the end of all other consultations with a "rule-out" orientation.

Discussions with the resident revealed that Mrs. McA. had had two hospitalizations for severe anorexia accompanied by marked depression when she was 20 and 21 years of age, respectively. At that time, both the eating disorder and the affective syndrome responded well to a combination of psychotherapy and amitriptyline. The request concerning amitriptyline currently was because of a suspicion that Mrs. McA.'s current presenting complaints masked an underlying depression once more. (For a full discussion concerning the use of antidepressants during pregnancy, see Chapter 12.)

Mrs. McA. presented as a pale, fretful young woman with a rather puffy face and pressured speech. During the course of the direct consultation, she showed no signs of nausea or vomiting. She did confirm, however, the current description of her physical problem as described in the chart and by the nursing and medical staff. She seemed resentful and irritated that her obstetrician had insisted on hospitalization and bed rest because of her frequent vomiting. In fact, he apparently had informed her that, unless this could be brought under control, she would need to stay in the hospital for the remainder of her pregnancy.

Mrs. McA., although ostensibly anxious and irritable, was quite coherent and showed no gross signs of a thought disorder. She did seem mildly depressed and admitted to this but stated that this was more a reaction to her confinement than anything else. She added a fact that the staff had not emphasized previously. Her husband was an noncommissioned army officer stationed at a NATO installation somewhere in Western Europe. Because of her physical condition, she had not been able to join him, and she was feeling very isolated and unsupported in her marriage at this point. Also she described that her mother, who had been previously widowed, had recently remarried and had a 20-year-old stepson who is mentally retarded and requires much attention.

She seemed to emphasize that the two key people in her life, her husband and her mother, were unavailable to her. She made no connection between this and her physical condition. She expressed no concerns about the baby or about her diabetic status, feeling that both of these were under good control (and in fact, this was supported by the objective data available in the chart).

Her only request was to be discharged from the hospital so that she could return to her home where she felt more comfortable in spite of the vomiting.

Recommendations and disposition. Conferencing both with the resident and the attending obstetrician was used to shift the focus from what the consultant perceived as a search for a "quick fix" by the use of an antidepressant to a treatment plan that recognized the crisis nature of this patient's status. Recommendations were made for introduction of frequent counseling, not so much focused on her physical symptoms but her overall life situation. It was emphasized that this should start at once in the hospital and be continued upon discharge, particularly because the pregnancy was now in the third trimester and, although all signs were within normal limits, the introduction of a new baby with all of the constant attention and care that that would require appeared to be a precipitant that might very well worsen Mrs. McA.'s emotional status if she did not have adequate support and guidance from professionals.

The obstetrician agreed to give up the idea of using antidepressants and to organize a plan, using both a clinical nurse specialist available in the hospital and visiting nurses to implement a professional support structure for Mrs. McA.

While this plan was being organized, Mrs. McA.'s husband appeared unexpectedly in the hospital on compassionate leave of absence. Mrs. McA. had requested this, and her family physician, someone who was not directly communicated with by the obstetrician, had certified it. Mrs. McA. had informed no one of this action.

Her nausea and vomiting stopped almost immediately, and she was discharged from the hospital. The consultation and liaison service was not notified about this until 2 days post facto. No follow-up is available at this writing.

The elaborate plans that we had developed and "sold" to the obstetric staff were left as words on paper. Later information indicated that the remainder of Mrs. McA.'s pregnancy was uneventful but details are sketchy.

Comment. This experience sent the psychiatric attendings and house officers scurrying to the literature. Was Mrs. McA. malingering? How could the sudden appearance of her husband result in such a magical disappearance of what had been a grave and intractable symptom? The literature proved to be simultaneously helpful and confusing, depending upon which studies one relied on. Since the late 1950s, both positive and negative correlations between hyperemesis gravidarum and hysteria, gall bladder disease, alienation from the patient's own mother, unconscious rejection of the pregnancy, and a whole host of other variables have been described. In the aggregate, these seem to cancel each other out and to suggest that we still know comparatively little about this "disorder." In the event that the consultants neglected to remember this fact, Mrs. McA. emphatically reminded us!

Case 7

Type of referral. Request for emergency psychiatric evaluation.

Consultation request. At 6 days postpartum, Mrs. S. was referred for emergency psychiatric evaluation because she "became hysterical" when speaking to her obstetrician by phone. She was crying unconsolably and screamed: "I've already called five places trying to get help! You've got to do something to help me!" The obstetrician was alarmed but also puzzled because Mrs. S. had a normal pregnancy, delivery, and 3-day hospital stay. She had always been a pleasant, cooperative patient.

Data collection. Mrs. S. was a 26-year-old white married woman who had delivered a healthy male infant 6 days prior to evaluation. The patient gave a history that suggested the postpartum blues, with onset of spontaneous weeping, restlessness, anxiety, irritability, difficulty concentrating, and insomnia that reportedly began 4 days after delivery. Her major complaint was marked anxiety. Fortunately, she had excellent support from her family who were able to help considerably with the infant's care.

Education regarding the transient nature of postpartum blues and a prescription of benzodiazepine were given to the patient in the psychiatric emergency room. Upon follow-up evaluation at 9 days postpartum, the patient's symptoms had increased. She experienced marked sedation and dysphoria in the morning after taking the benzodiazepine. Additional history from the patient and her husband revealed that she had experienced significant symptomatology during her pregnancy: 2 to 6 hours per day of sadness, insomnia, diurnal variation in mood with sadness and marked irritability in the morning, anergia that resulted in the patient remaining in bed or sitting on the couch for prolonged periods, and feelings of guilt for not being ecstatic with her planned pregnancy as she had been during her first pregnancy. She had experienced anxiety, palpitations, and tachycardia (about 100 bpm) during the first trimester, which was accompanied by hyperdefecation. These symptoms diminished in intensity over the second and third trimesters.

Upon examination at 9 days postpartum, the patient was tearful and quite distressed: "No one believes me!" was her comment regarding the reassurance she had received in the emergency room that the "blues" were transient. She denied suicidal ideation and thoughts of harming her children. She agreed to additional medical work-up, which included thyroid studies. Anxiety, insomnia, borderline tachycardia, and hyperdefecation suggested hyperthyroidism, which often is more active during the first trimester, subsides during the second and third trimesters, but flares postpartum.

Follow-up evaluation at 13 days postpartum revealed that she had not improved, a course that was unlikely for uncomplicated postpartum blues syndrome. The thyroid studies were "normal" with respect to the immediate postpartum state in which elevated total serum T_4- but lower T_3-uptake values are found, with resultant normal free T_4-index. The patient appeared to be suffering from a major depression, which had its onset with pregnancy. The postpartum period had intensified the patient's distress.

Recommendations and disposition. The recommendation was to begin antidepressant medication after establishing that the electrocardiogram, liver function studies, and blood count were normal. The patient was begun on nortriptyline, and she experienced significant reduction in her presenting symptoms within 2 weeks.

Supportive therapeutic work for the patient and her husband was recommended because they had planned to have a large family and they were appropriately concerned about whether she would experience depression with subsequent pregnancies.

Comment. Although this patient had both pre- and postnatal depression, her presentation illustrates several important points. The symptom of marked anxiety in the postpartum period is often the most troubling to women who have a *major depression.* Frequently, the early signs of postpartum depression are mistaken for a "normal reaction," anxiety disorder, or the "baby blues." Often medications such as antianxiety agents or barbiturates are prescribed to treat the insomnia, and reassurances are given. Although benzodiazepine hypnotics are appropriate for symptomatic treatment of the blues, the key point in this case is the need for close follow-up in the immediate postpartum period to distinguish the blues from major depression.

Mrs. S. made a full recovery and was motivated by her experience to write an account of her illness. She wrote:

> When the baby was 4 days old, I started to cry. I don't know why. I was sitting, talking to my parents, and the next thing I knew I got an overwhelming urge to cry. I couldn't snap out of it, I was so down. I had a pit in my stomach. Butterflies. I kept wringing my fingers. Sometimes I held my head, knowing that at any second it was going to explode. I was petrified to get up with my baby. I also feared the morning. I would cry at a drop of a hat. Absolutely no control over that. I was scared. I didn't know what was happening. I wanted to go—constantly. I got upset because my body couldn't keep up. I felt guilty because I couldn't control myself. I could not bring myself to eat. I had to force my mouth to chew. Forget housework. I couldn't care less what a mess the house was. My concentration was nil. I couldn't sleep even though I was exhausted. I thought: Isn't there anyone who can help me?

Case 8

Type of referral. Request for advice about the use of lithium during pregnancy.

Consultation request. This consultation was requested from the inpatient staff of a psychiatric hospital. The physicians were concerned about the teratogenic effects of lithium and haloperidol.

Data collection. Mrs. Y. was a 35-year-old woman with bipolar affective disorder who was admitted to the hospital with delusions, hallucinations, and "abdominal swelling." Evaluation of the swelling by obstetrical consultants revealed that the patient was 11 weeks postconception. Her medication had been lithium, 1200 mg/day, and haloperidol, 10 mg/day. She had been non-compliant, and the lithium level upon admission was 0.2 mEq/L. When the pregnancy was dis-covered, all medications were withdrawn "to prevent harm to the fetus." The patient became progressively more psychotic and required seclusion because of aggressive outbursts. Haloperidol was reinstituted because "the risk outweighed the benefit." The patient's aggression had dimin-ished since reinstitution of the haloperidol.

Mrs. Y. and her husband greeted the consultant with an angry outburst in which Mr. Y. demanded to know why his wife's medication had been held upon admission to the hospital. He was upset that "she got real sick" and questioned why she "didn't get her medicine," even though he brought her "because she was starting to get sick again." Although he was aware that she was pregnant, he said, "She was on the same medicines during the last pregnancy, and the baby was okay."

Clinical evaluation of Mrs. Y. revealed that she continued to experience hallucinations but did understand that she was pregnant and demonstrated some attachment to the fetus. She told the consultant the names she had selected and admitted to omitting doses of her medication because she thought she might be pregnant. The couple stated firmly that they wished to continue the pregnancy.

Review of the chart revealed no documentation of discussions with the couple regarding the options for treatment and the risks and benefits of these options.

Recommendations and disposition. The major intervention was targeted toward the resident and attending physicians who were caring for Mrs. Y. The physicians admitted to being concerned about a "lawsuit." Consultation included review of clinical considerations for the use of psycho-tropics during pregnancy and practical information about teratogenicity of lithium and haloperidol (see Chapter 12). The use of participant prescribing as a maneuver that builds physician/patient (and husband) relationships was emphasized. Fear of the lawsuit was precipitating behaviors that were alienating the patient and her husband and were increasing the risk of what the physicians feared. Ongoing consultation was offered. Mrs. Y. and her husband favored reinstitution of her lithium and haloperidol regimen, and Mrs. Y.'s mental status improved dramatically. Mrs. Y. gave birth to an infant who appeared normal at birth.

Comment. This case raises several issues. Prescribing medication to a pregnant patient involves considerable anxiety upon the part of the physician. In this case, there was a "knee-jerk" reaction to hold medication because of the pregnancy. There was no risk/benefit discussion with the wife and husband. The woman predictably became more psychotic until her state "justified" reinstitution of medication, again without risk/benefit discussion with the couple. It is likely that a greater total dose of medication was given to the grossly psychotic woman than if she had been treated in the significantly less disorganized state in which she presented, and this resulted in increased exposure to the fetus. The major focus of this consultation was not the question that the physicians generated but an intervention focussed on the physician/patient relationship. This type of consultation requires skillful diplomacy and avoidance of criticism or blame.

The fetus had been exposed to lithium during the first 11 weeks of gestation; the major concern was regarding lithium cardiovascular malformation. Because the tricuspid valve and heart are formed prior to the time at which the patient presented, the withdrawal of medication at 11 weeks is unlikely to significantly diminish the risk of this anomaly. In this type of situation, it is easy to focus on fear of errors of *commission* (such as the giving of medication in situations of risk) versus errors of *omission* (such as withdrawing medication in a psychotic woman).

Case 9

Type of referral. Request for opinion regarding the use of psychotropic medication during pregnancy.

Consultation request. Mrs. W. was a 22-year-old married woman who was hospitalized during the fifteenth week of her first pregnancy with severe new-onset systemic lupus erythematosus with cerebritis. The consultation/liaison team was asked to assess the patient to decide "which medication would be the most appropriate in the management of her agitation and hallucinations." She had been hospitalized since 10 weeks gestation for multiple complications that included sepsis; however, according to the obstetrician, the fetus was viable and was normally sized for age of gestation.

Data collection. Upon examination, the patient exhibited classic signs of delirium with rapid alterations in the level of consciousness, rapid changes in affective state from withdrawn and somnolent to fearful or euphoric. She identified the interviewer as her sister and had obvious visual hallucinations of people to whom she spoke. Her speech varied from appropriate answers to questions to total lack of response. Her attention span was limited. Despite this level of symptomatology, the patient remained in her hospital bed and did not raise her voice to a level that disrupted other patients on the ward. She accepted redirections of her behavior and orienting statements from an aide who was present in the room.

Recommendations and disposition. The question to be addressed in this case is *whether* medication is indicated. Because of her minimal agitation, she could be managed on the hospital ward with close observation by a familiar aide, removal of harmful objects, and other routine measures for the management of delirium. Appropriate medical management of her lupus cerebritis resulted in marked improvement of her clinical picture, and a normal gross mental status exam within 3 days. If the level of agitation had increased and the patient had exhibited violent behavior or self-harm, our recommendation would have been to add small doses of haloperidol to the regimen. Frequent small doses, with careful attention to evaluation of symptom response, are more favorable than infrequent large doses that bolus the fetus and increase the likelihood of side effects (see Chapter 12).

Comments. Many interesting staff reactions to Mrs. W.'s situation occurred. Some of the staff were attempting to defend against anxiety created by medicating a pregnant woman by casually stating, "She had so many medications already, the baby's probably damaged anyway. It's not too late for her to have an abortion."

After Mrs. W.'s mental status improved, brief supportive therapy of the patient was undertaken by an interested psychiatric resident. Mrs. W. had experienced the delirium as a "lapse in time" and had no recall of events for that period. She said, "They said I was crazy." Historical information and interview revealed a psychologically well-functioning woman with no previous psychiatric history. She stated emphatically that she wished to continue her pregnancy and that she had already bought clothes and nursery items. During the second visit, she became tearful and expressed several appropriate concerns: Does the "crazy episode" mean that she was crazy and will she need psychiatric hospitalization? Would "lupus" mean that she would always have difficult pregnancies, and, what is most important, did the medications that she was taking mean that her child would have "no fingers or toes"? A joint conference with the psychiatric consultant, obstetrician, and internist with the patient in order to answer her many appropriate questions was accomplished. Continued work with the complexity of her situation. Follow-up revealed that she delivered a normal infant, and she appeared to adapt well to motherhood, despite postpartum exacerbation of her lupus.

Case 10

Type of referral. Request for psychiatric examination following a reproductive catastrophe.

Consultation request. The obstetrical staff initiated a request for consultation because Mrs. R., a 34-year-old married woman, had suffered her second episode of abruptio placentae with intrauterine fetal death, toxemia, and dissemination of intravascular coagulation. She was hostile to the obstetrical staff postoperatively, and a nonspecific request for "psychiatric evaluation" was initiated. Clarification of the consultation request was difficult. Although the obstetrician was concerned about the hostility of the patient and her husband, he was also obviously upset at the loss of the infant and the critical medical status of Mrs. R.

Data collection. Mrs. R. had been hospitalized at a psychiatric facility following the first episode of abruptio placentae. She had suffered a prolonged grief reaction and major depression that required antidepressant medication. Mrs. R. was very pleased about the current pregnancy and elected to discontinue her antidepressant medication at the time she confirmed her pregnancy. She began to exhibit depression about 1 month after discontinuing the medication that she had used about 3 months into gestation. Although offered medication, Mrs. R. chose to manage her increasing depression with frequent sessions with her therapist. Approximately 1 week prior to the second abruption, the patient began to experience suicidal ideation; however, she refused medication and hospitalization because "I'm 34 weeks pregnant—I only have a few weeks before my baby will be born, and I don't want to do anything to hurt it." Mr. R. was a chronic alcoholic who had deteriorated markedly after the first fetal death.

At 2 days postoperatively in the ICU, clinical examination of Mrs. R. revealed a woman who was experiencing a mild delirium and was difficult to interview; however, she voiced fears of the staff's "trying to hurt" her and responded that she wanted to "jump out the window" when asked about suicidal thinking. Constant observation was recommended. At 3 days postoperatively, the patient was "cooperative and pleasant," according to the nursing staff. She was stabilized medically and transferred out of the ICU. Curiously, she did not appear to exhibit signs of major depression, which were well documented prior to the fetal death. Mrs. R. continued to be a model patient during the remainder of her stay. Mr. R. visited frequently and behaved appropriately but smelled of alcohol.

When given an opportunity to discuss the death of the fetus, Mrs. R. responded, "It makes me sad to think about it," and changed the subject. She had refused several opportunities to hold the dead infant. She refused to look at pictures of the dead infant that the social worker had given her.

About 10 days after the fetal death, the consultant was called at night because "Mrs. R. was screaming hysterically about the baby." The obstetrical resident wished to know "what medication to give." Review of the situation with the resident revealed the Mrs. R. had screamed after a dream and was crying! A senior obstetrical nurse had entered Mrs. R.'s room and was holding her hands while Mrs. R. sobbed about the "unfairness of losing two babies." The resident was asked to check the current situation and found that Mrs. R. was sobbing softly and speaking with the nurse. The resident was given information about the process of grief and advised against the use of medication.

Mrs. R. did not speak further about the dead infant(s), and continued to state that she did not wish to discuss it. Although she previously admitted to suicidal ideation, she denied it when the possibility of psychiatric inpatient admission was discussed with her.

Recommendations and disposition. Because of the concern about suicidality, her well-documented depression prior to the abruption, the need for support in her grief, and the unsupportive marital relationship, psychiatric admission was recommended and reluctantly accepted. The patient appeared cooperative on the inpatient unit and denied all symptoms of depression except mild sleep disturbance. She spoke about the death of the infant without affect. After 10 days, she insisted upon leaving the hospital. When the patient resumed treatment with her previous therapist, she admitted to him that she had to act appropriately "so I could get out of the hospital because all those doctors and patients were following me and planning to kill me." She believed that she had caused an elevator to break down because she was in the building. Mrs. R. refused medication but continued seeing the trusted therapist. After approximately 1 month, the paranoid symptoms diminished, and Mrs. R. began to exhibit progressively increasing signs of grief and depression. She spontaneously requested medication as an adjunct to her psychotherapy. Although she had responded well to treatment, Mrs. R. made an appointment with her obstetrician to review the course of events during the abruption and to ask about another pregnancy. The therapist stated that Mrs. R. feels that Mr. R. will "stop drinking" if she "gives him a child." Mr. R. is unwilling to pursue treatment.

Comment. This sad and complex case required multiple interventions that included a lengthy "listening" to the obstetrician about his sadness at his inability to save the infant's life. Points that should be emphasized are the patient's suicidal ideation and plan in the face of a mild delirium and the need for obstetrical staff to deal with grief over perinatal loss, as did the wise obstetrical nurse (see Chapter 11).

Case 11

Type of referral. Adolescent pregnancy—crisis over the question of keeping or relinquishing baby for adoption. Although it is not at all unusual for an adolescent to experience serious conflicts over the decision about keeping the baby, most of these are dealt with by expert counseling on the part of hospital personnel and/or social workers from the appropriate community agency. At times, the problem becomes so entangled with the internal dynamics of the adolescent's development, her family system, her self-esteem, and her problems with reality testing that the mental health consultant may be called upon for assistance.

Consultation request. Alice is a 15-year-old white female who is currently in the sixth month of her first pregnancy. Although the father of the baby is known, he has removed himself from the situation and is totally uninvolved. Alice is experiencing tremendous pressure from her own parents to relinquish the baby for adoption. There have been innumerable family battles over this during the past 2 months, often ending with Alice's decision to run away. Each time she has been brought back and is now placed in a community agency that serves troubled adolescents.

The referral was actually originated by the director of this agency whose staff feels that Alice, previously an excellent student and popular teenager, is now becoming disorganized, failing in school, and refusing to plan in any rational way for the baby's future.

Data collection. Alice was brought to the office by the agency social worker and remained present during the first part of the interview. When it was clear that the patient was more comfortable and had established some level of communication, the social worker was asked to let the interview continue on a more confidential basis. Only then was she able to disclose the storminess of her feelings. She viewed her mother as overinvolved, controlling, and always treating her like a baby. She saw her father as her mother's agent and the peacemaker in the family.

She could talk about how frightened she was and how aware she was of her unreadiness to care for a baby and the loss she knew she would experience when it came time to relinquish her normal adolescent activities to a large degree. But she insisted that she had always been able to meet challenges in the past, that this was her baby, and that she fully intended to keep it and take care of it. She would not finish school. By the time the baby was born, she would be 16 and legally able to drop out of school at which point she would get a job, put the baby in day care, get a small apartment, and take care of it. These, in essence, were her plans.

She described many dreams in which she was taking care of the baby alone. She stated that she wished to have nothing more to do with her parents except in superficial ways because they would not accept her present state, would not accept the baby, and would not make it their grandchild.

She knew that the agency social worker was trying to help her, but she felt she was biased in the direction of putting the baby up for adoption "because they don't have enough white babies."

Alice displayed many assets. She was quite articulate, intelligent, had a good track record in school, and had demonstrated age-appropriate social skills. She had an excellent singing voice and was an accomplished musician.

Medically, her pregnancy had gone well. Beyond the type of planning described here, she had done very little of the specific concrete type of thinking necessary to care for a baby. She had little or no fantasy life about the fetus as such. She was an only child and had no experience with taking care of younger children, not even baby-sitting. She had made no arrangements for clothing, for medical care, or for any of the special needs of a newborn infant.

She pictured herself working in a fast-food chain, picking the baby up at the end of each day, and taking it to her apartment to care for it. She had no idea what her earnings might be, what it would cost to support the baby, what apartment rent would be, or any of the other daily living expenses that she might accrue. She stated that she could get no help from her parents and did not want any.

She had already experienced quickening and did not find it particularly pleasant. She knew that it meant that the baby was alive, but she had no further questions about it. She was frightened of labor and delivery and had discussed this with the social worker but not with the physician who was taking care of her.

She had no contact with the father of the child. She felt he was too much of a baby himself to assume any responsibility and that she could expect nothing from him or his family.

In summary, she seemed bent on a single-minded, determined pursuit of independent motherhood despite any cost to herself.

With her permission, we subsequently spoke to both parents by telephone and met again with the agency social worker. Essentially, they confirmed most of the facts that Alice had communicated. The social worker informed that the agency was about to start a new program that would provide residential support and partial independent living for teenage mothers and their babies and that there would be a close liaison with special classes being developed by the school system so that the mothers could bring their babies with them to the special school and care for them intermittently during the day while pursuing their education. In fact, events seemed to move in the direction of supporting Alice's rather magical wishes to be a teenage super mom. This was the point at which the "consultant" began to assume a rather atypical role (at least for him).

Recommendations and disposition. What emerged from these relatively brief contacts was that the issues had much less to do with pregnancy and the care of the coming infant than with intrafamilial issues of dependency, autonomy, and emancipation. Alice was literally imprisoning herself in order to be free!

At this point in the process, I almost refused to discuss the pregnancy at all and insisted on focusing on the family system and its current dysfunctioning as a child-rearing mechanism. The agency social worker was assisted in meeting with the family as a whole and with acting as a kind of mediator, negotiator, and referee in developing a graded system of increasing levels of freedom and privileges for Alice. Her mother was to focus more on gratification from her marriage and from watching her bright and talented daughter develop as a young adult. Although that process took many weeks, the consultant was not directly involved in any face-to-face contact with Alice or her family and functioned largely by telephone in consultation with the agency social worker.

Within 1 month, Alice had made a decision for relinquishment for adoption and, although there were many signs that her relationship with her mother was still that of much sparring for advantage, much defensiveness, and frequent backtracking; at the same time, there was a greater emergence of positive affect on the part of each, a willingness on Alice's part to reaccept her adolescent status and begin to enjoy it, and a greater acceptance of age-appropriate parental authority in her life.

This particular case is an excellent illustration of the unwitting use of pregnancy as a device to thrust the adolescent almost by jet propulsion into a state of adulthood in opposition to what is perceived as inappropriate parental authority and control. Focusing strictly on pregnancy and the baby to come may be a disservice to all. Resolution of the family system's issues and the intergenerational conflict is of paramount importance.

Case 12

Type of referral. Adolescent pregnancy occurring in a juvenile offender. Connie is a 14½-year-old black, Catholic girl now held in the local juvenile detention center because she was one of a group of four youngsters apprehended, trying to break into a parked car apparently for the purpose of stealing it. After she was remanded to the detention center by the juvenile court Judge, it was discovered during a routine examination that she was approximately 10 weeks pregnant. The hearing during which her case will be adjudicated has not yet occurred so that at the point of consultation, her future status with respect to the juvenile justice system had not been determined.

Consultation request. Because of a service contract between the juvenile court and the psychiatric institute, consultations were frequently requested on adolescents who were suspected of suffering from some form of emotional or mental disorder. In this instance, the request for consultation for Connie was made by the director of the juvenile detention center because this was her fourth arrest within a period of 18 months, because she was requesting an abortion, and because her parents were vehemently protesting any such action on a religious basis, indicating that they were prefectly willing to assume responsibility for Connie's baby.

On direct examination, Connie proved to be a well-developed, mature-looking young woman who was angry, solemn, and relatively uncommunicative. She did indicate that she had strongly suspected that she was pregnant prior to her arrest and had attempted "to bring on my period" on two occasions by taking some pills a girlfriend had given her. She could not identify them.

She did not know for certain who the father of the baby was and expressed little interest in that subject. She had no wish to have the baby and understood the seriousness of her position because she had already been arrested several times for rather serious offenses. On each occasion, her probation had been extended. This time, she feared incarceration, even though she had simply "gone along" with some boys who wanted to "borrow" a car and go for a ride. She stated that she had done nothing herself but accompany the youths.

With respect to her pregnancy, she stated that she had missed her last two menstrual periods, that she had noted some beginning breast changes, and that on three or four occasions she had experienced some morning nausea. Beyond this, she felt pretty much as she usually did. She could say very clearly that she did not feel pregnant and that the whole idea was unreal and crazy to her.

Connie was the youngest of five siblings. All of the older children were now out of the house. Her father was a letter carrier and her mother a full-time homemaker. She described her father as a "weekend drunk"; during these periods, he drank steadily and silently, annoying no one and staying pretty much to himself. Her mother was very active in their local parish and considered herself a devout Catholic.

In a meeting with members of the juvenile detention staff, I was informed that the judge was ready to "support" an abortion for Connie if the family would agree and if I would indicate that it was in the best interest of her "mental health." I wondered whether such a judgment was entirely legal but did not question it because it seemed clinically irrelevant. Despite Connie's repeated offenses, the staff predicted that she would not be sentenced to detention because there had been no violence and because the facts of the case rather clearly indicated that she had not been one of the primary perpetrators. Their best guess was that Connie was not receiving adequate supervision at home and that the judge would make quite a point of this because the parole officer was concerned about it.

A telephone contact with Connie's mother revealed that she was militantly opposed to any idea of abortion and that she was more than ready to assume responsibility for Connie's child until Connie could do so for herself. She did indicate that her husband was either working or likely to stay "to himself most of the time" and that she had become very active in church affairs because most of her children had left the house. Much blame was assigned to Connie's having selected "bad company" for herself.

Recommendations and disposition. This psychiatric consultant was not inclined to certify that unless Connie received an abortion, her "mental health" would be adversely affected. In a follow-up contact with Connie, the consultant made a strong point that Connie's mother was a most experienced mother herself, was willing to take care of the baby, and that this would provide an opportunity for Connie to return to the normal life of an adolescent girl, to make a fresh start, and to learn something from her mother about how to take care of babies.

Connie gave herself away when she responded, "Well, maybe if we have a baby in the house now, things will go back more to normal. My mom will be around more, and my dad will stop drinking!" Although there was no opportunity for prolonged contact with Connie in order to explore whatever unconscious motivations may have been operating in her becoming pregnant, it was clear that the pregnancy and the coming baby did in fact provide an opportunity for reestablishing a status quo in her family and for recreating a more nurturant environment, one of which she could now partake.

The staff's prediction concerning the decision of the juvenile court judge on the case proved to be most accurate. Connie was remanded to the custody of her parents under strict supervision. She was instructed about the conditions for continuing probation that included school performance, keeping her mother informed as to her whereabouts, assisting in the care of the baby when it was born, and working with her probation officer on career planning and on long-term planning for her child.

Long-term follow-up on this case was possible because of the relationship between the psychiatric institute and the juvenile court proved possible. Connie's pregnancy proceeded well within normal limits. She gave birth to a 7-lb baby girl to the delight of the maternal grandmother, and the family's life cycle began once more with the process of child care now under the supervision of the grandmother but with Connie's serving a long-term apprenticeship as she completed her education.

Comments. These two adolescent pregnancy consultations are different in many ways but share much in common. On the surface, one adolescent wanted to keep the child, whereas her parents pushed for adoption. In the second case, the adolescent wanted an abortion, but the grandparents wanted to care for the baby. Yet in both instances, the pregnancy proved to be a stress contingency in the family system and the role of the consultant proved to be a significant force in the using the pregnancy not simply on its face value but as a catalyst to shift the interaction in the family to a more adaptative mode—one that, at least on preliminary assessment, seems to have been more supportive of the goals of adolescent development.

Case 13

Type of referral. Request for psychiatric evaluation for ability to care for the newborn.

Consultation request. At 2 weeks postpartum, the patient was referred for evaluation in order to provide an opinion about her ability to care for her newborn daughter. The referral was generated by the child welfare agency, and the woman had been charged with recklessly endangering a minor.

Data collection. Ms. Q. was a 20-year-old single woman who became pregnant with her fourth child and attempted to hide the pregnancy by wearing large clothes and only gaining 4 lb. She gave birth to the child in secrecy. She cut the umbilical cord and wrapped the infant girl in a sheet. Ms. Q. then put the infant in a shoe box and placed it outside the home of a friend. Upon hearing the child's cries 20 hours later, a neighbor called the police. The newborn was in good condition at a local hospital. At the time of consultation, the child was in the custody of child welfare.

A friend suspected that the baby belonged to Ms. Q., and the police requested that she be examined by an obstetrician-gynecologist. She consented to this procedure but continued to deny that the child was hers. Upon examination, it was clear that Ms. Q. had recently delivered and that she was in good physical condition. Ms. Q. admitted to the details of the birth when confronted with the results of the evaluation.

Upon examination, Ms. Q. was an attractive woman who looked older than her years. She was cooperative in answering the interviewer's questions. She stated that she had not told anyone that she was pregnant because she was ashamed of having her fourth child so young. During the birth, Ms. Q. said that she was concerned about "what people would think." She stated that she had some thoughts about the baby on the day of the birth but that when she considered calling to ask about the baby, she felt foolish and did not do so. She admitted to being aware that the infant might have died. After the birth, Ms. Q. joined her family for a picnic but ate very little. Ms. Q. could not say why she did not have an appetite but denied that it was related to being upset about the birth. She had no difficulty sleeping on the evening of the birth.

Ms. Q. was able to describe the infant's birth in detail and denied any memory impairment or lapse of consciousness. Although she displayed a range of affect during the interview, her affect was notably constricted during the discussion of the birth events. She denied any depersonalization, derealization, or any symptoms that were consistent with psychosis, depression, or the baby blues (see Chapter 6). She had no personal history or family history of neurological or psychiatric disorder. Ms. Q. was a high-school graduate who had obtained above-average grades. She had no history of legal involvement. None of her pregnancies was planned, and they were the result of liaisons with four different males.

Ms. Q. maintained her own home. The child welfare worker had made a home visit and described the environment as "neat and pleasant." The worker had evaluated Ms. Q.'s three other children, who were well-groomed, reportedly happy children who were playing nicely together at the time of the visit. Ms. Q. described her children in positive terms and noticeably brightened when discussing them during the visit. No previous reports to the child welfare agency had been generated.

When asked how she understood the events on the day of her fourth child's birth, Ms. Q. said, "I was afraid that my friends and family would be hurt and wouldn't care about me anymore if I had another baby. If I could relive that day, I would tell everyone about the pregnancy and keep the baby." Ms. Q. considered allowing the baby to be adopted but decided to seek return of the baby to her care at the urging of her friends and family. She had not selected a name for the infant. At the time of the interview, legal charges were pending, and the patient had no contact with a lawyer. She was informed that her records could be subpoenaed.

Recommendations and disposition. The immediate recommendation was for continued placement of the infant with child welfare but with liberal supervised visitation. The function of these
visits would be to allow further evaluation of the mother–infant interactional process. A second
recommendation was for further evaluation of Ms. Q.'s three other children and her interactions
with them. With Ms. Q.'s approval, interviews with her best friend and mother were arranged to
obtain further information regarding the pregnancy and birth of the fourth child. Finally, it was
recommended that Ms. Q. obtain individual psychotherapy. The focus of the therapy would be to
explore details of the conception and obtain information about the father of the baby as well as to
examine Ms. Q.'s fear of rejection if she had a fourth child. Further understanding of the psychological factors that allowed fear of rejection of herself to take priority over the newborn's well-being
was strongly advised as an important aspect of therapy.

Comments. The patient was clearly not suffering from any of the commonly described illnesses
that occur postpartum. Such illnesses can interfere markedly with the ability to parent. She also
clearly fit criteria for competency. The patient had been regularly attending psychotherapy sessions,
and the outcome of the legal charges are pending at the time of this writing.

Conclusion

It is clear that this chapter cannot be all inclusive. We have attempted in presenting
this broad variety of cases to demonstrate how diverse in nature referrals for consultation
can become, and how, as we have stated many times, it becomes necessary to modify the
more classical medical consultation model when attempting to intervene in childbirth
settings. For specific references and other supportive material that may be helpful in
dealing with these and similar situations, the reader is referred particularly to Chapters 5,
6, 7, 12, 14, and 17.

10

Staff Education, Liaison, and Program Consultation

RICHARD L. COHEN

Introduction

In whichever context the reader chooses, the contents of this chapter have the potential for stimulating conflict or controversy among any group of mental health and childbirth professionals. Depending on what kind of end-point data one wishes to select, there may be much or little documentation that the activities and programs herein described are (1) cost-effective; (2) clinically beneficial, or (3) likely to have any long-range impact on the developmental outcome of the infant who is the product of the pregnancy.

One is faced either with waiting until all of the hard data are in or continuing to plan and develop new programs that have a pilot design, or, better yet, a research design so that a more convincing body of evidence can be collected over time to demonstrate either the usefulness or lack of it of these activities.

However, this volume could not be considered complete without reference to the many efforts of innovative clinicians who have attempted these programs in the past and who continue to do so under difficult professional and fiscal circumstances.

We will proceed from the more straightforward types of liaison, to mental health program consultation for existing traditional services, to consultation for the development of new services, and finally to consultation for the development of nontraditional, alternative health system programs not based in medical hospitals. As the reader will quickly note, the supportive data base for each of these loci exhibits a sharp decremental curve as we move along the programmatic scale.

Richard L. Cohen • Department of Psychiatry, Western Psychiatric Institute and Clinic, University of Pittsburgh, Pittsburgh, PA 15213.

Educational and Liaison Activities

It is a truism that all direct case consultations should contain at least latent educational components for the consultee. Beyond this, the consultant should be consistently available to expand, to explicate, to widen horizons, and to interpret the significance both of his or her findings and his or her recommendations beyond the words on the written page. This kind of work is best done at the nursing station, in the hallway, and over the telephone. In these modes, it is best done with house officers and attending physicians.

Simultaneously, an investment in more direct and organized teaching using the "trickle-up" theory is likely to yield many dividends. Staff nurses, in particular, are hungry to understand the behavior and often unpredictable emotional responses of the patients they must care for day and night. Physicians, as a rule, are not exposed to, or even aware of, these phenomena.

The process should begin with a few "needs assessment" meetings with the leadership of the nursing staff to identify content areas that may be useful to increase both the knowledge base and skill of the nursing staff in targeted areas. These should assist the consultant in addressing subjects that are of immediate interest.

Sometimes, presenting a list of possible topics may be helpful in directing the attention of the nursing staff to deficit areas. Such a list might include the following:

- The developmental tasks of pregnancy and the postpartum period.
- Recognition of early signs of emotional disorder in pregnancy.
- What are some of the high-risk stressors that have been identified as influencing the frequency of complications?
- Postpartum depression: its recognition in treatment.
- Latest findings concerning sibling visitation.
- Sleep disorders during pregnancy.
- Pregnancy, work, and emotional development.
- Physical birth trauma and long-term development of the child.
- Psychological factors in infertility.
- Physical abuse during pregnancy.
- Latest findings concerning the effects of alcohol and drug use during pregnancy.
- The use of psychotropic medications during pregnancy: risks and benefits.

This list is virtually endless. These are a few examples of topical areas in which nursing staffs have expressed particular interest during recent years. Much of the content material for such classes is contained in this volume and in the references that appear at the end of each chapter.

Live interviews with pregnant or postpartum women, both normal and problem oriented, are extremely helpful to nursing and other ancillary personnel because they demonstrate techniques for eliciting relevant material that may not be within the repertoire of non-mental health personnel.[1-3]

It has been my experience that persistence at such teaching results in considerable discussion among nurses, begins to be reflected in patient care, and begins to be noticed both by nursing administration and by the medical staff.

Referrals for psychiatric consultation are not only likely to increase under such circumstances; just as important, they are likely to become more appropriate, more focused, and more goal directed.

There are no studies that indicate that basic attitudes of obstetricians toward psychiatry and psychiatrists will be fundamentally altered by such efforts. What is likely to happen is that there is better use of psychiatric expertise, a noticeable improvement in staff morale, with reduced burnout and a tendency on the part of nursing personnel to urge more collaboration with both social workers and mental health professionals at early stages of problem development (rather than as a last resort).[4]

Nursing administration must be prepared to give "release time" for these activities so that nurses are not giving up lunch hours or staying extra time in order to participate. The message should be clear that the activities are important, are valued by the leadership, and should be used in daily clinical practice. This represents an economic investment on the part of the obstetric hospital that is equal to or greater than the investment of time of the mental health professional.

Program Consultation to Conventional or Traditional Childbirth Services

If one is to reach yet a wider segment of the population in need, the next step in the process of involvement of mental health consultation in childbirth programs is to begin to introduce a "public health" approach. By this, we mean introducing a model that (1) does not depend on consultation to a referred population already displaying pathology; (2) is prospective in nature rather than retrospective; (3) that has more of a preventive rather than an interventive approach; and, finally (4) in which ancillary or collateral professionals, not necessarily trained in the mental health specialties, can be oriented toward identifying at-risk populations and developing strategies for improving the level of risk both for the pregnancy itself and for the infant.[5-7]

It is important at this juncture to recall the data and the concepts that have been outlined in Chapters 4 and 6 (those having to do with the epidemiology of disorders and their nosology). One should keep in mind that the actual percentage of pregnant women who display frank or gross psychiatric disorders is relatively low if one recalls the "iceberg" picture (see Figure 1, Chapter 6). Beneath the surface, there is an ever-expanding spectrum of risk levels that render the woman and her family more prone to maladaptation or subsequent frank illness, depending on the balance between environmental stresses, support systems, and maternal assets.

What is clear is that if one relies totally on intervening with referred populations, this is the proverbial bailing out of the ocean with a bucket. One must develop more comprehensive approaches to vulnerable target populations if there is to be a significant and long-lasting impact on the final outcome of the mental health status of this group.

One of the best ways to demonstrate the need for such an approach is to select, at random, a group of women volunteers in any private obstetrical practice or in any prenatal clinic and to interview them in an open-ended, semistructured interview (see Chapter 5) that is aimed at looking at their support systems, their past and current stresses, and their preparation for childbearing and child rearing.

When, at one point in the development of a spectrum of services, I randomly selected over time 125 pregnant women from a university-based prenatal clinic, the following startling results were demonstrated to the clinic staff:

1. Forty-three percent of the women reported inadequate or distorted preparation for sexual activity childbearing or child rearing.
2. One out of five reported no previous experience with caring for children, even baby-sitting.
3. Almost 10% reported that they were already experiencing some behavioral or developmental problem in one of their existing children.
4. In 29% of the women, there was reported a significant loss by death or separation during the 2 years immediately prior to the interview.
5. Although 83% of the women had already experienced quickening, only 65% of that group reported a positive response to it, whereas 21% experienced it as a negative process.
6. Only 22% of the women experienced any fantasies at all about the fetus. Of these, only one in five reported that the fantasies were pleasurable, whereas half of the 22% experienced them as neutral.
7. Approximately one-third reported that they had no sources of gratification or reward outside of their experiences in childbearing and child rearing.
8. One in five was concerned that some prior experience or condition might adversely influence the baby's development, and the same number (one in five) feared that some condition existing during pregnancy would have an adverse effect on the baby.

These were revelations to the obstetric and nursing staff who, for the most part, were not aware of these situations. In fact, there was little or nothing in their standard history taking or data collection that would be likely to reveal such information unless it was volunteered by the patient herself. In most instances, this was unlikely.

The consultant should offer a conceptual model on which the staff can base its thinking about how to approach patients. For better or for worse, there is no dearth of such models (see Chapter 5). In fact, there is no overarching model that is broadly applicable, and there is no unifying theoretical approach on which standard clinical procedures can be based. Each consultant tends to select from the "menu" of generally accepted theoretical approaches a kind of eclectic orientation that, in his or her opinion, incorporates the best of all models and is likely to provide a screening mechanism for identifying at-risk situations.

From among the many theoretical approaches that can be useful in formulating screening procedures (which are necessary before any other activities can take place) are the crisis-orientation model developed by Caplan[8] as early as the 1950s and by many others; an approach to identification of psychopathology in various forms, particularly through the use of depression scales or anxiety rating scales[9,10]; the life events type of approach developed by Holmes and Rahe[11] of which there are many modifications extant[12–15]; the locus of control theoretical model originally developed by Rotter[16–19]; the theoretical and practical work of Garmezy,[20] particularly in the area of identifying vulnerability; and many others. The advantages of combining these is that, indeed, this presents the possibility of approaching the woman from many vantage points and of identifying either latent psychopathology or risk factors that might be missed by one particular approach.

Unless one is developing a formal, well-designed research project, it is not necessary to have a highly complex, lengthy protocol or to have specially trained research assistants administering such questionnaires.

It is important to remember that obstetrics is basically a surgical specialty, that it is procedure-oriented, and that obstetric practice is extremely busy and hectic. Therefore, any instruments developed to identify at-risk populations should be straightforward, concrete, easily read or scored, and perhaps most important of all, able to be administered by non-mental-health professionals and incorporated into the normal data-gathering process rather than as a separate interview.[5,9] They should not add unduly to the length of the examination but should, in fact, hopefully shorten the clinic day by screening out those particular women who need special attention and by permitting the staff to pay a bit less attention to those women who demonstrate excellent support systems and low stress.

Basically, what one expects to uncover with such screening instruments are early signs of maladaptation to pregnancy. This is most likely to be reflected in one of three or four major areas[2]:

1. Excessive maternal concerns about adverse previous experience in childbearing or child rearing.
2. Conflicts in or defects in marital, kinship, or social support systems.
3. Inadequate preparation for childbearing or child rearing.
4. Concerns about maternal health that may be adversely affected by the pregnancy or by labor and delivery.

Admittedly, there are many other areas that may be tapped in order to identify risk factors, but, for purposes of simplicity, brevity, and efficiency in office operation, our experience has been that concentration in these areas is likely to reveal most of the danger signals. The nature of the exercise refers back to our original developmental milestones of pregnancy (see Chapter 5) and the impact on these of either excessive stresses or inadequate supports. Signs of rejection of the pregnancy beyond the first trimester, signs of lack of emotional attachment or affiliation with the fetus, signs of deficient nesting behavior following quickening later on in pregnancy, and, finally, during the neonatal period, signs of inadequate attachment to the new infant are all useful "red flags" in the screening process.

It is possible to develop a series of relatively simple, nonleading, straightforward questions that will help to uncover maladaptive responses. We have found, for example, that the questions listed in Table 1 can be quite useful in screening.

It is very likely that any woman who is perceiving stresses in the absence of adequate supports may respond to any of the questions in Table 1 (plus others that are relatively easy to formulate) with "indicators" that should heighten the awareness of clinic or office personnel that this is a situation that may need some additional attention. A few examples may be useful.

Case 1

During psychosocial screening, Mrs. B. was asked, "Has anything happened to you during your pregnancy that causes you concern about how the baby will be?" The mother, after a

**Table 1. Sample Questions and Responses to Elicit "At-Risk" Responses
for Maladaption to Pregnancy**[a]

Sample questions	Illustrations of "at-risk" responses
1. Identification of adverse previous experience in childbearing or child rearing	
Has anything happened (to you) in the past (or during this pregnancy) that might affect the baby?	1. "Mother died giving birth to me."
	2. "Sexual intercourse caused the baby to 'ball up.'"
	3. "My sister had a retarded baby."
	4. "My last baby was born dead."
	5. "My husband's ex-wife called me and said she hopes the baby dies."
	6. "Watched a horror movie on TV. Think the baby might be deformed."
2. Major conflict with support system	
Do you plan to raise your children any different from the way you were raised?	1. "I won't send my kids away to school like I was."
	2. "My mother was always sick or tired."
	3. "Yes. My mother never approved of anything I did."
Is your husband (father of the baby) much help to you?	1. "Are you kidding? He's like another child to take care of."
	2. "He's angry because I got pregnant."
	3. "I'm beginning to wonder if I married the right man."
3. Lack of prior experience in infant and child care (for primagravidas)	
How much experience did you have as you were growing up in taking care of children?	1. "None, I'm really terrified."
	2. "I guess I was sort of spoiled. My mother wouldn't ever let me help around the house."
	3. "I grew up in a house full of adults. There were never any kids around."
4. Maternal health concerns	
Do you have any condition that you think might be made worse by being pregnant?	1. "I had rheumatic heart disease when I was a teenager."
	2. "Not really. Just nerves, I guess."
	3. "I'm usually crippled up for months with my back after I have a baby."

[a]From Cohen RL: Maladaptation to Pregnancy, in Taylor PM (ed): *Parent-Infant Interaction.* New York, Grune & Stratton, 1980, p. 59. Reprinted with permission.

significant pause, said, "Yes, I had a very disturbing telephone call from my own mother a few weeks ago."

On the surface, such a response has a paralogical overtone to it that may lead the clinician to think this mother may be either irrational or mentally ill. Follow-up inquiry of this mother once the screening had been evaluated led her to reveal information that she had not disclosed previously.

She indicated that her own mother had told her that she had not been the firstborn child (as she had always believed) but that there had been an earlier pregnancy in which the offspring had been born with several congenital deformities and had died at 3 weeks of age. The mother had been "protected" from this information all of her 24 years, believing that she had been the firstborn child. The maternal grandmother had chosen this moment to reveal this "family secret." The patient was in a panic over this and yet had revealed nothing about the telephone call either to her husband or the obstetrician until the previously stated question was asked of her. Her entire attitude about the pregnancy had changed following the telephone call, and she was now in a constant state of fearful apprehension about what would go wrong, whether or not the baby would be intact, and, even if it appeared to be so, whether or not it would harbor some secret defect that she would not be able to discern until it was older.

Case 2

Mrs. G. was asked the same question as noted in Case 1 and responded, "Yes, my husband is in jail on a drug charge."

Again, the manifest content is perplexing if taken only at face value. Mrs. G. was questioned in more depth at her next prenatal visit: Why indeed would this affect the baby? She explained at some length that she had read a newspaper article indicating that drugs and alcohol had an adverse effect both on the liver and brain. She had learned following conception of the extensive nature of her husband's proclivity for substance abuse. Would this not, she reasoned, be transmitted in some way to the baby, causing it to be "mentally ill" (her exact words)? She felt she would know immediately on looking at her newborn if it were mentally ill. Indeed, during a follow-up interview 48 hours postnatally she stated that the baby had "a bad disposition" and that it had "snapped back" when she had attempted her first breastfeeding.

Case 3

Mrs. T. was asked, "Do you plan to raise your child any differently from the way you were raised?" Her unhesitating response was, "Yes. My mother worked all the time."

Here, perhaps, the physician may safely assume that the answer means exactly what it seems to mean. Further questioning revealed, however, that Mrs. T.'s mother removed herself from the house for many reasons other than required working hours; that she had an unbridled temper and that the children had to tiptoe about the house when she was within earshot; and that she often lost control and abused the children, especially Mrs. T. Now, pregnant herself, Mrs. T. felt irritable, short tempered, and unready to accept responsibility for an infant. She feared that she would not know what the baby wanted and that the inevitable result would be explosive and abusive behavior on her own part.

Case 4

Mrs. J. was asked the simple screening question, "What was your reaction when you found out that you were pregnant?" She answered, "Oh boy. You don't want to know. I'm going to sue the drug company that makes those birth control pills!" [Nervous laughter]

Follow-up inquiry revealed that Mrs. J. had conceived when she believed herself to be "on the pill." She had been angry because the pregnancy was inconvenient and untimely. She was just beginning to accept the idea that she was pregnant when a neighbor in whom she had confided told her that if she had conceived while taking oral contraceptives her child would be born sterile. Mrs. J. was now depressed but was masking her mood with a jocular, flippant approach to the whole matter.

The varying results of large-scale screening procedures in prenatal clinics are reported in the literature. Obviously, these results depend on the nature of the instruments being used: whether they are generic-type screening devices, or whether they are specifically geared to the phenomena of pregnancy; whether they are searching for specific types of psychopathology or risk factors; or whether they are broader-based screening instruments; and the rigor of reliability checks for the staff. All of these factors will clearly influence the nature of the final "product."

Instead of attempting, therefore, to quote statistics or to give percentages about various types of categories that emerge from screening, it seems more useful to attempt to conceptualize what has emerged, at least from my experience. There appear to be six broad categories of "problems" that can be conceptualized and that lend themselves to specific kinds of referrals and intervention procedures.

These are schematically represented in Figure 3, Chapter 6, and, as one might expect, they appear to decrease in prevalence as they increase in severity and in the difficulties they present for intervention. One proceeds from simple straightforward problems arising from maternal anxiety about inadequate preparation for the coming experience, through chronic deficits in support systems to crisis events in life supports, and so on, as indicated in the figure.

What is also indicated schematically is the kind of intervention that tends to be most indicated for that problem category. Although this is rather simplistic and overly condensed, it is quite useful to busy clinic personnel to have this outlined in this way because it helps them organize information that they collect through screening; it helps them place the nature of the problem in a specific risk level, and it helps them to direct their attention toward particular resources for intervention purposes. It is likely to lead to the most efficient use of psychiatric or mental health professional time that should not be spent on identifying and treating problems that other intramural or community-based personnel can do as well or better.

Finally, and again with the understanding that this tends to be rather oversimplified and contains the usual dangers associated with such concrete checklists, it is often helpful to provide clinic personnel with a list of "red flags" that should serve the purpose of raising their early warning system to at least yellow if not red. I have found the most useful markers or indicators to be the following (this list has been adopted from the early work of Rose[21]):

1. History of loss of the mother's mother before her own puberty and without adequate replacement by a substitute maternal figure.
2. Chronic conflict with or alienation from one's own mother and other female relatives.
3. Previous birth of a damaged child.
4. Parents report older child to be emotionally disturbed or behaviorally disordered.
5. Chronic marital discord, especially if focus of conflict is around childbearing or child rearing.
6. Parents have had virtually no preparation for sexual experience, childbearing, or child rearing.
7. Parents report prior activity or exposure to "toxin" that they fear will damage baby (especially if they do not respond to simple, direct explanation and reassurance by physician).

8. Behavior indicating overt or disguised rejection of pregnant state as late as third trimester.
9. Absence of nesting behavior (especially in primigravidas) in third trimester.
10. Inability to show early signs of identifying baby's individual characteristics during early weeks of extrauterine life.

For those students (for instance, social work students or psychology trainees) who may be interested in learning how to do more in-depth interviews with pregnant women in clinic or office setting (in contrast with more superficial screening procedures) or for those who are interested in following-up on screening procedures that reveal women to be at high risk, it is useful to provide a structured outline for interviewing pregnant women in more depth. An example of such an outline is sketched in Table 1 in Chapter 5.

Program Consultation to Special Projects or Services

As the consultant demonstrates his or her contribution and expertise in facilitating the various conventional hospital service delivery programs, there may be opportunities to have input into (or even to initiate) other types of efforts. There is now a growing body of data that demonstrates that these kinds of programs, if they do not incorporate a significant mental health component, are likely to be less successful. Some examples of these types of program include (1) the planning and implementation of special clinics for teenage pregnant girls[22-26]; (2) the development of a program for obstetrically high-risk women who may be much more vulnerable to the fears and anxieties that accompany pregnancy, labor, and delivery, anyway[27]; (3) special clinics for women addicted to alcohol and/or drugs, incurring special risks both to themselves and their offspring (see Chapter 13); (4) more advanced prenatal classes that incorporate information about the psychological processes and the neonatal period (see Chapter 5); and (5) early parenting or child development classes for first-time parents (see Chapter 5).

All of these represent high visibility areas in which the mental health consultant, with relatively low investments of time and energy, can make contributions that are significant both to the staff and the patient population. Because all of the programs mentioned involve psychosocial risk in one form or another, the expertise of the mental health consultant in developing inclusionary and exclusionary criteria for acceptance into the program, for developing appropriate rating scales and screening techniques for measuring levels of risk, for planning curricula for special classes for consumers, and for developing procedures for measuring behavioral change over time all represent skill areas that one cannot expect to find even among the most advanced obstetric and childbirth staffs.

Program Consultation for Extramural Programs and Out-of-Hospital Nontraditional Services

The branching out of the consultant into community resources and contacts is a major step that should occur at some point in the development of a truly comprehensive approach. This effort has to be a long-term one and is likely to develop only over a 5- or 10-year period of continuous investment. The invitations to speak before community groups, the opportunity to join and advise in childbirth education programs at both regional and local levels will provide experiences and interactions with families who might not ordinarily use traditional health systems.[3]

Exposure to this type of population is less likely to occur in conventional hospital settings because most of these women are of low-risk nature, tend to be quite self-sufficient, have excellent support systems, and may even be antagonistic toward traditional, medically dominated, tertiary care systems. It takes considerable skill and imagination to tailor approaches that are geared to their particular needs.

These are areas where the consultant is not likely to be called upon unless he or she has become identified as a major regional expert or national figure. Nevertheless, the consultant has considerable to offer in the planning and implementation of programs for (1) nurse-midwife birthing centers; (2) home delivery programs where these are socially acceptable and medically supported, and (3) birthing rooms in community hospitals that do not have experience in the development of such facilities and wish to attract a more nontraditional population of young parents.

Summary

The sum total of all of these efforts that may take between 5 and 10 years for the consultant to develop is potentially enormous. The numbers of families that can be reached and the potential benefits toward reducing complications of labor and delivery and improving the quality of the early child-caring efforts is almost incalculable. It must be recognized both by the consultant and by the facility that many of these activities cannot be billed for and are not reimbursable by any current stream of medical care payments. These must be seen at this stage of the game either as major investments in the quality of care that will impact on length of stay and the eventual end product of obstetric service, or they must be financed as pilot projects or research projects through other funding streams besides traditional clinical reimbursement systems. It is important to develop a baseline data pool and then to keep this current to demonstrate both to the administration of the hospital and to professionals that this is indeed a cost-effective component in the total spectrum of professional services which is offered.

References

1. Cohen RL: Some maladaptive syndromes of pregnancy and the puerperium. *Obstet Gynecol* **24**:562–570, April 1966.
2. Osofsky HJ, Osofasky JD: Normal adaptation to pregnancy and new parenthood, in Taylor PM (ed): *Parent-Infant Relationships*. New York, Grune & Stratton, 1980, pp 25–48.
3. Cohen RL: Parental experiences in out-of-hospital birth centers, in Taylor PM (ed): *Parent-Infant Relationships*. New York, Grune & Stratton, 1980, pp 189–209.
4. Pasnau RO: Psychiatry and obstetrics-gynecology: Report of a five-year experience in psychiatric liaison, in: *Consultation Liaison Psychiatry*. New York, Grune & Stratton, 1975, pp 135–147.
5. Horsley S: Psychological management of the prenatal period, in Howells JG: *Modern Perspectives in Psycho-Obstetrics*. New York, Brunner/Mazel, 1972, pp 291–313.
6. Gloger-Tippelt G: A process model of the pregnancy course. *Hum Dev* **26**:134–148, 1983.

7. Mercer RT, May KA, Ferketich S, et al: Theoretical models for studying the effect of antepartum stress on the family. *Nurs Res* **35**:339–346, 1986.

8. Caplan G: General introduction and overview, in Caplan G (ed): *Prevention of Mental Disorders in Children*. New York, Basic Books, 1961, pp 3–30.

9. Kumar R, Robson KM, Smith AMR: Development of a self-administered questionnaire to measure adjustment and maternal attitudes during pregnancy and after delivery. *J Psychosom Res* **28**:43–51, 1984.

10. Lips HM: A longitudinal study of the reporting of emotional and somatic symptoms during and after pregnancy. *Soc Sci Med* **21**:631–640, 1985.

11. Holmes TH, Rahe RH: The social readjustment rating scale. *J Psychosom Res* **11**:213–218, 1967.

12. Helper M, Cohen RL, Beitenman ET, et al: Life-events and acceptance of pregnancy. *J Psychosom Res* **12**:183–188, 1968.

13. Paykel ES, Emms EM, Fletcher J, et al: Life events and social support in puerperal depression. *Br J Psychiatry* **136**:339–346, 1980.

14. Nuckolls KB, Cassel J, Kaplan BH: Psychosocial assets, life crisis and the prognosis of pregnancy. *Am J Epidemiol* **95**:431–441, 1972.

15. Barnett BEW, Hanna B, Parker G: Life-event scales for obstetric groups. *Journal of Psychosomatic Research* **27**:313–320, 1983.

16. Rotter JB, Seeman M, Liverant S: Internal versus external control of reinforcement: A major variable in behavior theory, in Washburne NF (ed): *Decisions, Values and Groups*. Oxford, Pergamon Press, 1962, pp 473–516.

17. Riley E: What do women want?: The question of choice in the conduct of labor, in Chard T, Richards M (eds): *Benefits & Hazards of the New Obstetrics*. Philadelphia, JB Lippincott, 1977, pp 62–71.

18. Shapiro MC, Najman JM, Chang A, et al: Information control and the exercise of power in the obstetrical encounter. *Soc Sci Med* **17**:139–146, 1983.

19. Lefcourt HM, Martin RA, Saleh, WE: Locus of control and social support: Interactive moderators of stress. *J Pers Soc Psychol* **47**:378–389, 1984.

20. Garmezy N: Vulnerability research and the issue of primary prevention. *Am J Orthopsychiatry* **26**:330–339, 1971.

21. Rose JA: The prevention of mothering breakdown associated with physical abnormalities of the infant, in Caplan G (ed): *Prevention of Mental Disorders in Children*. New York, Basic Books, 1961, pp 265–282.

22. Leynes C: Keep or adopt: A study of factors influencing pregnant adolescents' plans for their babies. *Child Psychiatry Hum Dev* **11**:105–112, 1980.

23. Lewis CC: A comparison of minors' and adults' pregnancy decisions. *Am J Orthopsychiatry* **50**:446–453, 1980.

24. Schneider S: Helping adolescents deal with pregnancy: A psychiatric approach. *Adolescence* **17**:285–292, 1982.

25. Vernon MEL, Green JA, Frothingham TE: Teenage pregnancy: A prospective study of self-esteem and other sociodemographic factors. *Pediatr* **72**:632–635, 1983.

26. Hardy JB, King TM, Repke JT: The Johns Hopkins adolescent pregnancy program: An evaluation. *Obstet Gynecol* **69**:300–306, 1987.

27. Cohen RL: Pregnancy stress and maternal perceptions of infant endowment. *J Ment Subnormality*, **22**:18–23, June 1966.

Additional Readings of Interest to the Liaison Psychiatrist

Many important topics are covered in chapters already cross referenced in the text. Others include

Parent–Infant Bonding

Klaus MH, et al: Human maternal behavior at the first contact with her young. *Pediatr* **46**:187–192, August 1970.

Campbell SBG, Taylor PM: Bonding and attachment: Theoretical issues, in Taylor PM (ed): *Parent-Infant Relationships*. New York, Grune & Stratton, 1980, pp 3–23.

Taylor PM, Hall BL: Parent-infant bonding: Problems and opportunities in a perinatal center, in Taylor PM (ed): *Parent–Infant Relationships*. New York, Grune & Stratton, 1980, pp 315–334.

Sibling Participation

Isberg RS, Greenberg WE: Siblings in the delivery room: Consultations to the obstetrical service. *J Am Acad Child Adolescent Psychiatry* **26**:268–273, 1987.

Ballard JL, et al: Sibling visits to a newborn intensive care unit: Implications for siblings, parents, and infants. *Child Psychiatry Hum Dev* **14**:203–214, 1984.

Working during Pregnancy

American College of Obstetrics & Gynecology: Pregnancy, work, and disability, Technical Bulletin No. 58, May 1980.

Murphy JF, Dauncey M, Newcombe R, et al: Employment in pregnancy: Prevalence, maternal characteristics, perinatal outcome. *The Lancet,* May 26, 1984, pp 1163–1166.

Saurel-Cubizolles MJ, et al: Work in pregnancy: Its evolving relationship with perinatal outcome (A review). *Soc Sci Med* **22**:431–442, 1986.

Chamberlain G: After office hours: Effect of work during pregnancy. *Obstet Gynecol* **65**:747–750, 1985.

Mahone ME, Wilkinson WE: Women, work and pregnancy: Implications for occupational health nursing. *Occup Health Nurs* **33**:343–348, 1985.

Zuckerman BS, Frank DA, Hingson R, et al: Impact of maternal work outside the home during pregnancy on neonatal outcome. *Pediatr* **77**:459–464, 1986.

Morbidity in Fathers

Gerzi S, Berman E: Emotional reactions of expectant fathers to their wives' first pregnancy. *Br J Med Psychol* **54**:259–265, 1981.

Liebenberg B: Expectant fathers. Paper presented at The American Orthopsychiatric Association. Washington DC, March 1967.

Fawcett J, Bliss-Holtz VJ, Haas MB, et al: Spouses' body image changes during and after pregnancy: A replication and extension. *Nurs Res* **34**:220–223, 1986.

Fawcett J, York R: Spouses' physical and psychological symptoms during pregnancy and the postpartum. *Nurs Res* **35**:144–148, 1986.

Shapiro S, Nass J: Postpartum psychosis in the male. *Psychopathology* **19**:138–142, 1986.

Clinton JF: Expectant fathers at risk for couvade. *Nurs Res* **35**:290–295, 1986.

Infertility

Rosenfeld DL, Mitchell T: Treating the emotional aspects of infertility: Counseling services in an infertility clinic. *Am J Obstet Gynecol* **135**:177–180, 1979.

Kraft AD, Palombo J, Mitchell D, et al: The psychological dimensions of infertility. *Am J Obstet Gynecol* **50**:618–628, 1980.

Lalos A, Lalos O, Jacobsson L, et al: Depression, guilt and isolation among infertile women and their partners. *J Psychosom Obstet Gynaecol* **5**:197–206, 1986.

Edelmann RJ, Connolly KJ: Psychological aspects of infertility. *Br J Med Psychol* **59**:209–219, 1986.

Prepared Childbirth

Joy LA, Davidson S, Williams TM, et al: Parent education in the perinatal period: A critical review of the literature, in Taylor PM (ed): *Parent-Infant Relationships*. New York, Grune & Stratton, 1980, pp 211–237.

Katona CLE: Approaches to antenatal education. *Soc Sci Med* **15A**:25–33, 1981.

Doering S, Entwisle D: Preparation during pregnancy and ability to cope with labor and delivery. *Am J Orthopsychiatry* **45**:825–837, 1975.

Charles, AG, et al: Obstetric and psychological effects of psychoprophylactic preparation for childbirth. *Am J Obstet Gynecol* **131**:44–52, 1978.

Olive D, et al: Patient education in a woman's hospital: Attitudes of the medical and nursing staffs. *Obstet Gynecol* **65**:686–690, 1985.

Beck NC, Hall D: Natural childbirth: A review and analysis. *J Obstet Gynecol* **52**:371–376, 1978.

Beck NC, Geden EA, Brouder GT: Preparation for labor: A historical perspective. *Psychosom Med* **41**:243–258, 1979.

Smoking during Pregnancy

Enkin MW: Smoking and pregnancy—A new look. *BIRTH* **11**:225–229, 1984.

Gender Differences in Caretakers

Zambrana RE, Mogel W, Scrimshaw SCM: Gender and level of training differences in obstetricians' attitudes towards patients in childbirth. *Women Health* **12**:5–24, 1987.

Premature Birth

Pederson DR, Bento S, Chance GW, et al: Maternal emotional responses to preterm birth. *Am J Orthopsychiatry* **57**:15–21, 1987.

Hibbard B: The aetiology of preterm labour. *Br Med J* **294**:594–595, 1987.

Omer H, Elizur Y, Barnea T, et al: Psychological variables and premature labour: A possible solution for some methodological problems. *J Psychosom Res* **30**:559–565, 1986.

Newton RW, Webster PAC, Binu PS, et al: Psychosocial stress in pregnancy and its relation to the onset of premature labour. *Br Med J* **2**:411–413, 1979.

Physical Abuse during Pregnancy

Adams Hillard PJ: Physical abuse in pregnancy. *J Obstet Gynecol* **66**:185–190, 1985.

Elective Nulliparity

Kaltreider N, Margolis A: Childless by choice: A clinical study. *Am J Psychiatry* **134**:179–182, 1977.

Daniluk JC, Herman AL: Children: Yes or No, a decision-making program for women. *Personnel Guidance J* **62**:240–243, 1983.

11

Psychiatric Services in the Neonatal Intensive Care Unit

KLAUS K. MINDE AND DONNA E. STEWART

Introduction

The psychological problems of infants, parents, and staff members who are patients, visit, or work in an intensive care unit have been the focus of increasing attention. For example, mental health professionals more than 30 years ago highlighted the psychological difficulties parents experience when they have a small premature or sick newborn.[1-3] Since Barnett and his colleagues[4] wrote their article on the effect the separation of a premature infant from his or her mother may have on her parenting ability, much effort has been made to humanize the highly technological environment of these units.[5] This has included around-the-clock visiting hours, support groups for parents of premature infants,[6] and lately, an extension of free visiting for other relatives, including siblings.[7]

These administrative changes have made neonatal units more accessible and allowed parents to feel that they have a definite role to play during the early weeks of their small infants' lives. However, these changes do not address the more fundamental dilemma of a medical unit whose staff is constantly confronted with severe illness or death of their patients and the accompanying tensions of grief and mourning. Because most pediatric deaths still take place in the neonatal intensive care unit (NICU) and the death of an infant is not easily accepted in our society, all staff in such units are under extremely high pressure to perform daily miracles.

The emotional needs of physicians and nurses who work in the NICU and possibilities of dealing with stresses inherent in such work have been variously addressed.[8,9] Unfortunately, much of this work has been published in nonmedical journals, and for this

Klaus K. Minde • Department of Psychiatry, Pediatrics, and Psychology, Queen's University, Kingston, Ontario, Canada K7L 3NG.   **Donna E. Stewart** • Department of Psychiatry, Obstetrics, and Gynecology, University of Toronto, Toronto, Ontario, Canada M5G 1X8.

reason it may be less known to physicians who direct the day-to-day functions of intensive care units.

The present chapter will therefore

1. Outline the commonest problem areas contributing to parental and staff stress in an NICU.
2. Define the role of the psychiatrist in an NICU arising out of these problems.
3. Discuss the difficulties and rewards encountered by mental health specialists who work in an NICU.
4. Describe a consultation—liaison model that is designed to assist neonatologists and nurses as well as the infants' families in their competence to work or to parent.

Each of these issues will also be highlighted by short case vignettes.

Common Sources of Parental and Staff Stress in an NICU

Parental responses to an NICU can best be divided into immediate and later reactions. Early on, most parents experience a sense of failure that they have given birth to a less than perfect baby. Mothers have often just acknowledged their pregnancy but have not yet attended childbirth classes and, therefore, are relatively poorly informed about the demands and,challenges associated with childbearing. Superimposed on this poor preparation is the often overwhelming technical environment of an NICU that parents of such babies initially experience. This environment as well as the size or physical status of their infant often causes parents to fear that their infant will die or grow up with a developmental handicap. Yet after a premature delivery, there is no time to mourn the loss of the perfect baby before the demands of the new sick infant must be met. As it is often difficult for parents in the beginning to obtain and comprehend appropriate information about their infant, unreasonable expectations of the baby's future may be quite prevalent. For example, many parents worry that their children will not be sufficiently attached to them because of the anomaly of their neonatal experience. In addition, mothers are frequently criticized by their relatives who suggest that they have "failed" their families by giving birth to such a tiny infant.[10] The ensuing feelings of guilt, anger, and despair are exacerbated when mothers have given birth in an outside hospital and are separated from their infants during the initial days of their lives. The acute agony and yearning for their infant that many mothers in outlying hospitals experience during this time is the reason why about 10% sign themselves out of the hospital before their obstetrician feels this to be appropriate.[11] The father is often the only readily available parent and conveyor of information to the mother of the infant; he therefore becomes a special source of comfort to the mother during this period. However, the burden placed on the father is heightened when he, too, is young, may not be married to the mother, and finds himself a reluctant go-between the referral center and the mother who remains at the distant outlying hospital. Physical exhaustion at a time like this may further decrease the father's coping ability. He may also become highly protective of his wife or partner and screen out information that he feels she should not hear yet.[12]

After the initial survival of the infant seems assured, other concerns and feelings surface within the parents. Many center around their new total preoccupation with their baby. In our experience, some 50% of all mothers during the first 4 to 6 weeks can think of little besides their infant. They will want to visit and observe the staff's interactions with the baby for hours each day and yet will call the ward again as soon as they have arrived home after an 8-hour visit. They often sleep poorly, eat little, show quick mood changes, and may avoid talking to relatives or friends about their baby's progress. Thus behaviors during this period are very similar to those commonly associated with the initial phases of a mourning process. During this stage, frequent repetition of information may be necessary for assimiliation. Parents may also ask the neonatal staff the same questions over and over again, seeking a source who gives information compatable with their need for an optimistic prognosis.

Although most mothers and fathers become "more reasonable" by the second month, that is, are able to take in and remember reassuring medical information, begin to appreciate the work of the staff in the NICU, and become true members of the caretaking team, a minority of parents continue to translate their worries and concerns into a heightened vigilance over the staff caring for their babies. Thus they may read their infants' chart several times a day, forever count the drops of IV fluid the baby gets, and, after comparing the number with the doctor's orders, complain if the infant gets 32 rather than the prescribed 30 drops per minute. Although it initially appears that these parents want to find fault with the nursing or medical staff, they often simply fear that they are relegated to be visitors rather than parents of their children. By checking on everyone, they, therefore, primarily attempt to take control of their infants' day-to-day activities and assure coherence of the self in face of overwhelming trauma and perceived helplessness.

Other parents seem to have developed their own set of milestones for the improvement of their infants. When feeds are stopped or oxygen levels need to be increased, even temporarily, such parents feel they have lost control of the situation, and anxiety may turn into anger directed at the medical staff or the hospital in general.

If an infant remains critically ill for more than 6 weeks, parents often become increasingly anxious and depressed. What is more important, however, is that they may seem to become so preoccupied with their child's illness and possible later handicap that they do not perceive and respond to medical improvement when it does occur. Thus, rather than augment their interactions with their increasingly healthy and competent infant, they continue to treat him or her as if he were still seriously ill.[13]

Case 1

Angela was born by caesarean section after 27 weeks' gestation, weighing 920 g. Her mother, an Italian-born 34-year-old secretary, had lost four previous infants during the first and second trimester and had stayed in bed for almost 20 weeks during this pregnancy so as to "hold-on to the baby this time." Angela was transferred from her local hospital to a neonatal intensive care unit immediately but developed serious pulmonary problems, requiring high-pressure ventilation, within 4 days after birth. The mother, who had been delighted to have "a real baby," became terrified when her husband initially told her about Angela's need for ventilation. Fearing her overconcern, Mr. A. did not talk about Angela's illness to his wife anymore, and Mrs. A. was afraid to call the ward to find out about it. After her discharge from the hospital, she visited Angela immediately but found her so tiny and beset by tubes and machines that she left just after 10 minutes and did not return. At home, she reportedly cried for many hours a day but would neither call the hospital nor visit her baby. Mr. A. got angry at his wife for seeming so helpless but felt better once he was back at work. He visited the baby three to four times a week but told his wife little about Angela's progress that was quite slow. In fact, he would often spend the evening with his parents and siblings after visiting Angela and would return home only late at night. During his visits, he would spend much time looking at other infants and talked to other parents about their difficulties with doctors and nurses. Three weeks later, Angela's key nurse asked Mr. A. why he did not bring along his wife for his visits. This seemed to upset Mr. A. and coincided with his accusing the medical staff of caring poorly for Angela and being responsible for her recently developed heart condition. At that point, the responsible physician called a consultation meeting attended by the key nurse of Angela, the unit's social worker, neonatal fellow, and the consulting child psychiatrist.

The stress experienced by the NICU staff comes from various sources. Nurses or physicians need to almost intuitively sense at which stage in the process of dealing with the crisis of having a premature or ill baby a parent or family functions at the moment. This is a difficult task, especially if nurses have not received training in this area and if physicians, because of short-term rotations, meet parents whose infants have been on the NICU longer than they have. In addition, to be faced with the death of many young infants and with the pain of grieving parents is extremely stressful for any professional. Many nurses cope by using institutionalized support structures, such as in-service training courses or seminars, where difficult experiences are shared and validated by their colleagues. Nurses can also change their affiliation and move from an NICU to a less demanding ward.

Physicians, who may find their careers much more fixed, may not have this option, yet they are expected to weather emotionally draining experiences. As a result, they will often shield themselves against the painful aspects of their work by concentrating on the technical aspects of neonatology and by withdrawing from the healing and comforting parts inherent in any physician's role. Tensions between nonmedical staff who see the need to respond to parents and infants on an emotional as well as a practical level and physicians who avoid this commitment are, therefore, commonly encountered in the NICU. This can powerfully affect the work of the consulting psychiatrist as he or she may be tempted to side with the "emotionally sensitive" against the "technical" physician or staff person and inadvertently contribute to staff divisions within such a unit. Important dynamics within individual physicians working with infants, such as the need to be in total control of one's patients or to be a true savior of life, can further complicate the struggle between those who are primarily interested in providing good physical care and those who also consider the emotional needs of the infant and his or her family.

The Role of the Psychiatrist in the NICU

The role of the psychiatrist in the NICU is a nontraditional one as his or her major work is often with the staff involved in the care of the neonates, dealing only indirectly with parents and even more distantly with the actual patients. This creates its own set of logistic and personal difficulties.

In our experience, the best way for the psychiatrist to be helpful to staff and parents is to function as

1. An educator who helps parents and staff understand their different roles and needs vis-à-vis the infant and each other.
2. An advocate who is able to explain specific behaviors of a parent or staffperson to others and thus facilitate communication between individuals or groups.
3. A therapist who can assist parents to understand their feelings or actions and help them regain control over their lives.

As an advocate of the sick neonate, the psychiatrist has other roles. They are based on his or her intimate knowledge of child development and the psychosocial conditions necessary for optimizing the developmental process. Therefore, it is the psychiatrist's task to

1. Suggest and help implement policy changes that will assist the emotional, social, and cognitive growth and development of a premature or ill infant.
2. Engage in teaching and research that can lead to a better understanding of the complex interplay of psychosocial and biological forces affecting development.

Case 1 Team Discussion

The team reviewed Angela's present medical condition and discussed her parents' behaviors. The following hypotheses were advanced:

1. Both parents are frightened that Angela may die. Mrs. A. copes by avoiding seeing Angela and "not attaching herself" to a baby she may lose. Mr. A. copes by avoiding to be with his crying wife and blaming others for Angela's suffering.

2. The nurse's question about Mrs. A. was perceived by Mr. A. as a direct attack and increased his projection and anger.

The suggested management was as follows: The responsible physician and psychiatrist would meet with Mr. A. and point out to him that they understood why he was angry and upset about Angela's slow medical progress. They would also stress their own disappointment with her slow recovery but at the same time mention how they had much hope and had not given up on her. They would then focus on Mr. A.'s hard life, the pain he must feel about his crying wife at home, and offer the assistance of the NICU staff to help Mr. A. in his predicaments.

During the meeting, Mr. A. did begin to talk about his concerns for both Angela and his wife and agreed to take a new polaroid picture of Angela home to her mother. On the next day, the responsible physician called Mrs. A. and asked her to come and see him with her husband. Both parents did keep this appointment and then visited their baby. The key nurse had placed a little sign on the incubator, saying "Hi, mum and dad," that greatly moved Mrs. A. and established a first positive link between her and the NICU staff.

Difficulties and Rewards Encountered by the Psychiatrist Working in the NICU

The practical difficulties a psychiatrist may encounter in working in an NICU are many. Psychiatrists work within a time frame that is very different from the day-to-day demands typical of an NICU. They sit down with their patients, listen to them, and probe gently for areas of conflict or for information that patients do not readily volunteer. They often need several interviews to reach a solid diagnosis. Neonatologists, on the other hand, usually need to make rapid decisions whose effects are often immediately evident. Their understanding and expectations of what psychiatrists have to offer may, therefore, often be distorted and can lead to conflict and failure of communication. There are also psychiatrists, however, who take great pride in their "special" understanding of human nature and its operations and who burden their pediatric colleagues with jargoned explanations of why Nurse A may have said B to Mother C. Such psychiatrists often find it difficult to provide concrete suggestions to their more practical pediatric colleagues, adding to the danger of misunderstanding between the two specialties.[14]

On a dynamic level, there are more differences between child psychiatrists and intensive care physicians. Child psychiatrists think in terms of ecological systems and have learned to live with anxiety and uncertainty in their day-to-day work. Intensive care physicians, on the other hand, frequently find it difficult to acknowledge the feelings of personal helplessness a very small sick neonate can engender. They often cope with these feelings by becoming medically more active rather than initially assessing a situation calmly or examining the "traditional goal" of saving every life. These differences in basic philosophies can make the work of the psychiatrist difficult, especially when he or she tries to institute changes that may affect some part of the administrative structure of the neonatal unit (such as getting space on the NICU where mothers can sleep with their infants, prior to discharge). It is on those occasions that neonatologists as well as administrators often ask for controlled prospective long-term outcome studies and detailed cost-efficiency estimates "to validate" the psychiatrist's suggestions. As a consulting psychiatrist obviously works on a neonatologist's territory, he or she has to rely on persuasion, personal integrity, and clinical ability to change the administrative system of an NICU if that should be necessary. If the psychiatrist yields to the challenges inherent in cost-efficiency estimates and does not assert the principles that underly his or her understanding of development,[15] his or her effectiveness will remain limited.

Another common problem encountered by mental health specialists is the previously mentioned tendency of neonatal staff to avoid more emotionally based interpersonal encounters. In practice, this may result in some physicians or nurses regarding as abnormal parent or staff behaviors that may be quite appropriate considering the unusual environment of the NICU. Thus the mother who is angry about getting insufficient information about her infant's medical condition or who feels she can develop a special relationship with her baby by visiting him late at night or singing to him or her may be referred for psychiatric consultation instead of being given an opportunity to explain herself to her infant's caregivers. In fact, there is a general resistance in such units to obtaining a good family and social history, partly because the infant is often admitted without an accompanying adult or the NICU staff are too busy to sit down with a parent and explore unusual behaviors. Frequently, parents are so upset initially that they are unable to reflect on their past. They must therefore be seen a number of times to obtain a valid assessment of their early life history that may be crucial in helping them in their later parenting competence.

Case 2

Ms. B. had given birth to twins weighing 1250 and 1340 g. She was a 26-year-old highly verbal unemployed Caucasian artist. The infants' father was a West African student who had returned to his native country 3 months prior to the infants' birth. Both infants had been given traditional African names.

Ms. B. visited her children daily for many hours and talked freely to the nursing staff about the day-to-day events of her life. Although she was on welfare, she wore fancy leather boots and would often come by taxi to the hospital. She would also often bring along a pillow and sit on the floor in front of her babies' incubator singing contemporary songs to them. When the nurses objected to her behavior, she would calmly reply that there were no rules against singing and sitting on pillows. At the same time, she would point out how a nurse had forgotten to close an incubator on the day before or fed a baby so that it choked.

Two weeks later, the head nurse contacted the psychiatrist and suggested shortening visiting hours on the ward. She also reported that her staff did not want to work in the room that the B. twins shared with three other babies.

In two group discussions, attended by the head nurse, the nurses who worked with Ms. B's babies, the child psychiatrist, and the responsible physician, it became obvious (1) That Ms. B. was a concerned, intelligent mother who was sensitive to the needs of her babies and competent in the care of them; and (2) that Ms. B's disdain for conventional middle-class behaviors had annoyed and possibly even frightened many nurses who saw it as an incursion of "wildness" into their highly organized working environment.

It was decided to actively involve Ms. B. in the ward routines. As she was able to express her thoughts and feelings extremely well, she was invited to participate in two lectures that the child psychiatrist gave to medical students and newly hired nurses and that dealt with the emotional impact of prematurity on parents. This allowed Ms. B. to establish an intellectual bond with the psychiatrist and the nursing staff. It also permitted the psychiatrist to let her talk about her pain and worries and opened the door to later private discussions that dealt with her feelings of being deserted by her parents and by the father of her infants.

Nurses who are in close contact with the infants' families during their work at times see mental health professionals as rivals and resent it when parents choose a mental health nurse or a social worker rather than one of them to ask for personal advice. However, nurses in the NICU's often work 12-hour shifts; hence they are on the unit only three times a week and therefore provide little continuity of care for an individual infant. In fact, Minde and his group[16] reported that in their unit small premature infants who had an average hospital stay of 49 days were cared for by an average of 72 different nurses. It is understandable from these figures that some parents may find it difficult to reveal personal concerns to the nursing staff, at least in large neonatal units. On the other hand, the long stay of these babies gives some nurses a very intimate view of a developing parent–child relationship. Both parents and nurses at times have trouble finding the type of relationship with each other that will permit a mother to see herself as both a legitimate and autonomous parent and at the same time somebody who can cooperate fully with the necessary routines and treatment procedures prescribed by the hospital authorities.

Finally, there are often some tensions between the medical and nursing staff on an NICU. Nurses who work on these wards are usually highly competent and independent. Many medical members of these units, however, are junior physicians in training who are grappling with their own feelings of incompetence vis-à-vis the field of neonatology and are just beginning to realize the emotional implications of this specialty. This can lead to struggles of control, that is, whether the "experienced nurse" or the "inexperienced physician" knows best how to deal with the infants and their families. The child psychiatrist consultant, who is a physician and is often inexperienced in neonatal care, for this reason is also at times received with some suspicion by the nurses of such a ward. To minimize the ensuing difficulties, it is advisable to use competent senior clinicians for the work on such units.

Difficulties among the two disciplines can also arise because NICU nurses, like the neonatologists, are action-oriented people whose sense of efficiency may clash with the working style of a mental health professional. Because many NICUs now also have nurses who are delegated to deal with mental health problems and because virtually all such wards have a complement of social workers, the psychiatrist may unwittingly become involved in a territorial struggle between these professionals that may cost him or her part of his or her effectiveness.

Finally, there are the parents of the small or ill infants. Their difficulties are usually responsible for the psychiatrist's entry into an NICU. Yet the great majority of parents who are identified as troubled are not psychiatric patients but fathers and mothers who are overwhelmed by events surrounding their infants' births. To find a way of recognizing their competence and yet to provide them with the assistance they need to deal with their special infants provide the main reward and the true challenge for the psychiatrist in an NICU. At the same time, it must be remembered that about 5% to 10% of parents with children in an NICU can be expected to have significant problems in parenting later on. The highest possible number of these parents must be identified and provided with much needed support early on.[17] To establish procedures that will allow for the identification and treatment of such high-risk families is clearly difficult and requires tact and clinical expertise from the mental health professional.

Case 3

Mrs. C., a 25-year-old receptionist, had given birth to a twin boy and girl weighing less than 1100 g. The boy died after 72 hours of an intracranial hemorrhage without having been formally named. His sister Esther developed severe chronic lung disease and required long-term low-flow oxygen therapy.

Both parents appeared concerned and interested in Esther, although during their regular visits, it was the father, a teacher in a local college, who usually handled and played with Esther while her mother watched them silently. Mrs. C. also never visited Esther alone, but the father came by almost every day for a short period. When Esther was 3½ months old, the responsible physician wanted to discharge her to her home despite her chronic lung condition. However, Mrs. C. refused to have Esther come home, stating that Esther might get sick too easily in their new house and that it would cost too much time to bring her the 3 miles to the hospital.

When further discussions with the responsible physician and the social worker did not change Mrs. C.'s opinion, a psychiatric consultation was requested.

Mrs. C. began the interview with the psychiatrist by saying "this has been coming for a long time" and then talked at length about her parents' concentration camp experiences. Further interviews revealed her to have strong fears about harming children, serious marital problems, and many unresolved conflicts with her parents. While the psychiatrist continued to support Mrs. C. and helped her to accept the discharge of her daughter 3 months later, she also referred her to an analytic colleague for more intensive treatment.

One Model of a Consultation–Liaison Service for an NICU

The practical implementation of a psychiatric consultation–liaison service to an NICU depends both on the size of the unit and whether the unit is located in a pediatric or a general hospital. If the unit is small, that is, has 20 or less intensive-care beds, certain parent-support measures that may be based on group meetings cannot be set up for lack of infants who are at the same developmental stage. Likewise, when the unit is situated in a pediatric hospital, the patient population will tend to be more mixed and will include full-term infants with congenital abnormalities or with other serious neonatal illnesses as well as preterm infants. This will necessitate a somewhat different administrative structure and also be accompanied by different types of psychological problems among parents and staff. Nevertheless, we feel that there are a number of basic administrative principles that the consulting psychiatrist should aim to implement in all types of neonatal intensive care units. Specifically, we suggest the following:

1. A neonatal intensive care nursery should be limited to 20 beds, as larger units require so much personnel that meaningful personal interactions among staff, parents, and their families become extremely difficult. The administration of such a unit and the cohesiveness of the staff likewise present problems in bigger units. This may compromise the support staff members can get from each other and in turn can give to the parents of their infant patients.

2. Each intensive care nursery should have facilities that make visiting for parents a comfortable task. For example, there should be rocking chairs, and the opportunity for breastfeeding or pumping in a special area where a parent can be alone with her infant.

3. All professionals who work in a neonatal intensive care unit should be carefully selected and provided with opportunities for regular in-service training. The physician in charge of the infant should be identified to the parents,and he or she should actively approach the parents and regularly tell them of the infant's progress. This task should not be delegated to junior staff as their frequent rotation makes consistency in the type and style of information given to the parents more difficult to achieve. Each unit of 20 beds should also have available the services of one full-time social worker. The social worker should review all new cases and be more involved in some than others.

4. Each infant should have a primary nurse assigned to him or her for his or her total hospitalization. Each primary nurse looks after a small number of patients for a prolonged period of time and provides the necessary continuity of care. As the nurse spends many hours every day with "her" patients, she can monitor the parents' visiting patterns and also learn something about the family's personal and social backgrounds. This may give important clues about their parenting abilities and will allow the nurse to alert other professionals if additional support is needed. Because parents will develop trust more easily in a primary nurse, it will also give the nurse the opportunity to teach parents more about the care such an infant requires.

5. All parents should receive literature on prematurity (for example, *The Handbook for Parents of Premature Infants,* by Shosenberg)[18] right after the delivery or during their initial visit to the nursery. Parents should be welcomed to the NICU and, from the first visit, be given every opportunity to partake in the care of their infants. Breastfeeding should also be encouraged when wanted.

6. Parents of premature infants should have the opportunity to sleep 1 or 2 nights with their infants, in a room separate from the nursery, prior to the infants' discharge from the hospital. This will familiarize them with the night routines of their babies and will diminish the parental fears so commonly encountered after an infant's transfer from hospital to home.

7. The psychiatrist, like the social worker, should be introduced to the parents as just

another team member. This can be done by pointing out that it is extremely stressful for any family to have a premature or sick infant and that such an event may trigger some of the symptoms of parental stress outlined in this chapter. Families may also be told that premature babies often show unusual behaviors early on in life, that is, that they may have jerky movements or poor feeding and sleeping habits and that mental health professionals can help with such matters.

Such an introduction eliminates much of the stigma traditionally associated with a psychiatric consultation, and, in our experience, is readily accepted by a great majority of families.

The psychiatrist should also be called to assess and treat families who appear likely to develop a parenting disorder. Two types of parental behaviors are especially indicative of possible later difficulties in the parent–infant relationship:

Lack of Parental Visiting

There is much evidence that parents who do not visit their infants are more likely to show other parenting difficulties later on.[5,17] However, it is important to investigate the reasons for this behavior (e.g., distance between the hospital and home, maternal ill health, other children, the fear of attaching to a sick baby) and institute remedial measures as soon as possible. The procedure we have found useful is to ask parents who have not visited their infant within a few days of admission to the NICU to come to a "formal" meeting with the neonatologist. This meeting should be set up with the primary aim of informing the parents about the medical status of their infant. However, it also allows the physician to address the parents' reluctance to visit and their possible wish to participate actively in the care of their baby. After the meeting, the neonatologist and the parents can visit the baby together and, in this way, make it easier for the parents to get over the initial hurdle of seeing or touching their infant. If such a "consultation visit" does not stimulate parental visits, the family should be referred to a social worker or psychiatrist to obtain a more detailed psychosocial history. Parents who seem depressed, unrealistic, or in other ways out of tune with their infants during the initial interview should likewise be referred for a more detailed investigation. Although some of them will show characterological difficulties, others will suffer from an abnormal grief reaction. Such parents may refuse to visit their infant, claiming they must prepare themselves for the death of the baby. They may also show a severe sleep and appetite disturbance. When forced to be with their infant, they may initially feel a "lack of bonding" and show more interest in other babies than their own. A substantial number of these parents in our clinical experience are immigrants from countries with less sophisticated neonatal care systems who still assess the chance of their infants' survival on a scale appropriate for their country of origin.

Postpartum depression may be another reason why mothers do not visit the nursery. Because mothers of sick infants are especially at risk for this condition[19] and the accompanying psychological unavailability of a depressed mother during her infant's first year of life is significantly associated with later behavior and developmental difficulties,[20] the early diagnosis and treatment of this condition is critical for the psychological survival of the infant. It is especially important to be aware of "minor" depressive episodes that last longer than 3 weeks because family members often consider these to be "normal" and see no need to assist such a mother. Yet recent data[21] have shown that mothers with minor depressions do not recover readily without assistance and that their children at age 1 show more sleeping, eating, or other behavioral disturbances than do children of mothers who were seriously depressed postnatally.

Parental Insensitivity to the Developmental Needs of the Special Infant

There is a substantial minority of parents (about 5%, in our experience) who are quite insensitive to their infants' developmental needs. Such parents may be difficult to detect because a psychiatrist rarely observes a mother's actual interactions with her infant in the nursery. Nurses must, therefore, be trained to record obscure and obviously incorrect attributions a parent may make about his or her infant's behavior (e.g., a mother's saying, "You really look as if you hate me today" or "Don't look so mean") and report them to the responsible physician.

Parents who exhibit the following characteristics may also find it difficult to assess their infant's developmental needs:

1. Any parent who either constantly stimulates or never touches or talks to his or her infant in the nursery and seems unable to respond in his or her ministrations to changes in the baby's state of alertness.
2. Any parent who attributes motives and intentions to his or her child that are outside the infant's developmental abilities. Examples here would be the attribution of hate, revenge, or "being spoiled" given to a child below the age of 6 months.
3. Any parent who does not perceive or appreciate the social cues a baby above the age of 6 weeks sends out to those around him or her. This might include parents who have failed to develop private little games with their babies, have no sense of their infants' uniqueness, and are unable to note when their babies may be frustrated, angry, or unhappy.

Although, the sources for a parent's difficulties in "reading" the infant's state or needs are obviously complex and multidetermined, one can usually differentiate between (1) parents who are aware of their difficulties but seem unable to change them; (2) parents who are oblivious to the distorted image they have of their infant; and (3) parents who are temporarily "out of phase" with their baby because of fatigue or other acutely stressful life events.

Services Provided by the Child Psychiatrist

In our experience, a child psychiatrist working in an NICU should:

1. Be a geographically full-time clinician who is able and willing to see parents referred to him or her within 48 hours.
2. Participate in routine activities of the NICU such as ward rounds but also at social occasions.
3. Be involved in teaching nurses and residents and other staff on such issues as psychosocial aspects of development or parental grief reactions.
4. Actively participate in orientation programs for new nursing staff and residents.

We have found it useful to separate the day-to-day services the psychiatrist provides to an acute neonatal intensive care unit (NICU) and to a transitional care nursery. The former unit is generally so heavily oriented toward crisis management that the most acceptable way to have some psychiatric input is by seeing and treating specific referred cases. It is important to insist, however, that parents be notified by their primary physician of his or her wish for them to see a psychiatrist and that they agree to this referral. Social workers should ideally have seen all parents who have particular "high-risk" characteristics (e.g., all single or teenage parents, those who have had no, or poor, prenatal care, and those with known previous mental disorders) and provide background social data for the psychiatrist. The psychiatrist should write a short note directly after seeing the patient and, in addition to a later longer consultation summary, should also communicate his impressions to the referring physician verbally. This will maintain good interprofessional communication and satisfy the action-oriented neonatologist in a manner more compatible with his or her traditional working style.

Once an infant is transferred to the transitional care nursery, acute medical procedures become less frequent and the psychiatrist is generally able to organize some type of regular meeting with physicians, nurses, and other health care practitioners during which psychosocial issues of individual infant patients and their families can be discussed. As various paramedical professionals such as physical or occupational therapists or public health nurses are frequently involved in the care of the infants at that stage, it is extremely important to involve them in these meetings. Specific nurses as well as members of the house staff should also participate, as, in addition to the problems of a particular family, minor administrative changes or more general topics relevant for the development of premature or ill infants may be discussed. Postdischarge follow-up arrangements for each infant that will insure ongoing support for high-risk families should also be an important topic of these meetings. The exact format of such rounds may be decided in conjunction with the senior attending staff member. On our unit, some staff members prefer psychiatrists to go on rounds with the pediatrician; others want to sit down and discuss individual families in more detail; and others again prefer to have regular weekly psychosocial rounds.

Another effective way to assist parents who have trouble conceptualizing their proper role in the caretaking process and to help them cope with the birth of their premature or ill infant is to provide them with the opportunity to formally meet with each other. In our unit, such meetings take place once per week in the evening and are led by a mother or father who has had a premature infant in our unit within the last 12 months. Groups consist of 8 to 10 parents. The "veteran" parents invariably establish a rapid and intense relationship with the new parents, allowing them to work through some of their own grief within 3 to 4 weeks. Once this has been achieved, the meetings can become more educational. For example, a public health nurse or a physiotherapist may talk about community resources for high-risk infants or how to stimulate a difficult baby. Although these group meetings are best organized by an active perinatal parent organization, the psychiatrist should be available to provide support for the group leader.

Some authors have suggested that parents who show obvious psychological problems in the nursery should be encouraged to begin intensive psychotherapy at that time.[22] We have been very reluctant to suggest such a course of action but have preferred to approach our parents as important albeit troubled allies who help us in the care of their sick or small infants.

Furthermore, the psychiatrist can make valuable contributions to any discussions about physical changes in the NICU by highlighting areas of concern for parents that administrators may not be aware of. For example, the furnishings of a care-by-parent unit or the lighting of an NICU may be important factors in determining how frequently or eagerly parents visit their infants. Likewise, the consulting psychiatrist should always participate in discussions that lead to administrative or policy changes as these can affect the total psychological milieu of an intensive care unit.

Finally, it can be of considerable benefit for the NICU if the psychiatric consultant engages in some research project in conjunction with members from the unit. Research is an academic activity that is valued and shared by all physicians and that can bring different specialties together on yet another level in their common pursuit of better patient care. Although some of the preceding suggestions will take time to come to fruition and some may be less relevant in small neonatal units, their implementation will no doubt contribute greatly toward improving staff morale and care for all infants and their families.

References

1. Prugh D: Emotional problems of the premature infant's parents. *Nurs Outlook* 1:461–464, 1953.
2. Kaplan DM, Mason EA: Maternal reactions to premature birth viewed as an acute emotional disorder. *Am J Orthopsychiatry* 30:539–552, 1960.
3. Caplan G, Mason E, Kaplan DM: Four studies of crisis in parents of prematures. *Comm Ment Health J* 1:149–161, 1965.
4. Barnett CR, Leiderman PH, Grobstein R, Klaus MH: Neonatal separation: The maternal side of interactional deprivation. *Pediatrics* 45:197–205, 1970.
5. Klaus MH, Kennell JH: *Parent-Infant Bonding*. St. Louis, CV Mosby, 1982.
6. Minde K, Shosenberg N, Marton P, et al: Self-help groups in a premature nursery—A controlled evaluation. *J Pediatr* 96:933–940, 1980.
7. Maloney J, Ballard JL, Hollister L, et al: A prospective controlled study of scheduled sibling visits to a newborn intensive care unit. *J Amer Acad Child Psychiatry* 22:565–570, 1983.
8. Schmidt C: Emotional stress in the NICU. *Perinatal Neonatal* 1:37–44, 1977.
9. Sherman M: Psychiatry in the neonatal care unit. *Clin Perinatol* 7:33–46, 1980.
10. Minde KK: The impact of prematurity on the later behavior of children and on their families. *Clin Perinatol* 11:227–244, 1984.
11. Minde K: Parenting the premature infant: Problems and opportunities, in Taeusch HW, Yogman MW (eds): *Follow-Up Management of the High-Risk Infant*. Boston, Little Brown, 1987, pp 315–322.
12. Marton P, Minde K, Perrotta M: The role of the father for the infant at risk. *Amer J Orthopsychiatry* 51:672–679, 1981.
13. Minde K, Whitelaw A, Brown J, et al: The effect of neonatal complications in premature infants on early parent-infant interactions. *Developm Med Child Neurol* 25:763–777, 1983.
14. MacMillan H: Behavioral pediatrics: What has it achieved and where is it going? A resident's perspective. *J Developm Behav Ped* 6:100–103, 1985.
15. Sameroff AJ, Chandler MJ: Reproductive risk and the continuum of caretaking casualty, in Horowitz FD (ed): *Review of Child Development Research*. Chicago, University of Chicago Press, 1975, pp 187–244.
16. Minde K, Ford L, Celhoffer L, et al: Interactions of mothers and nurses with premature infants. *Can Med Assoc J* 113:741–745, 1975.
17. Hunter RS, Kilstrom N, Kraybill EN, et al: Antecedents of child abuse and neglect in premature infants: A prospective study in a newborn intensive care unit. *Pediatrics* 161:629–635, 1978.
18. Shosenberg N, Minde K, Swyer P, et al: *The Premature Infant. A Handbook for Parents*. Toronto, Hospital for Sick Children Foundation, 1982.
19. Stewart DE, Gangbar R: Psychiatric assessment of competency to care for a newborn. *Can J Psychiatry* 29:583–589, 1984.

20. Ghodsian M, Zajicek E, Wolkind S: Maternal depression and child behavior problems. *J Child Psychol Psychiatry* **25**:91–109, 1984.
21. Cox JC, Connor Y, Kendell RE: Prospective study of the psychiatric disorder of children. *Br J Psychiatry* **140**:111–117, 1982.
22. Zeanah CH, Conger CI, Jones JD: Clinical approaches to traumatized parents: Psychotherapy in the intensive-care nursery. *Child Psychiatry Hum Dev* **14**:158–169, 1984.

12

Psychopharmacologic Agents and Electroconvulsive Therapy during Pregnancy and the Puerperium

KATHERINE L. WISNER AND JAMES M. PEREL

Introduction

The treatment of pregnant and lactating women with psychopharmacologic agents requires skilled decision making on the part of the psychiatric consultant. The physician must consider the benefits of pharmacotherapy compared to the risks it involves not only for the mother but also for the developing fetus. In assigning weights to the factors that enter the risk/benefit equation, the physician must be aware of data from the literature regarding medication administration during pregnancy. The objective of this chapter is to provide an overview of currently available data with respect to pharmacologic treatment during pregnancy and lactation for the major classes of medications used in psychiatric practice: antipsychotics, antidepressants, lithium, and antianxiety agents. Information on the use of electroconvulsive therapy (ECT) during pregnancy will also be reviewed.

Factors that must be considered in the risk/benefit analysis are teratogenicity, maternal side effects or toxicity, and side effects in the newborn. Unfortunately, there are few controlled treatment studies of psychiatric disorder in pregnant women. Data available for treatment of psychiatric disorder in the general population must be applied to pregnant women; this may not be a valid generalization.

Katherine L. Wisner • Department of Psychiatry, Western Psychiatric Institute and Clinic, University of Pittsburgh, Pittsburgh, PA 15213.   James M. Perel • Departments of Psychiatry and Pharmacology, Western Psychiatric Institute and Clinic, University of Pittsburgh, Pittsburgh, PA 15213.

Physiologic Changes during Pregnancy

The state of pregnancy is characterized by major physiologic changes that should be considered when prescribing psychotropic medication. Pregnancy is a dynamic physiological state that influences the disposition of the drug and the maternal response to therapy.[1] The emptying rate of the gastrointestinal tract is decreased by 30% to 50%, and there is decreased gastric acid and increased mucus secretion.[1] The pregnant woman is predisposed to constipation; therefore, adding medication with anticholinergic side effects may create additional discomfort. There are significant increases in total body water volume during pregnancy, which result in lower serum concentrations than in the nonpregnant woman. Orthostatic hypotension may be a significant side effect in the pregnant patient.

Placental Transfer of Medication

Research has demonstrated that the placenta is not a "barrier" to pharmacologic agents, and all medications traverse the placenta to some degree.[2] There are several factors that influence the ease with which agents gain access to the fetal compartment; Mirkin[3] has summarized these factors:

1. *Lipid solubility and the degree of ionization.* If an agent is highly lipid soluble, it will access the fetus more readily. Highly polar compounds are impeded, but pharmacologically active amounts may cross the placenta, as is the case for the ion lithium.
2. *Protein binding.* This is particularly important for compounds that are polar because diffusion is the rate-limiting step in access to the placenta for these compounds, and binding will diminish the amount available for diffusion.
3. *Molecular weight.* Compounds with molecular weights of 200 to 500 cross the placenta readily. Most psychopharmacologic agents are in this range of molecular weight.
4. *Placental blood flow.* The uteroplacental flow is reduced during contractions. The pH of the umbilical vessel blood is 0.1 to 0.15 units lower than maternal blood; consequently, the concentration of an un-ionized basic drug is higher in the maternal circulation than in the fetal circulation. This promotes transfer of a drug from the mother to the fetal compartment.
5. *Placental maturation.* The thickness of the trophoblastic epithelium decreases in the last trimester, so that the width of the tissue layers interposed between the fetal capillaries and maternal bloodstream decreases from 24 microns early in gestation to 2 microns at birth.
6. *Placental metabolism of drugs.* Some metabolism of agents occurs in the placenta, although this is much less than transformations that occur in the maternal or fetal liver. Placental enzyme systems may metabolize drugs into reactive intermediates that may be cytotoxic, mutagenic, carcinogenic, or teratogenic substances.[4]

Fetal Metabolism

Recent research has shown that the fetus possesses the capacity to metabolize drugs to an extent through its own hepatic enzyme system, which appears in early development and reaches a plateau by midpregnancy.[5] Most of the blood entering the fetus through the umbilical vein perfuses the fetal liver parenchyma before gaining access to other fetal organs[6]; however, when a woman takes *repeated* doses of a drug to sustain plasma level concentrations, the drug will likely be equal in the mother and fetus.[2] There is no mechanism to prevent fetal exposure to a drug taken regularly by the mother when the agents are lipid soluble and of average molecular weight, as are the psychotropic agents discussed in this chapter.

During pregnancy, it is particularly important to monitor both treatment response and toxicity. Although clinical evaluation is the main mechanism of assessment, therapeutic serum levels have been established for some of the agents to be considered (particularly lithium and antidepressants) and are of value in the careful monitoring of the pregnant patient.

Teratogenicity

In considering the risks of drug treatment, a major concern is morphological teratogenicity, which has meant that its presence during gestation, particularly the first trimester, will increase the risk of physical deformity in the fetus. It is impossible to guarantee that a pharmacological agent is not a teratogen, and low levels of teratogenicity are difficult to separate from the spontaneous occurrence of anomalies.[7] It is an unwise policy to reassure a woman that her infant will be normally developed when she has been exposed to a pharmacological agent, even if the agent is not known to be a teratogen. The incidence of major birth defects in the United States is 2% to 4% and the cause of 65% to 70% of these defects is unknown.[7] Only 3% are attributed to environmental causes, including drug exposure.[7]

The capacity of a drug to act as a teratogen depends upon multiple factors. In his classic chapter, Wilson[8] culled from the literature a series of six principles (here paraphrased):

1. The susceptibility to teratogenesis varies with the developmental stage at the time of exposure to the agent; organogenesis is a particularly vulnerable time in the production of anatomical lesions.
2. Susceptibility to teratogenesis depends upon the genetic constitution of the conceptus and its interaction with environmental factors.
3. Teratogenic agents act in specific ways on developing cells and tissues to initiate abnormal embryogenesis, that is, malformations are not "agent-specific," and multiple etiologic agents may act in common ways to initiate abnormal developmental outcomes.
4. The final manifestations of abnormal development may be death, malformation, growth retardation, or functional deficits.
5. The access of adverse environmental influences to developing tissues depends on

the nature of the influences; for example, access of medication to the fetus depends upon its metabolism within the maternal organism, whereas radiation reaches the fetus directly through the maternal tissues without major modification.

6. Manifestations of deviant development increase in degree as dosage increases from the no-effect to the lethal level. What is important is that the presence or absence of *maternal* toxicity is not a reliable indicator of embryotoxicity.

Principle No. 4 deserves expanded consideration. Teratologic effects include "functional" deficits, which encompass delayed behavioral maturation, impaired rates of learning, abnormal activity, and impaired problem solving.[9] The term *behavioral teratology* first appeared in the early 1960s to describe deleterious changes in the behavior of offspring exposed to teratogens during fetal development.[10,11] Animal research has shown that psychoteratogenic agents are CNS teratogens or those classified as psychoactive.[9] Therefore, the psychotropic agents have come under particular scrutiny as behavioral teratogens.

Research in behavioral teratology, or psychoteratology, has expanded rapidly in recent years. The principles delineated by Wilson have been adapted to the field of psychoteratology.[9] The type and magnitude of the behavioral response is a function of the type of agent administered, dose of the agent, stage of development at which the agent acts, genetic milieu of the target organism, and environment of the target organism. Psychoteratogenesis is a manifestation of abnormal development that is demonstrable at doses of the agent at or below which morphological malformations are induced. The period of maximum susceptibility to psychoteratogenesis corresponds to the period of maximum susceptibility to structural and physiological abnormalities of the central nervous system (CNS); however, conclusive gestational timing studies with many agents have not been done. The effects of behavioral teratogens are not limited to the period of closure of the neural tube.[12] Not all agents that are capable of producing physical malformations are psychoteratogens.

Monitoring the production of physical deformities by chemical agents is not an effective screening strategy for behavioral teratogenicity. Vorhees[9] has formulated a theory of the spectrum of embryologic toxic reactions, in which there is increasing toxicity to the embryo (Figure 1). With increasing dosage, the response includes behavioral dysfunction, growth impairment, physical malformation, and finally embryonic death. Most CNS-active drugs have a low potential for producing physical malformations in animals, but their potential as psychoteratogens is pervasive.[9] Exceptions to this generalization are alcohol, thalidomide, and anticonvulsants. It is particularly disturbing to consider that if physical malformations due to these agents had not suggested their teratogenicity, the associated behavioral aberrations would almost certainly have been missed.[9]

Because of these suggestive and concerning findings in subhuman behavioral teratology research, it is unwise to presume that because a psychotropic agent has not been demonstrated to be a physical teratogen, it is "safe" during pregnancy. However, the public health significance of behavioral teratogens in human populations is largely unstudied.

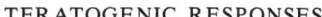

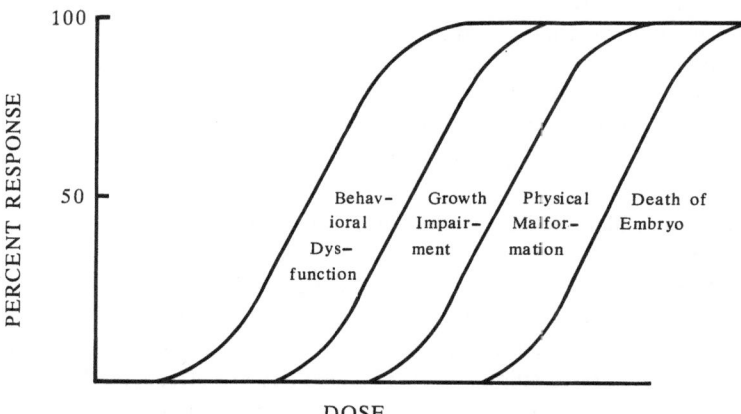

Figure 1. Theoretical set of dose-response curves showing the relationship between the four primary manifestations of teratogenesis. Figure modified from Vorhees CV, Butcher RE: Behavioral teratogenicity, in: Snell, K *Developmental Toxicology*. New York, Praeger Publishers, 1982.

Teratology is a difficult research area for many reasons.[7] Animals have been used as models of teratogen testing, because it is unethical to expose human fetuses to teratogenic agents. An obvious problem is that of cross-species validity; the initial lack of demonstration of teratogenicity of thalidomide in the rat serves as a grim reminder of this principle. Anecdotal case reports are a very important source of information about possible teratogenicity and have been valuable in generating interest in more definitive studies. However, case reports are not conclusive because of the problems of isolating the drug as the critical etiologic agent and the difficulty of generalizing beyond the single case. Epidemiologic techniques are necessary to investigate the association between the drug and the abnormality; however, it is also difficult to isolate effects of the medication from other variables. Brent[13] identified criteria that are necessary in order for epidemiologic studies to demonstrate teratogenicity; these are excerpted below:

1. Epidemiological studies should repeatedly show a statistically significant association between exposure to the agent and an increase in congenital malformations, either a unique syndrome or a group of malformations.
2. A mammalian animal model for the teratogenesis was developed, and doses comparable to the therapeutic range in humans were utilized.
3. A dose–response curve for teratogenicity in the animal model was demonstrated.
4. A plausible mechanism of teratogenesis can be established, and/or the teratogenic result makes biologic sense.

Unfortunately, there are relatively few empirical studies available that address the teratogenicity of agents described in this chapter. The previously mentioned requirements are rarely fulfilled because of lack of information. With these methodologic concerns in mind, the available data on teratogenicity will be reviewed in this chapter. Data from prospective or retrospective studies will be presented in preference to case reports. The interested reader is referred to the excellent reviews[14,15] for a consideration of epidemiologic principles of drug exposure during pregnancy.

Prescription drugs must include information about the teratogenic effects of agents. In order to summarize material regarding teratogenicity of drugs, the FDA developed categories of risk.[16] A reference guide that categorizes pharmaceutical agents according to this scheme is available.[17] The five categories to indicate the teratogenic potential of a drug follow:

A. Drugs for which well-controlled studies in women fail to demonstrate a risk to the fetus. *Notably, such studies can never entirely exclude a risk to the fetus.*

B. Indicates either (1) that animal studies have not demonstrated a fetal risk but that there are no adequate studies in women, or (2) that animal studies have uncovered some risk that has not been confirmed in controlled studies in women.

C. Either (1) studies in animals have revealed adverse effects on the fetus and there are no adequate controlled studies in women, or (2) studies in women and animals are not available.

D. This category includes drugs that human experience shows to be associated with birth defects, but the potential benefits of the drugs may be acceptable despite their known risks. A category D drug will generally be one indicated for use in a life-threatening situation or serious disease for which safer drugs cannot be used or are ineffective.

X. This category includes drugs for which fetal abnormalities have been demonstrated in animal or human studies and the potential risks of the drugs clearly outweigh their potential benefits; these agents are contraindicated for use during pregnancy.

Although this categorization is useful, and perhaps reassuring, it is simplistic and has been criticized for multiple reasons, which include the following: lack of identification of the performer of the risk/benefit analysis, inability to prevent the introduction of teratogens, creation of a population of women who are therapeutic orphans, miseducation of physicians and laypersons, and causation of unnecessary abortions.[13]

The following physician responsibilities have been defined in prescribing drugs for pregnant women[7]: avoid unnecessary drug use and select the drug with the most favorable risk/benefit ratio; inform patients about the implications of drug exposures during pregnancy; with necessary or inadvertent drug exposures, advise patients on the priority for birth control measures; and, when birth defects are observed, determine exposures and report them. The reader is referred to excellent reviews of the issues involved in prescribing psychotropic agents, such as enlisting the patient to be a co-participant in the decision to use medication[18] and prescribing psychotropic agents to female patients.[19]

Antipsychotic Agents during Pregnancy

Pregnancy Testing

Some commercially available pregnancy tests may yield false positive results for women who take antipsychotic agents. Hillard and Hillard[20] reviewed this phenomenon and used the human chorionic gonadotropin (HCG) beta subunit assay to confirm an early pregnancy in a woman who had experienced a psychotic decompensation due to her fear that she might be pregnant.

Choice of Antipsychotic Agent

Information on the use of antipsychotic agents and the treatment of schizophrenia must be extrapolated to the pregnant patient; a recent comprehensive review is available.[21] There are few systematic data to justify the preferential use of a particular antipsychotic agent during pregnancy. We prefer high-potency agents because they have minimal autonomic effects and less sedation, hypotension, and cardiovascular difficulties than their low-potency counterparts. Despite this, more studies during pregnancy are available for the low-potency agents, particularly chlorpromazine, which have been in clinical usage for a greater period of time.

Morphological Teratology

Little research has focused on the use of these antipsychotic agents by *psychotic* women during gestation, compared to their use for hyperemesis in nonpsychotic women.[22] A reanalysis of data from the California Child Health and Development Project,[23] which evaluated antiemetics in nonpsychotic women, suggested a trend toward an increase in congenital heart disease when phenothiazines were prescribed during the fourth to tenth week of gestation. The data were particularly valuable because they offered information on the timing of the exposure. The congenital anomalies targeted in this study were those that would impair a child's development, such as congenital heart disease or mental retardation.

Chlorpromazine (Thorazine). Kris[24,25] reported the results of 52 children whose mothers had been treated with chlorpromazine throughout pregnancy and concluded, after following the children for 2 to 4 years, that the exposure did not result in morphological defects or adverse effects on the child's development. The maintenance doses were relatively low (50 to 150 mg per day).

Sobel[26] studied 52 women who received chlorpromazine during pregnancy and found the incidence of fetal damage to be similar to that observed in a control group of untreated women who delivered in the same psychiatric hospital as the treated women. He noted that the infants of three women who received daily doses of chlorpromazine of 500 to 600 mg were born with respiratory distress and cyanosis, and one infant died. There were no similar severe outcomes in the remaining 49 cases treated with lower doses of medication. These findings do not justify generalized conclusions; however, the importance of careful consideration of dosages is demonstrated by this study.

Slone and colleagues[27] reported the results of the Collaborative Perinatal Project, which was a large prospective study of outcome following drug exposure during gestation. There were 142 mothers exposed to chlorpromazine during the first trimester. No evidence was found for effects on the following outcome measures: malformations, perinatal mortality rate, birth weight, or IQ score at 4 years of age.

In a prospective French study,[28] the relationship of phenothiazine ingestion to malformations was evaluated. Malformations were defined as an abnormality of appearance or function evident at birth or within the first 4 weeks of life. Phenothiazines were taken by 315 pregnant women either once or several times during the first 3 months after the last menstrual period, and there were 11 newborns with malformations; this finding was significantly different when compared to the group of non-phenothiazine-exposed women who bore malformed infants ($p < .01$). The authors found that the phenothiazine with a 3-carbon aliphatic side chain (including chlorpromazine) were significant at the $p = .01$ level, whereas other phenothiazine groups were not associated with this significance level. Of particular interest would be whether the women who received the 3-carbon side chain agents, such as chlorpromazine, were receiving the drug for symptoms related to psychiatric disorder as opposed to hyperemesis, which might introduce other confounding variables, such as poor prenatal care.

Trifluoperazine (Stelazine). Trifluoperazine was reported to be associated with limb reduction anomalies in the early 1960s[29]; however, later studies have not supported this association. Moriarty and Nance[30] retrospectively studied 480 treated pregnant women, and the incidence of live births with congenital malformations and stillbirths was comparable to that of the control group. In the majority of cases, the medication was given for nausea and vomiting. Rawlings, Ferguson, and Maddison[31] treated 341 women beginning at 5 weeks gestation with trifluoperazine and found that the incidence of congenital anomalies in the offspring was the same as the general population. The Collaborative Perinatal Project[32] monitored 42 pregnancies with first trimester exposure to trifluoperazine. There was no evidence of association between exposure and malformations, perinatal mortality rate, birth weight, or IQ score at 4 years of age.

Thioridazine (Mellaril). Scanlan[33] studied the offspring of 23 women exposed to thioridazine during pregnancy and noted no anomalies. In the Collaborative Perinatal Project,[32] 13 mother–child pairs were exposed to thioridazine, but specific data regarding malformations are presented as grouped data with other phenothiazines; there is no evidence of malformations for the entire group of agents.

Triflupromazine (Vesprin). The Collaborative Perinatal Project[32] collected data on 36 first-trimester exposures to triflupromazine; no association with malformation, perinatal mortality rate, birth weight, or IQ score at 4 years of age was observed. The small sample size dictated avoidance of generalizations.

Perphenazine (Trilafon). Data from the Collaborative Perinatal Project[32] studied 63 first-trimester exposures and 166 exposures at any point in pregnancy and noted no association with malformations, perinatal mortality rate, birth weight, or IQ score at 4 years of age.

Fluphenazine (Permitil, Prolixin). The only data available on exposure during pregnancy are found in case reports. Cleary[34] described a woman with schizophrenia who was treated with fluphenazine decanoate throughout pregnancy. The patient was also taking benztropine mesylate sporadically, drinking four or five cocktails per evening, and smoking a maximum of four packs per day. A healthy male child was born. Four weeks postnatally, a pediatrician thought the infant had "minor extrapyramidal manifestations," which were treated with diphenhydramine elixir. Phone and letter follow-up to the age of 2 revealed that the child was apparently healthy. Donaldson and Bury[35] reported a newborn with multiple congenital anomalies born to a woman with schizophrenia who was treated with fluphenazine enanthate throughout pregnancy. The defects were located in the eye, palate, anus, genitalia, and cranium.

Haloperidol (Haldol). The birth of an infant with multiple congenital limb anomalies to a mother who ingested haloperidol (15 mg per day) and multiple other medications was reported in the 1970s.[36] To investigate this possible teratogenic effect, Hanson and Oakley[37] performed a retrospective study of medication intake during pregnancy in women who had borne infants with limb reduction deformities. The mothers were shown a sample of the dosage forms of haloperidol and were asked to recall if they had taken it during pregnancy. Of the sample of 38 women, 31 were interviewed and did not recall taking the drug. Records of the remaining 7 cases were reviewed and did not contain evidence that the haloperidol was prescribed. The number of cases in the study is small, and the dependence on recall is a methodological problem.

To evaluate the safety of haloperidol for treatment of hyperemesis gravidarum in the first trimester, 100 women and their offspring were evaluated.[38] No effects were noted on birth weight, duration of pregnancy, sex ratio, fetal, or neonatal mortality, and no malformations were found in abortuses, stillborns, or neonates. However, this treatment is often instituted beyond the critical period for limb development, and the doses may be smaller than those used for psychiatric indications.[38]

Reports of the use of haloperidol for the treatment of chorea gravidarum have appeared in the literature.[39,40] The exposures (1 to 2 mg/day) generally occurred in the second trimester when the disorder develops. No abnormalities in the offspring were indicated.

Summary: Teratogenicity

Evidence from the prospective Collaborative Perinatal Project and most other studies reveals that the antipsychotic agents as a general class do not produce a rate of malformation that is readily distinguishable from that in the general population, and no specific organ malformation is repeatedly identified. However, little research has focused on the use of these drugs (particularly the phenothiazines) by *psychotic* women compared to their use by nonpsychotic women for hyperemesis. Data regarding dosage and timing is not often reported in epidemiologic studies.

Pharmacological and Behavioral Effects in the Newborn

Jaundice and anticholinergic side effects have been described in phenothiazine-exposed infants. An infant with jaundice, hypotonicity, lethargy, and depressed reflexes was born to a mother who had received 8000 mg chlorpromazine during the 10 days prior to term.[41] Other medications (including lithium) were also given. Jaundice in newborns who were exposed to phenothiazines during labor has also been described.[42] Small left colon syndrome (a functional intestinal obstruction) occurred in two newborns who had been exposed to chlorpromazine and other anticholinergic agents during late pregnancy.[43]

Extrapyramidal syndromes have been reported in infants exposed to chlorpromazine prenatally.[44-46] Hill[46] described the infant offspring of a woman with schizophrenia who had received phenothiazines during pregnancy. The infant exhibited hypertonicity, tremor, "flapping" arm movements, and abnormal hand posturing that persisted for at least 5 months; the hypertonicity persisted for 10 months. Follow-up at 32 months revealed no abnormalities. The child entered school at the age of 6 and "did well." Interestingly, the same mother had another pregnancy that resulted in an infant exposed to chlorpromazine with similar symptoms for 6 months.

Abnormal behavior has been observed in infants born to women who had consumed antipsychotic agents during pregnancy.[47] Infants whose mothers had received combinations of major or minor tranquilizers in large doses throughout pregnancy had deep skin creases and persistence of intrauterine position, which they suggested might be due to diminished movement *in utero*. A biphasic response with initial postnatal depression and subsequent agitation was described. Depression was characterized by diminished spontaneous movement and cry, brief response to stimulation, vasomotor instability, thermolability, and difficulty with oral feeding. This phase lasted 1 to 5 days. The subsequent agitated phase was characterized by excessive motion and crying, alerting behavior, hyperreflexia, hypertonicity with tremor, excessive sucking drive with increased intake, vasomotor instability, low-grade fever, and hyperacusis. Less frequent findings were abnormal hand posturing, prolonged tongue protrusion, uncoordinated suck and swallow mechanisms, hyperperistalsis, and seizurelike movements. The duration of the agitated phase was 1 to 7 months and was characterized by varying levels of intensity.

One of the issues raised in considering the behavioral teratology of long-acting medications is whether behavioral effects noted in the neonate are due to alterations in the embryologic unfolding of the neurological substrate or to retained drug. Madsen[48] attempted to address this issue by studying labeled haloperidol distribution in the brains of neonatal rats. The data suggested that the persistence of prenatally acquired neuroleptics may account for behavioral and biochemical alterations in the neonatal rat as an alternative explanation to developmental aberrations in the central nervous system. Unfortunately, there are no published systematic data on the long-term behavioral consequences of human antipsychotic medication exposure *in utero*.

Breast-Feeding

Very little data is available to guide the clinician in making decisions regarding breast-feeding during the ingestion of antipsychotics. Whalley[49] reported data from a mother who had established breast-feeding and who developed "puerperal hypomania" on Day 16 postnatally. She was admitted to the hospital and treated with oral haloperidol (15 mg twice daily). She continued to breast-feed her infant during the time she was treated, which was the third to the sixth week of the infant's life. Haloperidol was continued at the same dosage, and measurements were obtained. The concentration of haloperidol in the mother's milk was measured twice and was found to be an average of 64% of that in the maternal serum on days 6 and 7 of treatment. When the drug was discontinued on Day 21, the mother's milk contained 81% of the plasma level. The question of whether the drug concentration in the milk would have continued to increase compared to the plasma level if treatment had continued is unanswered. Clinical observation of the infant revealed no sedation, normal feeding, and achievement of expected developmental milestones at 6 months and a year. There were no behavioral or motor abnormalities noted.

Haloperidol excretion in human milk in a 33-year-old woman with psychotic depression has been studied.[50] Levels of drug in the breast milk of the patient were 5 ng/ml after an average dose of 30 mg/day and 2 ng/ml following a 12-mg dose. Figuring 1,500 ml of milk ingestion per day, the dose would be 0.0075 mg/day. The physiological significance of chronic ingestion of low doses of haloperidol in the newborn is unknown.

The Pharmacological Management of Postpartum Psychosis

Careful differential diagnostic evaluation is important in the management of postpartum psychoses because the majority are affective psychoses, and other agents such as lithium or antidepressants may be appropriate (please refer to Chapter 6).

In the 1960s, Kris[24,25,51] addressed a clinical problem that has yet to be studied in a systematic fashion. She presented data on women with schizophrenia who had multiple pregnancies who had been maintained on chlorpromazine for the *prophylaxis* of psychosis. In one case,[24] a 21-year-old woman delivered a child while no medication was being taken; she developed a psychosis at 2 weeks postpartum. She conceived and gave birth to another child, but this time was treated prophylactically with 100 mg of chlorpromazine throughout the pregnancy, and she did not develop a postpartum psychosis. Although these data are suggestive, they are not convincing because they are essentially from an A–B single case study design,[52] and other intervening variables may have been responsible for the change in outcome. Another case[24] is more convincing because it represents an A–B–A single case study design.[52] A mother delivered a child while no medications were taken during pregnancy and suffered a postpartum psychosis at 10 days. In the next pregnancy, the mother took 75 mg of chlorpromazine throughout pregnancy and did not suffer a postpartum psychosis. For a subsequent child, the mother refused to take medication because she felt well, and she again suffered a postpartum psychosis at 2 weeks. Although it is not valid to generalize findings from a single case, these data are certainly quite interesting, and the question of prophylaxis for postpartum psychosis deserves further research.

Brown[53] stated that there are no established guidelines for the use of antipsychotic medication on a preventive basis for women with psychotic illnesses outside of or during the puerperium. In the face of this uncertainty, he felt that a reasonable clinical approach was to begin antipsychotic medication following delivery in any woman who has had two or more consecutive postpartum psychoses. The choice of medication should be determined by the medication to which she has responded in the past. He stated that haloperidol in a dose of 5 to 10 mg orally at night or the equivalent dose of another antipsychotic drug is the usual dose range required for maintenance treatment. This dose is somewhat higher than the dose used by Kris, which was 50 to 150 mg of chlorpromazine, or about 0.5 to 1.5 mg of haloperidol as an equivalent; however, Kris's patients were treated throughout pregnancy. In the absence of a recurrence of psychosis, Brown[53] recommended discontinuation of the medication after 6 months.

Kris's astute clinical observations raise another interesting point, that is, that the focus in most articles has been the negative aspects of treatment of pregnant women with neuroleptics, such as morphological and behavioral teratogenicity. The benefit must not be underemphasized. She raises the issue: Does a mother on pharmacotherapy provide a better environment for the development of children? By her anecdotal report, "Several of the mothers stated that they themselves were less nervous while under pharmacotherapy in the postpartum period and that this reflected on the children, who, they felt, were much easier to manage than their previously born children."[24] The point is that the decision about risk/benefit must not only focus on toxic physiologic effects for both mother and fetus but a consideration of the interactional capabilities of the mother with her family as well.

Kris also gives an interesting example of a woman who received her dose of chlorpromazine at night and could not hear her infant.[25] The time of administration was made earlier in the day with the remediation of the problem.

Antiparkinson Agents and Diphenhydramine during Pregnancy

Because these agents are commonly used to treat the side effects induced by the antipsychotic agents, their use during pregnancy will be addressed. It is optimal to reduce the dosage of the antipsychotic to the lowest effective level in order to minimize side effects and the need for additional medication; however, acute dystonic reactions may occur.

Diphenhydramine (Benadryl). This antihistamine may be used to treat extrapyramidal symptoms related to antipsychotic agents. An apparent interaction between diphenhydramine and temazepam resulted in stillbirth near term, and a high incidence of fetal stillbirths with the combination of drugs in rabbits was produced.[54] It is unknown whether diphenhydramine and other benzodiazepines carry this risk, but the combination of agents should be avoided.

Saxen[55] reported an association between diphenhydramine usage in the first trimester and the occurrence of cleft palate in newborns. The Collaborative Perinatal Project[32] studied 595 mother/child pairs who had been exposed to diphenhydramine in the first trimester, and 2,948 mother–child pairs who had been exposed at any point during pregnancy. There were associations between first trimester exposure to diphenhydramine and genito-urinary malformations, inguinal hernia, eye and ear malformations, ventricular septal defects, malformations of the diaphragm, clubfoot, and other syndromes.

Withdrawal symptoms were reported in a neonate whose mother had taken 150 mg of diphenhydramine during pregnancy.[56] Tremulousness and diarrhea began on the fifth day postnatally. The excretion of diphenhydramine into breast milk has been described,[57] although levels have not been reported.

Benztropine (Cogentin), Trihexyphenidyl (Artane), and Biperiden (Akineton). The Collaborative Perinatal Project reported on 2,323 mother–child pairs in which exposure to parasympatholytics (as a general class of agents) occurred in the first trimester.[32] There was a statistically significant association between exposure and the occurrence of minor malformations. However, very few cases were exposed to these particular agents; nine exposures to trihexyphenidyl and four exposures to benztropine occurred. There is no information on biperiden.

Antidepressant Medication

Choice of Antidepressant Agent for the Pregnant Woman

Information on the therapeutic efficacy of individual antidepressants shows that none are convincingly more effective than any other, but they differ appreciably in side effects.[58] We prefer to use nortriptyline during pregnancy for the following reasons:

1. Nortriptyline has lower relative anticholinergic potency compared to most other antidepressant agents.[58]
2. There is a well-studied relationship between the plasma concentration and therapeutic effect. The "therapeutic window" is between 50 and 150 ng/ml, which may be of use in the clinical management of the patient under certain circumstances.[59] Plasma level studies may be of particular use in evaluating the pregnant depressed patient who appears to be a nonresponder without the risk of increasing dosage to levels that may create toxicity for the mother and fetus. However, dose-response curves have not been validated in pregnant women.
3. Nortriptyline is a high-potency tricyclic agent, and a lower total dosage is required to achieve an antidepressant effect. The total amount of drug available to produce teratogenic effects on non-CNS fetal tissues will be relatively less.

Although protriptyline is a more potent agent, it has a high relative anticholinergic potency,[58] and its plasma level/therapeutic response curve is not as well documented.[59] We avoid the use of maprotilene as an antidepressant in pregnant women because of data that suggest increased risk for the occurrence of seizures.[60] Theoretically, it would be unwise to prescribe this agent for a pregnant patient who is at risk for pre-eclampsia/eclampsia.

Morphological Teratology

Tricyclic Antidepressants. McBride[61] reported that a child with limb anomalies had been exposed to imipramine in utero; however, a review by the Australian Drug Evaluation Committee[62,63] failed to implicate imipramine as an important cause of limb abnormalities. Several practitioners reported case series of women who had been given imipramine or amitriptyline during pregnancy; all concluded that antidepressants did not result in increased risk of malformation.[64-66] The total number of women in the combined case series was 117; 110 of the offspring were apparently normal at birth. Of the remaining 7 pregnancies, 3 resulted in malformed infants, 1 resulted in a stillbirth, 2 spontaneously aborted, and 1 infant had unexplained swelling of the extremities that resolved. Sim[67] reviewed 211 cases of pregnant women who had "exhibited instability" during their pregnancies, and 81 of this group received imipramine for depressive symptoms; the dose was 150 mg total per day in three doses for at least 2 months, although the exact gestational timing is not given. Of the 211 cases, 9 were born with abnormalities, and all were in the unmedicated group of pregnant women. Although these anecdotal series are interesting and important, they lack methodological rigor.

The targeting of limb reduction anomalies as a teratogenic effect of antidepressants is likely to have been influenced by the specter of the thalidomide disaster. This focus resulted in retrospective studies[68,69] in which mothers of children with such anomalies were studied to determine exposure to tricyclic antidepressants. The tentative conclusion was that the medications were unlikely to represent a major cause of limb reduction anomalies.

A case-control study by Bracken and Holford[70] revealed that mothers of congenitally malformed infants were more likely than controls to have used an antidepressant; odds ratio $= 7.6$; $p < .01$. The odds ratio is a measure of the odds in favor of malformed infants being exposed to antidepressants in the first trimester divided by the odds in favor of controls being exposed. Exposure to antidepressants in the first trimester was associated with anencephaly, transposition of the great vessels, and other congenital syndromes. Transposition of the great vessels was also more common in infants whose mothers used antidepressants in the second trimester. The number of cases in this study was very small, and the most *common* antidepressant prescribed was amitriptyline ($N = 3$ cases, 0 controls for first trimester exposure).

The Collaborative Perinatal Project[32] is the only prospective study that examines the relationship of antidepressants to pregnancy outcome. There were 21 mother–child pairs exposed to amitriptyline during the first trimester, and no malformations were noted at birth. There were 20 mother–child pairs exposed to either imipramine (19) or nortriptyline (1), and 2 malformations were noted, although the authors concluded that the numbers were too limited to justify any comment on the teratogenicity of the antidepressant medications. It is quite unfortunate that the one prospective study of antidepressant use was inconclusive and that few comprehensive retrospective studies are available to include sound information into the risk–benefit equation for tricyclic antidepressants during pregnancy.

There are no case reports of malformations for the following agents: desipramine, doxepin, protriptyline, trimipramine, and the nontetracyclics amoxapine, maprotiline, and trazodone. Briggs and colleagues[17] generally rate the antidepressants in category C or D. Maprotiline is rated by the manufacturer in the B category; the authors state that they did not differ with this designation; however, limited data are available on this relatively new agent, and it is clinically unwise to conclude that lack of reported toxicity is synonymous with no toxicity.

Monoamine Oxidase Inhibitors. The Collaborative Perinatal Project monitored 21 mother–child pairs on various agents, and the most common was tranylcypromine.[32] There were three malformations, which resulted in an elevated relative risk of 3.4; but the authors pointed to the difficulty in interpretation with small numbers available. However, until (and if) further data become available, the use of monoamine oxidase inhibitors during pregnancy should be considered only if other options, such as tricyclic agents and ECT, have been exhausted.

Summary: Teratogenicity

Although there is little evidence to implicate tricyclic antidepressants as major teratogens, the studies upon which this tentative deduction is based are methodologically unimpressive. The data consist of case series, retrospective studies with small numbers of cases, and an inconclusive prospective study. This is unfortunate because major depression is the most common psychiatric disorder during pregnancy (refer to Chapter 6).

Toxic and Behavioral Effects in the Neonate

A neonatal withdrawal syndrome has been reported in the offspring of women treated with antidepressants. Eggermont[71] reported that three full-term infants whose mothers had ingested imipramine displayed slowed, jerky movements and seizures. Withdrawal symptoms in an infant whose mother had taken desipramine throughout her pregnancy consisted of cyanosis, tachypnea, tachycardia, irritability, feeding difficulties, and profuse sweating.[72] The child was symptomatic for 10 days and lost approximately 500 g; he gradually improved over the next 20 days. Withdrawal symptoms such as nausea, vomiting with dehydration, and abdominal cramps have been described upon abrupt withdrawal of amitriptyline[73] and imipramine[74] in older children. In a systematic retrospective study,[75] gastrointestinal complaints, drowsiness, decreased appetite, tearfulness, headaches, and agitation were significantly higher during a withdrawal phase than during a treatment phase in latency-aged children. Dilsaver and colleagues[76] examined evidence that supported a cholinergic overdrive hypothesis to explain antidepressant withdrawal syndromes, which included gastrointestinal, sleep, and movement disorders and behavioral activation in adults.

Anticholinergic effects have also been observed in neonates whose mothers were treated with antidepressants near term. Shearer[77] reported a case of a neonate with bladder distension at birth; the infant did not void by 30 hours of age and was again catheterized. The baby began to urinate spontaneously at 40 days of life. A cystourethrogram at 52 hours and an intravenous pyelogram at 7 months of age were normal. The authors stated that the retention was long-standing in utero because the bladder of the child contained remarkable quantities of urine. Although the maternal serum levels were not given, the dosage (100 mg/day) was within the usual range. It is curious that a report of *nortriptyline* toxicity should occur in the literature as compared to other tricyclics because this agent has a relatively low anticholinergic potency.[58]

In a woman who overdosed on nortriptyline 20 hours prior to delivery, the drug half-life in the mother and newborn were 17 and 56 hours, respectively.[78] The child had decreased muscular tone, appeared sedated, and had an abnormal electrocardiogram; however, he appeared to have normal psychomotor development upon follow-up. There are no long-term follow-up studies in the human literature that address the behavioral teratogenicity of antidepressants.

Breast-Feeding

Imipramine. Sovner and Orsulak[79] presented data on the breast-milk content of imipramine (IMI) and its metabolite desipramine (DMI) in a woman who was taking 200 mg/day on Day 14 of treatment. She stopped breast-feeding on Day 16 and collected milk samples for assay. The mother's plasma levels were less than those considered therapeutic; her level was 62 ng/ml of IMI + DMI (therapeutic = 200 to 250 ng/ml of IMI + DMI[59]). The authors concluded that the amounts of IMI + DMI in breast-milk specimens were similar to those found in plasma. They also stated that such investigations need to consider whether the patient has been taking medication chronically or whether samples have been collected after only a few doses of medication. Although the infant did not have any behavioral effects while breast-feeding, the maternal dose was subtherapeutic, and higher maternal serum levels might have resulted in a higher breast-milk content and greater exposure to the nursing infant. The authors recommended against breast-feeding if a mother is on antidepressant therapy because of concern about physiologic or behavioral effects.

This recommendation was challenged by Erickson and colleagues,[80] who presented a theoretical argument based on the amount of breast milk that an infant consumes and on the calculated amount that the infant would receive. With a maternal therapeutic level of 200 ng/ml, and a 5-kg infant who would consume about 1000 ml per day, the infant would ingest about 0.2 mg of IMI + DMI. They calculated this to be 0.04 mg/kg and compared this to the dose of IMI used for enuresis in a 6-year-old, which is 1 mg/kg. Sovner and Orsulak[81] responded by emphasizing the fact that the effects of chronic ingestion of very low doses of potent psychoactive agents such as tricyclic antidepressants in the neonate are unknown. Accumulation of such agents may result in subtle effects on neurologic or behavioral maturation. The authors concluded that the psychiatrist and pediatrician should weigh the risk/benefit ratio in each case.

We concur with this last point. Whether to breast-feed is a complex decision that involves a variety of factors that are weighted differently by different women (and their physicians). The decision must be case-specific, that is, decided after consideration of many factors by the individual woman with the assistance of her physician. The currently available data do not warrant any *absolute* recommendation.

Amitriptyline. Serum levels of AMI/NTP in a mother and her 2-month-old nursing infant were measured.[80] The mother had taken 150 mg of AMI daily for 3 weeks, and the serum concentrations were 90 ng/ml of AMI and 146 of NTP (236 ng/ml total tricyclics). No detectable amount of drug (less than 28 ng/ml of total tricyclics) was found in the infant's serum.

Bader and Newman[82] reported a case in which a breast-feeding woman had been on amitriptyline chronically for 10 years. Her usual dose was 150 mg/day, but the dose was decreased to 100 mg/day during pregnancy and lactation. Two measurements were performed to screen for detectable quantities of AMI and NTP in the milk. The first set of measurements was taken approximately 15 hours after ingestion of the drug. The concentration of drugs in the breast milk was very close to those in the mother's serum (serum values: 141 ng/ml AMI and 86 ng/ml of NTP). Because of this, the authors decided to take a second measurement, which would include maternal serum, breast milk, and infant serum. Despite being on the same dose, the mother's levels were significantly lower (AMI 83 ng/ml and NTP 59 ng/ml). The authors could not detect levels in the infant's serum with a measure sensitive to 10 ng/ml. Wisely, they added a known amount of drug to the breast milk and were able to recover it, which was a test of the ability of the technique to measure the drug from breast milk. They suggested that the mother breast-feed the infant, based on these results. However, infants may be breast-fed for extended periods, and the possibility exists that the agent is accumulating in the neonate, who has a limited capacity for excretion.[83]

An additional report on amitriptyline was presented by Brixen-Rasmussen and colleagues.[83] The mother was given amitriptyline at 3½ months postpartum. The mother's dose was 75 to 100 mg/day. A single sample of the infant's serum was obtained at 3 weeks after the beginning of the medication. The levels of medication in the maternal serum (AMT + NT = 121 and 111 at weeks 2 and 10 of treatment, respectively) were at the lower range of the therapeutic response.[59] The serum level for the infant was below the level of detectability (5 and 15 ng/ml for AMT and NT, respectively). The quantity of NT in the mother's serum was approximately the same as in the breast milk. The concentration of AMT was higher in the milk than in the serum; the ratio of maternal serum: milk AMT averaged 0.6:1. The infant showed no clinical signs of drug effects. Careful monitoring of the clinical status of the infant serum level determinations are advisable in mothers who breast-feed for extended periods while taking medication.

Trazodone. Verbeeck and colleagues[85] studied the presence of trazodone in breast milk after mothers were given a single oral dose of trazodone (50 mg). Although they concluded that the exposure of infants to trazodone through breast milk is minimal, the conditions under which the study was performed render the validity of this finding highly questionable. Much higher doses of trazodone are needed for antidepressant effects, and the medication is given chronically.

Other Agents. There are no data in the literature for infants breast-feeding when the mother is being treated with desipramine alone, doxepin, isocarboxazid (MAOI), nortriptyline alone, phenelzine (MAOI), tranylcypromine (MAOI), amoxapine, clomipramine, protriptyline, or buproprion.

The Pharmacological Management of Postpartum Depression

Postpartum depression is a common occurrence following childbirth (see Chapter 6). Despite the frequency of the disorder, there are relatively few empirical data regarding its pharmacological treatment. Kane stated that tricyclic antidepressants in standard doses are the initial pharmacologic treatment of choice for postpartum depression, except in seriously suicidal patients for whom ECT may be considered.[86] However, this is a subject of debate. Particularly in England, ECT is favored for the treatment of postnatal affective psychoses.[87,88] Hamilton[87] reported that ECT was very effective in his case series and emphasized the importance of psychotherapy as part of the treatment plan. There is no information on the use of monoamine oxidase inhibitors in the postnatal period.

Frank and colleagues studied women with recurrent major depression who had episodes of pregnancy-related illness compared to those who did not.[89] Women with histories of pregnancy-related episodes did not differ in the rapidity with which they responded to acute treatment (imipramine [150–300 mg/day] and interpersonal psychotherapy) compared to those whose past depressions were non-pregnancy-related. The index episode that was being treated in this study was not necessarily a postpartum episode.

Lithium

Pharmacological Considerations: Use of Lithium during Pregnancy

Management of lithium levels during gestation requires consideration of the physiology of pregnancy. Lithium clearance increases in the second half of pregnancy gradually by 30% to 50% until delivery, when it falls to prepregnancy values.[90] Close monitoring of serum levels in the pregnant woman shows a decrease in lithium concentration as the pregnancy progresses; the dosage must be increased to reestablish the desired serum level. With the rapid fall in lithium clearance that occurs at delivery, maternal levels can rise quickly, and toxic concentrations may occur if the dose is not rapidly adjusted.[91]

Several reviewers have expressed opinions regarding the management of pregnant women through late pregnancy, labor, and delivery. Schou[92] and Calabrese and Gulledge[93] recommended withdrawal of lithium several days before labor and resumption several days afterward. Linden and Rich[94] suggested that the dose be reduced at labor onset because of the short half-life of lithium, the risk of relapse, and the difficulty of predicting the delivery date. They recommended reduction of the lithium dose at onset of labor by one-half to parallel the reduction in creatinine clearance and subsequent adjustment, according to the levels obtained.

Weinstein[91] warned that signs of lithium toxicity may be attributed to the physiological changes of pregnancy. The usual corrective measures may worsen the toxic state; for example, sodium restriction for the fluid retention of mild lithium toxicity. Sodium restriction and diuretic use reduce renal lithium clearance and increase reabsorption of lithium, which results in rapid escalation of serum and tissue lithium. Weinstein[91] suggested the following (here paraphrased):

1. Avoid sodium-depleting diuretics and sodium-restricted diets.
2. Avoid weight reduction by exercise that produces excessive perspiration or saunas.
3. Monitor serum lithium levels closely in the presence of acute gastrointestinal disturbances and febrile illnesses that may lead to dehydration and/or sodium loss, which impairs renal lithium clearance.
4. Observe carefully the usual physiological upsets of pregnancy; early lithium toxicity may be present. If a rapid check of the serum lithium concentration is not possible, discontinue lithium until the problem is identified.
5. Keep maternal serum lithium levels at the lowest effective level.
6. Monitor serum levels closely; at least once a month in the first half of pregnancy and up to once a week toward the end of pregnancy.
7. Monitor thyroid function in pregnant women on lithium.
8. Avoid dose pulses, which are transmitted to the fetus; give lithium in three to five equal doses through the day. Probably no more than 300 mg of lithium should be

given as a single dose to a pregnant woman unless her total dose is over 1,500 mg per day.

Teratogenicity

Morphological Teratology. Nora and colleagues[95] and Weinstein and Goldfield[96] have discussed the cardiovascular malformations associated with lithium exposure during gestation. Weinstein and Goldfield cited information from the *Register of Lithium Babies,* which had the following as criteria for entry: lithium ingestion by the mother at least sometime during the first trimester of pregnancy and the availability of the infant or sufficient fetal tissue to permit identification of significant anomalies. Weinstein[91] summarized data from 225 cases within the lithium registry. Of the cases collected, 25 (11%) resulted in congenitally malformed infants. Congenital malformations were defined as "macroscopic abnormalities of structure attributable to a faulty development and present at birth."[91] A total of 18, or 8%, of the malformations were Ebstein's anomaly and other major cardiovascular malformations. Ebstein's anomaly was 150 times more frequent among the malformed infants reported to the *Register* than among malformed infants in the general population. Cardiovascular malformations of any type appeared about six times as often among the abnormal infants in the register as among malformed infants generally. Currently, the lithium registry has data on 250 subjects, and the distribution of malformations remains essentially unchanged (R. Lannon, personal communication, 1985).

Weinstein and Goldfield[96] emphasized that reports to a register will exaggerate the frequency of pathology, and the data gathered do not permit inferences or conclusions about the true incidence of any pathological state in the population. However, the ratios among *types* of cardiovascular pathologies should be similar to the corresponding ratios in the population. This is not the case in the *Lithium Registry* population, where Ebstein's anomaly is alarmingly frequent.

Ebstein's anomaly consists of downward displacement of an abnormal tricuspid valve into the right ventricle, which is divided into two parts by the abnormal valve.[97] The right atrial cavity is large, and the tricuspid valve has varying degrees of function. The effective output from the right side of the heart is decreased because of the diminished size of the right ventricle and poorly functioning tricuspid valve. Variable amounts of right to left shunting occur at the atrial level through the foramen ovale, which results in mild to severe cyanosis. The severity of symptoms depends on the degree of displacement of the tricuspid valve.

An important factor in the risk/benefit analysis of lithium use during gestation is the severity of the malformation. The prognosis for Ebstein's anomaly is extremely variable.[97] In many patients, symptoms are mild, and the only complaint is fatigue. Cardiac dysrhythmias are frequent. Newborn infants with Ebstein's anomaly may present with cyanosis, massive cardiomegaly, and long systolic murmurs. The reader is referred to reviews for a discussion of the physiology and natural history,[98] surgical intervention,[99] and morphological variability[100] of the disorder. Because Ebstein's anomaly represents a spectrum of anatomical dysmorphology that determines the severity of clinical manifestations, a definitive picture of the infant's possible impairment cannot be given to the mother who has been exposed to lithium.

According to Wilson,[101] the embryonic period of cardiac differentiation corresponds to days 20 through 45 in the human embryo; however, the timing of an exposure may not always correlate with an observed developmental deviation. Certain biochemical prerequisites that occur before the twentieth day of gestation may be altered or absent before the morphologic cardiac events appear. Also, because completion of ventricular septation normally occurs by the forty-fifth day after conception, incomplete septation during organogenesis often closes spontaneously later in gestation or during the early postnatal period. An agent introduced later in gestation could prolong or prevent this spontaneous closure. The period of formation of the tricuspid and mitral valves occurs on days 34 to 39 of pregnancy.[101] This is 20 to 25 days after the missed period in a woman with regular menses; therefore, prevention and early diagnosis of pregnancy are important.

Prenatal diagnosis of cardiac anomalies has been reported.[102] Cross-sectional echocardiography was used to evaluate two neonates whose mothers ingested lithium during pregnancy. One of the two infants had Ebstein's anomaly, and the other one was normal. The use of this technique was a highly accurate, noninvasive assessment of cardiac malformations in infants exposed to lithium prenatally. In another report, the diagnosis of Ebstein's anomaly was made at 23 weeks gestation with echocardiography[103] after cardiac enlargement had been suspected at a routine antenatal ultrasound examination.

In these reports, no mention is made of the possibility of abortion or the psychological preparation of the parent for the birth of a defective child. Progress in fetal cardiac echocardiography may allow early diagnosis of congenital cardiac abnormalities, which will raise complex ethical issues "when potentially remedial fetal anomalies are diagnosed prior to 20 weeks gestation."[102]

An issue that has been raised regarding the high incidence of cardiovascular malformations in lithium-exposed infants is that bipolar affective disorder itself may be associated with a higher incidence of cardiac anomalies in offspring. Kallen and Tandberg[104] studied the offspring of women with manic-depressive disease that had been significant enough to require at least one psychiatric hospitalization during the 1973–1979 period in Sweden. They collected data on 350 infants born during this period and compared the outcome in all deliveries that occurred during the same period. They found that women belonging to the manic-depressive cohort were older than expected and had higher parity than expected. After correction for these factors, the perinatal death rate was significantly increased. The difference in the number of congenital cardiac malformations was also increased significantly; however, no cases of Ebstein's anomaly were seen. The groups were broken down into (1) those who had no disease before pregnancy, (2) those who had the illness but took no drug, (3) those who took a psychotropic drug, but not lithium, (4) those who took lithium only, and (5) those who took lithium in combination with another drug. Of the total group, four cases of congenital heart defects occurred among the 97 women from the sample who had used drugs, and all four mothers had taken lithium. Infants with a serious heart defect were born to 7% of women who took lithium. Two other babies with heart defects were born to women in the cohort; one of the infants had Down's syndrome. The authors point out that the cohort is relatively small, but their data suggested that there is an association between the use of lithium in early pregnancy and the birth of an infant with a serious heart defect. The small number in the study may account for the lack of observation of cases of Ebstein's anomaly.

The data also suggested that women in the manic-depressive cohort may be subject to confounding variables.[104] There were a greater number of pregnancies of less than 36 weeks' duration and more infants of low birth weight than expected. The authors suggested that lower birth weight may be due to increased smoking in the cohort compared to the control group because smoking has been linked to low birth weight.

Behavioral Teratology. Schou[105] performed a follow-up study of children from the *Lithium Baby Register* who were not malformed at birth. Sixty-seven babies who had been reported to the Scandinavian registry and who were 5 years or older were assessed. The control group was nonexposed siblings. The data were collected by questionnaires sent to the psychiatrists or general practitioners who had originally reported the babies. These practitioners were asked to contact the mothers for recent information. None of the children was directly evaluated. The information requested was simply whether the development of the child was normal or abnormal, with additional details if the child was abnormal. Schou recovered 50 (75%) case questionnaires and 57 sibling control questionnaires. The difference in the number of developmental abnormalities between the lithium-exposed and control groups was not statistically significant. The author pointed out the weakness of the design in collecting subjective information from the mothers. The outcome measures of interest were not specified. This is the only follow-up study which considers the behavioral teratogenicity of lithium.

Summary: Teratogenicity. There is evidence from the *Register of Lithium Babies*[91] and from an independent investigation[104] that has established a comparable rate of occurrence (7% to 8% of exposed fetuses) for a similar pathological lesion, which is cardiovascular anomalies. The risk for serious cardiac malformations in lithium-exposed fetuses is about 1 out of 12 to 14 exposed fetuses, and this probably represents a ceiling value because reports to a register will overestimate the frequency of occurrence.

Recommendations for Women of Childbearing Age

Weinstein[91] recommended the following:

1. Women in the childbearing years should be given lithium only for *unequivocal indications*. The reader is referred to recent articles regarding the treatment of acute manic episodes,[106] psychotherapeutic issues in bipolar illness,[107] and the pharmacologic prevention of recurrences of mood disorders.[108]
2. Treated women should be informed of the probable teratogenic risk of lithium and the potential for toxicity. They should be encouraged to maintain effective contraception.
3. If the patient becomes pregnant, lithium should be withdrawn during the first trimester, unless there is convincing evidence that withdrawal would seriously endanger the mother or the pregnancy.
4. Therapeutic abortion is not routinely indicated.

There are no empirical studies to support recommendations for women who take lithium and who wish to become pregnant. Gelenberg[109] suggested that couples may choose to avoid conception, to pursue pregnancy and accept the risks, or attempt a temporary discontinuation of lithium treatment. For the last option, he recommended that the woman discontinue lithium at the beginning of the menstrual period on the cycle in which she hopes to conceive. Counseling on the times of maximal probability of conception should be given. The emphasis was upon decreasing the interval in which the woman remained lithium free. If lithium is avoided in the first trimester, the risk of major cardiovascular malformation is that of the general population.[109] He also recommended that the course of action to be taken if the woman relapses during pregnancy be discussed while the woman is in remission and that this discussion be carefully documented.

Toxic Effects in the Newborn

There are many case reports of transplacental fetal lithium exposure that has resulted in adverse effects on the newborn. Morrell and colleagues[110] described a case of severe transplacental lithium toxicity in a neonate. The mother had polyhydramnios at 35 weeks and signs of lithium toxicity two weeks later. Her lithium level was 2.6 mEq/L. The following day, she delivered a lithium-toxic infant whose level was 2.8 mEq/L. Symptoms were Apgar of 2 at 1 minute, with hypotension, pronounced general hypotonia, and gross cardiomegaly with sinus bradycardia. Cross-sectional echocardiography showed a structurally normal heart with marked left and right atrial enlargement, a poorly functioning left ventricle, and increased left and right ventricular wall thickness, which suggested a primary cardiac muscle dysfunction. The child had high urine output and became dehydrated despite adequate fluid replacement. She required therapy for diabetes insipidus. On exam at 1 year her cardiac and renal function were normal; however, delayed motor development was noted.

Karlsson and associates[111] reported their evaluation of a neonate who was born to a woman who had been successfully treated for lithium toxicity 16 days prior to delivery. The infant, who was 5 weeks premature, had transient muscular hypotonia during the first day of life. Cord serum concentrations revealed elevated thyroid-stimulating hormone, low triiodothyronine, and normal thyroxine. These concentrations were normal at 8 days, and no abnormalities were noted in the child through 6 months of follow-up. Transplacental lithium poisoning in the offspring of a woman whose levels of lithium were approximately 0.6 mEq/L has been reported.[112] The mother also took chlordiazepoxide. At 31 weeks gestation, she went into labor, and the fetal heart was found to be irregular until delivery. At 35 weeks, she delivered an infant whose serum lithium level was 0.32 mEq/L. The newborn had a cardiac arrhythmia that consisted of abnormal atrial beats; however, the child had no hypotonia or cyanosis. There were no clinical or electrocardiographic abnormalities beyond the twelfth day. Transient atrial flutter has also been reported in a newborn whose mother was maintained on lithium during her entire pregnancy.[113] She entered spontaneous labor at term and delivered a newborn who was bottle-fed. On the fifth day of life, the infant was noted to have atrial flutter with variable 2:1 and 3:1 atrioventricular block and an atrial rate of approximately 400/minute. The serum lithium concentration was 0.25 mEq/L. Forty-eight hours later she reverted to sinus rhythm. Echocardiography was normal.

A woman who was maintained on lithium and chlorpromazine throughout her pregnancy, which was complicated by gestational diabetes, gave birth to an infant with nephrogenic diabetes insipidus.[114] The disorder persisted for 2 months, despite removal of the lithium on the fourth day of life by exchange transfusion (which was done for hyperbilirubinemia secondary to ABO incompatibility). The authors cautioned that the lithium-exposed neonates be observed carefully for dehydration that may be due to this mechanism.

The serum half-life of lithium in the newborn has been estimated to be 96 hours.[115]

Breast-Feeding during Lithium Therapy

Toxicity resulting from exposure of the neonate to lithium through breast milk has been reported. Toxic symptoms in a term infant included multiple episodes of cyanosis, hypothermia, and hypotonia.[116] The child was born to a mother who took lithium and multiple other medications. The infant was breast-feeding and experienced cyanosis on Day 5 when the lithium level was measured at 0.6 mEq/L (maternal value 1.5 mEq/L). There were no data on serum level prior to Day 5, but the authors speculated that it may have been above the adult toxic range. The breast milk concentration was 0.6 mEq/L. Breast-feeding was discontinued, and by Day 8 the infant appeared to be normal. Sykes and associates[117] graphed the relationship of serum lithium values to infant serum and breast milk values. The breast milk values were about half of the maternal serum levels. The baby's serum level was similar to the mother's at birth but quickly fell to 0.03 mEq/L by the sixth day, with a slight rise when breast-feeding was well established at that time. The baby's urine was collected and revealed a concentration of 0.57 mEq/L, which was about 10 times the mean serum level, which demonstrated that the neonatal kidney was capable of excreting lithium against a concentration gradient. The infant was hypotonic during the first 2 days of life.

There is debate regarding the advisability of breast-feeding during lithium therapy. As an electrolyte, lithium passes easily into milk. Most data regarding lithium in milk reveal that milk levels average 40% to 50% of maternal serum levels and that infant serum and milk levels are approximately equal.[118] Long-term effects from exposure to lithium in breast milk have not been studied.

Schou and Amdisen[118] emphasized a joint decision about breast-feeding between the mother and physician but advised bottle feeding. After careful discussion of the risks and benefits, if the woman decides to breast-feed, the infant should be monitored for lithium toxicity. Berlin[119] concluded that lithium was contraindicated during breast-feeding. Ananth[83] has also strongly recommended that mothers on lithium *not* breast-feed their babies because the infant's regulatory and excretory mechanisms are not fully developed and tolerance of lithium in intrauterine life does not automatically prove that it will be safe in the neonatal period. We concur with this approach. The levels obtained in breast milk cannot be presumed to be pharmacologically inactive in the newborn if it does not reach levels that correspond to pharmacological effects in the adult, and adverse effects in some breast-feeding infants have been reported.

The Use of Lithium for Mania in the Puerperium

The postpartum period is one of high risk for the onset of mania in women with bipolar affective disorder who have been withdrawn from lithium during pregnancy.[120] (See Chapter 6.) The doses of lithium used and the therapeutic blood range appear to be similar to those used to treat mania in the nonpuerperal woman.[86]

Carbamazepine: A Brief Note

Post and Uhde[121] discussed the use of carbamazepine for treatment-resistant bipolar disorder and stated that although lithium has been implicated as a physical teratogen, carbamazepine has not been demonstrated to be a teratogen. According to the review by Briggs and colleagues,[17] the teratogenicity of carbamazepine has not been established, although there is some evidence for decreased head circumference in exposed infants compared to controls.

Electroconvulsive Therapy (ECT)

Indications for ECT during Pregnancy

ECT is useful for conditions such as delusional and severe endogenous depression, acute mania, and certain specific schizophrenic syndromes with marked affective symptoms.[122] ECT may be indicated as the initial treatment in situations of acute risk to life or in medical conditions in which the use of medication is hazardous. It should be considered in patients with severe depression or psychosis during the first trimester of pregnancy[122] and has been used safely during later pregnancy.[123-127]

The emergency use of ECT is indicated when the psychiatric condition of the mother presents hazard for the fetus, such as during states of severe agitation, catatonic withdrawal, dehydration, malnutrition, or violence.[128] Fink[129] stated that chronic exposure to agents such as lithium, antidepressants, or antipsychotics present the risk of teratogenicity, and avoidance of this risk is sufficient reason to use ECT in the pregnant manic, psychotic, or catatonic patient. Failure of other treatment regimens in the face of deteriorating psychiatric status is also an indication for ECT. Historical data that indicate previous successful treatment with ECT may also weigh heavily in the risk/benefit ratio for the pregnant patient.

Effects of ECT during Pregnancy

In later pregnancy, lying in the supine position can produce compression of the aorta and inferior vena cava, which reduces effective blood pressure and placental perfusion.[130] Use of a wedge under the right hip will displace the uterus to the left (or occasionally the reverse is necessary),[130] which reduces the occlusion of the large vessels by the gravid uterus.

Repke and Berger[123] described the case of a second-trimester pregnant woman in whom antidepressant therapy was complicated by cardiotoxicity. Successful treatment with ECT and subsequent (lower dose) antidepressant resulted in remission of the mother's illness. The authors observed a drop in maternal blood pressure during the first ECT procedure, which they attributed to decreased intravascular volume. Intravenous hydration prior to subsequent treatments prevented hypotension. Documented by continuous electronic heart rate monitoring, the fetal heart remained stable. Ultrasonography revealed insignificant changes in fetal movements during the procedure. Delivery of a normal full-term infant with favorable Apgar scores and neurological exam was accomplished.

Varan and colleagues[124] reported the successful treatment with ECT and chlorpromazine of a 33-year-old woman who was 18 to 20 weeks pregnant. She was diagnosed as having chronic schizophrenia and was felt to be catatonic with marked agitation and aggression. The fetal heart rate monitoring revealed that a bradycardia of 80 occurred during the tonic phase of the treatment and that the heart rate quickly returned to normal. No uterine contractions were observed during or after any of the ECT administrations. The child, a 4270-g male infant with excellent Apgar scores, was delivered vaginally at term, and no congenital anomalies were noted at birth.

Remick and Maurice[131] pointed to the lack of information other than case reports on the use of ECT during pregnancy. They suggested guidelines, which are summarized next:

1. A thorough physical exam, including pelvic exam if there has not been adequate prenatal care, which may be performed under anesthesia if the patient cannot tolerate the procedure otherwise.
2. Involvement of an obstetrician as a part of the team because of the need for ongoing assessment of the mother and fetus, which may involve special diagnostic techniques.
3. A high-risk pregnancy is a relative contraindication to the procedure; this factor must be weighed carefully into the risk/benefit ratio.
4. External fetal monitoring before and for several hours after the procedure, to study the maternal and fetal physiological changes that occur.

Wise and associates[125] reported the results of ECT during the third trimester in a woman whose pregnancy was complicated by insulin-dependent diabetes and major depression with marked psychomotor retardation, persecutory hallucinations, and suicidality. Successful remission of symptoms was accomplished, and a normal infant was delivered. The baby was developmentally normal at age 10 months. Based on their experience, the authors made recommendations for the management of ECT during high-risk pregnancy as follows:

1. Perform ECT in the presence of an obstetrician.
2. Endotracheal intubation.
3. Low-voltage, nondominant ECT with EEG monitoring.
4. Electrocardiographic monitoring of the mother.
5. Evaluation of arterial blood gases during and immediately after ECT. Adequate arterial blood gas analysis has been demonstrated during ECT in a pregnant patient given oxygen pretreatment and assisted ventilation until return of spontaneous respiration.[126]
6. Doppler ultrasonography of fetal heart rate.
7. Tocodynamometer recording of uterine tone.
8. Administration of glycopyrrolate as the anticholinergic of choice (see the section on medications used during ECT).
9. Weekly nonstress tests (to measure fetal well-being).

Medications Used During ECT

An advantage of ECT compared to the chronic administration of medication for a psychiatric disorder is the relatively brief administration of drugs for ECT[129]; however, medication is used following ECT to lower the rate of relapse.[122]

Succinylcholine. This drug is a neuromuscular blocking agent that is used to prevent muscular contraction during the induced seizure. The uterus itself does not contract with seizure activity, and lack of uterine contraction has been documented during ECT.[125] Succinylcholine is rapidly metabolized in by plasma pseudocholinesterase. Pregnancy is associated with a decline of serum cholinesterase activity to 60% of normal during the first trimester.[130] The decreased activity may represent a decreased rate of hepatic synthesis.[132] The level of plasma pseudocholinesterase activity returns to normal within a few weeks postpartum.[132] The diminished activity is not associated with any structural malfunction of the enzyme; it is doubtful that the reduction in activity of the normal enzyme leads to prolonged blockade in the absence of other factors.[130]

Data compiled by Foldes[132] regarding the frequency of atypical pseudocholinesterase revealed that the frequency of variants is approximately 4 per 100; 3 of these 4 are characterized by "intermediate" activity. Persons with intermediate activity may have prolongation of apnea by several minutes.[133] Pregnant women who have a reduction in plasma pseudocholinesterase activity because of the gravid state and who possess intermediate activity may be at particular risk for prolonged apnea due to less rapid metabolism of succinylcholine. Severe reduction in pseudocholinesterase activity ("atypical") is very rare (3 per 10,000).[132] This degree of reduction in activity results in prolongation of apnea to an hour.[133]

Because of the additional risk posed for the vulnerable maternal-fetal patient(s), we recommend that pregnant women be screened for pseudocholinesterase deficiency as part of the pre-ECT medical evaluation. This is particularly important for women with a personal or family history of postoperative symptoms suggestive of pseudocholinesterase deficiency. These precautions will protect the fetus from extended high levels of exposure to succinylcholine and the mothers from prolonged ventilatory assistance, when the mother is unable to metabolize succinylcholine rapidly. When administered to the mother in usual clinical doses, succinylcholine does not cross the placenta in demonstrable quantities, and infants do not appear to be affected.[134,135] However, even though this agent has a quaternary structure, prolonged exposure to high doses promotes its entry into the fetal compartment. When maternal cholinesterase activity is abnormal, succinylcholine use near term may affect the fetus with resultant muscle weakness at birth.[136]

Regarding the teratogenicity of succinylcholine, the Collaborative Perinatal Project[32] reported 26 normal pregnancies in which the drug was used in the first trimester. No malformations were noted, but the rate of occurrence of malformations could be quite high and not be detected with this small sample size.

Other Agents. According to the Collaborative Perinatal Project,[32] atropine exposure (401 cases, 25 malformations) in the first trimester did not produce elevated relative risk. Theoretically, glycopyrrolate is the anticholinergic drug of choice[125,134] because of its limited passage across membranes and better suppression of exocrine secretion. In the Collaborative Perinatal Project,[32] exposure to certain barbiturates during the first trimester was associated with cardiovascular malformations. There were 41 cases of prenatal exposure specifically to methohexital (Brevital), and 2 malformations were reported; this did not represent an excess of malformations.

Before using barbiturates, the physician should inquire about family history of porphyria or the symptoms that suggest this group of disorders.[137] Although acute intermittent porphyria is rare (1 or 2/100,000), patients with the disorder can present with psychiatric symptomatology.[137] Precipitation of an episode of acute intermittent porphyria during pregnancy is associated with significantly decreased birthweight compared to infants whose mothers did not experience an attack during gestation.[138]

Teratogenicity of ECT

Morphological Teratology. The largest sample that has been reported is that of Impastato and associates,[127] who compiled data on 318 patients. The procedure of using succinylcholine and oxygen supplementation was extant at the time of the study. Complications occurred in 18, or 5.6%, of the patients. Thirteen patients (4%) delivered damaged fetuses. Three patients had complications "not related" to ECT, such as premature labor that followed an enema. Four patients also received insulin coma treatments, which were most likely the cause of the abnormalities. In 4 patients, the ECT occurred after the sixteenth week of pregnancy, and the authors stated that ECT was unlikely to be the cause of the abnormalities. From these data, the authors concluded that there was no increased risk of fetal damage beyond that in either the general population or the population of psychiatric patients.

According to the same report,[127] 5 patients suffered from complications such as labor soon after treatment, abdominal pain, or vaginal bleeding. When the ECT procedure was stopped, these difficulties remitted, and the patients delivered normal babies at term. The authors suggested that these complications might have been due to inadequate relaxation of the abdominal musculature.

Behavioral Teratology. Forssman[139] studied 16 children whose mothers had received ECT (1 to 6 treatments) during the first and second trimesters of pregnancy. Outcome measures included interviews about psychomotor development and physical examination. He concluded that the 16 children were normal. Impastato and colleagues[127] followed 71 children born to mothers who received ECT. Children varied widely in age from 2 weeks to 19 years. At the time of examination, "they were all considered normal mentally and physically except two who were mentally defective and four who showed neurotic traits.[127]" The outcome measures were not specified in more detail.

Use of ECT in the Puerperium

In England, it is widely held that tricyclic antidepressants are not effective in the early puerperium, although there are no empirical data to support this belief.[88] ECT is believed to be an effective treatment for postpartum psychosis, but there are few empirical data to determine whether it is useful in all diagnostic subgroups, such as mania, schizoaffective disorder, and depression.[88]

The Benzodiazepines

Pharmacological Management of the Pregnant Woman

The benzodiazepines are used in the treatment of anxiety disorder. For the pregnant patient, nonpharmacologic intervention should be the initial consideration. The reader is referred to the following recent reviews regarding the psychotherapy of anxiety,[141] the relaxation response,[142] and exposure treatment for agoraphobia.[143]

Kanto[144] has thoroughly reviewed the pharmacokinetics of several benzodiazepines used during pregnancy and the puerperium. Because the benzodiazepines are lipid-soluble, undissociated medications with low molecular weight, they easily cross the placenta. Placental transfer is greater in late than in early pregnancy, because (1) the size of the placenta increases with advancing pregnancy, (2) the layer of cytotrophoblasts becomes discontinuous, (3) the lipid content of the placenta increases, and (4) the circulation and placental area of exchange of the uterus increase as pregnancy approaches term. Because these agents in general have long half-lives, or metabolites with long half-lives, repeated administration results in marked accumulation in the mother and fetus.[3]

Diazepam. The data for repeated administration during pregnancy, which is likely to be the regimen for treatment of psychiatric disorders, will be addressed first. Repeated administration in early pregnancy has been studied in aborted fetuses. Repeated administration of 15 mg/day of diazepam for a month produced fetal/maternal ratio of 0.4 for both diazepam and N-demethyldiazepam.[144] The lowest concentrations were present in the fetal brain, which receives circulation from the placenta through the liver.

Repeated dosing in late pregnancy was studied by Mandelli and colleagues.[145] The distribution in fetal organs of a 31-week premature fetus whose mother received repeated doses of diazepam (15 mg/day) from the twenty-seventh week of gestation for eclampsia was evaluated. Accumulation of N-demethyldiazepam was observed, and the highest concentrations were present in the lungs, heart, and brain. Kanto[144] stated that this distribution may account pharmacologically for the respiratory, cardiovascular, and central nervous system effects that have been observed in newborns. Moore and McBride[146] described an increase in the fetomaternal ratio of diazepam over the period of 6 minutes to 5 hours after administration, which was followed by equilibration between maternal and fetal compartments at 5 to 10 hours. Kanto[144] concluded that fetal levels of a lipophilic drug that rapidly crosses the placental barrier might be higher than the maternal concentrations until a steady state is reached. This is the concept of the "deep compartment," which equilibrates slowly with the maternal compartment because the fetal concentration lags behind maternal levels when the mother eliminates the drug. Kanto[144] summarized: "This pharmacokinetic curiosity explains the slow accumulation of diazepam in the fetus during continuous treatment and the long lasting persistence of diazepam and its metabolites in the fetal tissues after termination of treatment" (p. 363).

The disposition of diazepam is changed in pregnant women at parturition. The placental and fetal compartments are no longer present in which to distribute the drug, so that parturition is accompanied by an increase in plasma concentration.[144]

Chlordiazepoxide. The general principles that were discussed under diazepam apply to this agent as well: avoid prolonged administration of the agent to a pregnant woman in order to avoid fetal accumulation.[144]

Chlorazepate. For chlorazepate, there is an approximate 4-hour period of slow placental transfer because of low ability to cross biological membranes; however, the elimination of chlorazepate and its metabolite N-demethyldiazepam is greatly prolonged, which predisposes to long-lasting sequelae in the newborn or breast-feeding infant.[144]

Oxazepam. Oxazepam is an interesting agent because it is a derivative of diazepam that is metabolized through glucuronide conjugation and excreted through the kidneys.[147]

This drug also follows the same principle of distribution for benzodiazepines: After an oral dose of 15 mg of oxazepam, the total drug ratio between umbilical cord plasma and maternal vein is 0.6 in early (13–16 weeks) pregnancy, but in late (38–40 weeks) pregnancy, the same ratio is 1.1.[148] Kanto[144] stated that oxazepam may be superior to diazepam for use during delivery because it does not require metabolism in the liver. Oxazepam does have good anxiolytic properties and may be used in the treatment of anxiety disorders. However, its absorption may be erratic in some individuals.

Lorazepam. A considerably slower rate of placental transfer occurs than with diazepam; the only inactive conjugated metabolite reaches both the fetal circulation and amniotic fluid but less rapidly than the parent drug.[144] In theory, lorazepam may be the agent of choice during pregnancy because of its lack of active metabolites, glucuronide metabolism, high potency, and good absorption. The drawback of this agent is that there are few outcome data regarding its use in pregnancy. Neonates do appear to conjugate lorazepam slowly,[149] and the general principle of avoidance of chronic or high dose treatment applies to this agent.

Temazepam. Kargas and colleagues[54] reported the case of a woman who had been treated with a combination of temazepam and diphenhydramine near term. The 28-year-old woman had been taking diphenhydramine; for sleep disturbance, she was given one 30-mg capsule of temazepam. Following violent fetal movements, a stillborn infant was delivered. The authors reproduced a high incidence of fetal stillbirths with the combination of drugs in rabbits. It is unknown whether other benzodiazepines and diphenhydramine carry this risk, but this combination of agents should be avoided.

Flunitrazepam and Nitrazepam. These are used primarily as hypnotics. Single standard doses of these agents near term do not appear to have ill effects on the infants.[144]

In summary, we recommend the avoidance of these agents during pregnancy. Other means of treatment of anxiety disorder should be vigorously pursued. If circumstances dictate the use of an antianxiety agent, we would favor the use of lorazepam in the lowest effective dose for the least amount of time. Its use should be avoided near term. The chronic use of these agents for the sleep disturbances during pregnancy is contraindicated. Differential diagnosis of the sleep disturbance to rule out other disorders, such as major depressive disorder, is imperative. Sleep disturbances during pregnancy are common, and the degree of impairment must be carefully weighed against the risk of chronic treatment with these medications. The reader is referred to a discussion of the nonpharmacological treatment of sleep disorders[150] and a review of the pharmacological treatment of insomnia.[151]

Morphological Teratology

Meprobamate and Chlordiazepoxide. Several large epidemiologic studies are available that address the issues of the morphologic teratogenicity of these antianxiety agents. Unfortunately, the two major studies arrive at differing conclusions. Milkovich and van den Berg[152] used a carefully designed prospective study to examine the effects of these agents during early pregnancy in 1904 cases. Data on drugs were derived from physicians' notations in the mothers' medical records (combined hospital and clinic records). *Severe* congenital anomalies are reported in this particular paper, and the children were followed for at least 5 years. The mothers were treated for anxiety, tension, or mild depression. The medication was prescribed chiefly by physicians in departments of internal medicine or gynecology who were usually unaware that their patients were pregnant. The controls were women who were noted to be anxious, but no drug was given.

The findings were indicative of increased rates of congenital anomalies for both agents when prescribed during the first 42 days of gestation. For meprobamate, the rate of severe malformations for exposure in the first 42 days of gestation was 12.1, or four times the rate (2.7) if exposure occurred later in pregnancy ($p = .0025$). The rate of malformation was 2½ times the 4.6% rate for other drugs prescribed in early pregnancy ($p = .045$), and 4½ times the 2.6 percent rate for the no-drug group for which anxiety was recorded in early pregnancy ($p = .0278$). No differences in rates of severe congenital anomalies according to treatment group was found for treatment after 42 days. The pattern of congenital anomalies was interesting in that five out of eight of the severe congenital anomalies recorded in the meprobamate group were congenital heart disease, although not the same lesion.

For chlordiazepoxide, the trend appeared to be in the same direction, although the significance levels were slightly above $p = .05$. The rate of severe malformations was three times as great in the first 42 days as in later pregnancy for prescription of chlordiazepoxide. For less than 42 days, the rate for chlordiazepoxide was 2½ times the rate for prescription of other drugs and four times the rate for the no-drug anxious group.

In contrast, the study by Hartz and colleagues[153] did not reveal an association between the ingestion of these medications and congenital anomalies. In a total of 1870 children who were exposed to utero to meprobamate or chlordiazepoxide compared to children who were not exposed to these agents, no significant differences were found. They found similar rates of malformations when exposures occurred during the first trimester or later in pregnancy. They found no evidence that antenatal exposure to either drug increased the death rate through the fourth birthday. There were no differences in mental and motor scores at the age of 8 months or the intelligence quotient score at 4 years. The authors' explanations for the differing results from Milkovich and van den Berg were failure to miss associations by chance and the fact that the Hartz group controlled the analyses for potential confounding by a wide variety of risk factors for having a malformed child.

In a study by Bracken,[70] mothers of congenitally malformed infants were more likely than controls to have used a tranquilizer (usually chlordiazepoxide) in the first trimester than mothers of normal infants ($o.r. = 2.3; p < .01$). The use in case mothers was more common in the first or second trimesters. The malformations noted with first-trimester exposure were inguinal hernia, ventricular and atrial septal defect, and pyloric stenosis. Later exposure was more common among mothers of cases with hemangiomas, other heart and circulatory defects, and polydactyly or syndactyly.

Diazepam. Several studies have associated the ingestion of diazepam with increased risk of cleft lip and palate. Safra and Oakley[154] performed a retrospective study in which mothers of infants with selected malformations were questioned regarding the intake and timing of medication during pregnancy. The interview was conducted at approximately 4 months postpartum, and women were shown samples of the medications. First-trimester exposure for each drug was compared to exposure data in two control groups: One group comprised all interviewed mothers except those who had infants with the birth defect type being examined. The other control group was all mothers who had a child with Trisomy 21. Thus all mothers had an abnormal child, and the problem of recall bias of mothers with abnormal children should be similar in the study groups versus the controls. A statistically significant relative risk of 4.1 for first-trimester exposure to diazepam among the mothers of infants with cleft lip with or without cleft palate compared with the mothers of infants with all other defects was observed. Similar results were obtained using the Trisomy 21 control technique. The authors controlled for presence of a chromosomal disorder, race, family history of cleft lip and/or palate. They were concerned that a secular trend in the occurrence of the malformation might have occurred or that the problem of multiple comparisons might be present in their analysis.

More recently, Rosenberg[155] performed a retrospective study to evaluate the relationship of oral clefts to diazepam use during pregnancy. Infants with cleft lip with or without cleft palate ($N = 445$) and with cleft palate alone ($N = 166$) were compared with 2498 control infants having other birth defects. Information was collected by interview within 6 months after the birth of the child. The information was not verified by medical record. The control group was composed of all other malformed children. The authors did not find evidence for selection bias through their assessment of distribution of zip codes. The authors controlled for multiple factors: year of interview, elapsed time between birth and interview, maternal age, geographic area, maternal cigarette smoking, maternal history of infection during the first trimester, maternal history of convulsive disorder or use of anticonvulsants during the pregnancy, maternal history of diabetes mellitus, sex of the child, and history of cleft lip or palate in the mother, father, sibling, or half-sibling. Their data suggested that first-trimester exposure to diazepam was not associated with an increased risk of cleft deformity.

Other Agents. There are no case reports of congenital anomalies that have occurred after ingestion of the following agents: flunitrazepam, lorazepam, oxazepam. More recent benzodiazepine derivatives have just entered clinical usage.

Summary: Teratogenicity

The epidemiologic task of persistently demonstrating an anomaly, or group of anomalies, with exposure to chlordiazepoxide or diazepam has not been established. It has not been consistently demonstrated that exposure to these agents is associated with a rate of malformation that is beyond that in the general population. There is little information available regarding the teratogenicity of more recently marketed agents. We do not recommend the use of meprobamate during pregnancy because of the availability of safer agents and the suspicion of teratogenicity.[152]

Toxic and Behavioral Effects on the Fetus and Newborn

Diazepam has been used during pregnancy and labor to produce sedation and for treatment of the seizures of eclampsia. Maternal diazepam administration causes a reduction in the beat-to-beat variability in heart rate,[156,157] which is an important indicator of the adequacy of fetal oxygenation. As demonstrated by van Geijn and associates,[158] diazepam administered during late pregnancy and labor can produce this effect for several days in the newborn. The duration of the effect was found to be dependent upon dose and route of administration.

When given to women in labor, diazepam has little effect on the infant's condition if a total dose of less than 30 mg is given in the 15 hours prior to delivery.[159] Larger doses resulted in low Apgar scores at birth, apneic spells, hypotonia, and reluctance to feed. An impaired metabolic response to cold stress when compared to controls whose mothers had received medications other than diazepam was also noted. The glucuronidation of the metabolites of diazepam may competitively inhibit the conjugation of bilirubin, which may lead to hyperbilirubinemia in the newborn.[144]

There are two major types of neonatal toxicities related to the benzodiazepines: the "floppy infant syndrome" and a withdrawal syndrome. Gillberg[160] described the "floppy infant syndrome," which occurred after low-dose prolonged diazepam therapy. Symptoms were hypotonia, lethargy, sucking difficulties, hypothermia, and cyanosis. Speight[161] described additional cases. One woman had been given 5 mg diazepam three times daily throughout her pregnancy, and nitrazepam 10 mg for the last 9 weeks of gestation. An infant delivered by C-section was "floppy and unresponsive." He was unable to suck and required tube feeding for 4 days, after which he improved and was discharged at 10 days of age. Similar symptoms were noted in an infant whose mother received nitrazepam 10 mg at night for the last 8 weeks of gestation. Speight cautioned about the indiscriminate use of diazepam during pregnancy and stated that feeding problems due to this syndrome may result in difficulty establishing breast-feeding that may upset the mother and the emotional attachment process.

Passive addiction of the newborn to diazepam has been described only relatively recently, in the late 1970s.[162] Rementeria and Bhatt[163] described three neonates in whom a withdrawal syndrome from intrauterine exposure to diazepam was observed. The total daily dosages of diazepam ingested were 20 mg for the last 17 weeks of pregnancy, 15 mg during the last trimester except the final 2 weeks, and 10 to 15 mg in the final months. The intrauterine exposure to diazepam did not appear to affect the birth weights of the infants. The syndrome appeared 2 to 6 hours postbirth and consisted of tremors, irritability, hypertonicity, and vigorous sucking. Individual infants had cyanosis with feeding, vomiting, and dehydration. The symptoms were successfully treated with phenobarbital, but the tremors lasted from 10 days to 6 weeks. One infant died of sudden infant death syndrome, according to a coroner's report.

Mazzi[164] described a case in which a mother who had been taking diazepam 10 mg every other day for the last 4 months of pregnancy delivered an infant with marked hypertonia and hyperreflexia. Bloodwork, spinal tap, and viral titers were normal. An EEG at 9 days of age suggested a generalized convulsive disorder. At 16 days, the EEG showed excessive fast activity, which suggested a drug effect with no seizure activity. The muscular hypertonia persisted until 8 months of age, and the infant had normal developmental milestones.

Athinarayanan and colleagues[165] described a set of twins born to a mother who took chlordiazepoxide prior to and during her total pregnancy; the infants had a withdrawal syndrome that consisted of jitteriness and irritability at 21 days of age. Phenobarbital was not helpful, but administration of diazepam over a period of 9 days was markedly effective, and the infant subsequently did well. The long half-life of the agent likely resulted in delayed appearance of withdrawal symptoms.

Breast-Feeding

Because of concerns about pharmacological effects during long-term administration of high doses of diazepam, particularly in premature or sick newborns, Kanto[144] suggested that maternal doses higher than 30 mg of diazepam per day should be avoided during lactation. Erkkola and Kanto[166] made the clinical recommendation that women on diazepam refrain from breast-feeding their infants. The long-term consequences of neonatal exposure of the newborn to diazepam are unknown.

There have been several reports of infants who have been breast-fed while their mothers have taken diazepam. Patrick[167] reported a case of an infant whose mother was given 30 mg/day of diazepam, and the mother had received a total of 90 mg when the infant was observed to be lethargic. He had lost 170 g on the previous day. Breast-feeding was discontinued. An EEG showed bursts of fast activity in the frontal regions that the authors felt was consistent with sedative medication effects. Erkkola and Kanto[166] found that measurable quantities of diazepam and N-demethyldiazepam were present in maternal and fetal serum during breast-feeding. The maternal/fetal ratio changed from the fourth (2.8:1) to the sixth (8.1:1) days postpartum as the concentrations in three infants' sera decreased. This was attributed to the onset of the elimination mechanisms in the newborn that allowed more effective metabolism.

Lorazepam transfer into breast milk was "pharmacologically insignificant."[149] A mother who was breast-feeding required 2.5 mg lorazepam twice daily for 5 days after delivery, and her infant did not show a sedative effect; however, longer term follow-up was not given. "Clinically insignificant" amounts of flunitrazepam occurred in breast milk after a single dose.[144] There is no information on breast-milk content of these agents when the mother has taken them chronically.

Our opinion is that if the mother needs benzodiazepines on a prolonged basis postnatally, breast-feeding is inadvisable because of the opportunity for accumulation and the lack of data on long-term exposure through breast milk. The necessity for the medication and the possibility for alternative treatments should be carefully evaluated. If short-term administration is anticipated, it may be feasible to use other mechanisms to stimulate the breasts until the medication is discontinued.

Benzodiazepines in the Puerperium

Most of the literature on psychiatric disorder in the puerperium has focused on inpatient populations or upon women who exhibit the most severe pathology, such as major depression or psychosis.[168] There are few data on the occurrence of anxiety disorders and no data regarding the use of benzodiazepines in the postnatal period. Flunitrazepam may be used as adjunctive medication for sleep induction during the initial phase of treatment for major depression without effect upon serum antidepressant levels.[169]

Pregnant and Puerperal Women: Treatment Recommendations

Nurnberg and Prudic[170] provided guidelines for treatment of pregnant patients in the last 6 months of pregnancy and postnatally. Although the recommendations were written for the acutely psychotic pregnant patient, they are excellent and are worth considering for the general population of pregnant women with severe psychiatric illness. These guidelines are paraphrased here as a framework for discussion and expansion.

1. Hospitalization should be considered for the pregnant patient with severe psychiatric illness. The patient can be carefully evaluated for levels of symptomatology in a structured inpatient setting prior to the decision regarding initiation of medication.

2. If medication is required, high-potency agents should be administered at the minimum effective doses to control florid symptomatology. Complete resolution of all symptoms may not be a reasonable goal because this may require high doses. More modest and appropriate goals for the patient are reasonably good functioning and self-care. We would agree with this point and emphasize avoiding maternal toxicity. Striving to achieve the minimum effective dose, which is likely to be lower than a dose at which toxic effects are seen in the mother, is important in minimizing toxic effects in both mother and fetus. We would also agree that the specific targeting of symptoms is vital, so that improvement in symptoms that are known to respond to the medication may be monitored. Careful frequent monitoring of the patient is necessary to ascertain that the agent is effective. It is also feasible that no agent will be found to effectively control the symptoms, and it would then be unjustifiable to continue medication because the perceived benefit has not been demonstrated. The risk/benefit analysis is an *ongoing* one throughout the patient's treatment.

3. Document informed consent, which should be obtained from the patient and her partner. We would add, that if the clinician has the luxury of working with the pregnant patient while she is in remission, that the issue of management should the patient become ill be discussed prior to potential decompensation, so that the patient's wishes during a period of lucidity have been documented.[171]

4. Other medications should be used only if necessary; the prescribing physicians should be aware of all medications used and their indications.

5. Psychotropic medication should be discontinued as soon as possible. We would emphasize that the history of the course of the psychiatric disorder in the particular patient should be considered. For example, if a woman characteristically relapses 1 month after discontinuation of medication, the indication for continuing medication would be more compelling than for a woman with a previously good level of functioning who appears to have a brief reactive psychosis. The phenomenology of the disorder in the woman and careful diagnosis are imperative.

6. Supportive casework is imperative during the entire pregnancy and postnatally, when the relapse rate is increased. It is easy to become absorbed in management of the pregnant woman and neglect the importance of the family, who may be instrumental in supporting the patient and encouraging her cooperation.[53] Brown[53] emphasized the importance of asking the postpartum patient with psychotic disturbance if she has any thoughts about harming the infant; mothers with such symptoms should be carefully observed while caring for their infants. Brown[53] also recognized the importance of main-

taining the mother–infant relationship, and if inpatient treatment is necessary, hospitalization with the infant was his recommendation. In England, considerable experience has been gained with joint admission of mothers and infants into psychiatric mother and baby units.[172]

7. Maximum possible participation in prenatal educational programs should be encouraged for a mother whose pregnancy is complicated by psychiatric illness. This is an important point that is frequently neglected in the care of pregnant patients.

8. A close liaison between the psychiatrist and obstetrician is necessary throughout pregnancy. We would also encourage the psychiatrist and obstetrician to jointly consider the medical differential diagnostic work-up that is to be done. Certain illnesses present with significant psychiatric symptomatology and may be diagnosed during pregnancy and postnatally, such as acute intermittent porphyria[137] and postpartum thyroiditis.[173] Awareness of the woman's past obstetric and psychiatric history of both physicians facilitates appropriate medical management. Events such as previous intrauterine fetal death are important in the psychotherapeutic management of the patient.

9. Extended postpartum obstetrical hospitalization of 3 to 7 days should be planned because of increased risk for decompensation. Patients are at greatest risk for relapse during the first week postpartum, and the risk continues for several months (see Chapter 6).

10. Nurnberg stated that the reinstitution or initiation of psychotropic medication should be delayed until the mother's physiological fluid homeostasis is reestablished, which usually occurs 3 or 4 days postnatally. Supervision of the patient's medication in the hospital for several days was recommended. No rationale was provided for this approach. We understand the concern if the patient is being started on lithium, because a shifting fluid balance can make titration of the dose difficult but not excessively so if levels are checked frequently. We cannot justify the need to delay reestablishment of antipsychotic medication because the data suggest that the risk of relapse is quite high in the first postnatal week, and prevention (or diminution of florid symptomatology) would seem possible only with early intervention. This issue awaits empirical investigation.

11. Breast-feeding for patients on psychotropic medication is contraindicated. We feel that this recommendation should be somewhat tempered, in favor of a case-specific decision-making process without adherence to generalized rules.

In addition to the previously specified guidelines, we would add the following:

1. Pregnancy brings with it its own changes in physiological functioning that may complicate the use of psychotropic agents. We recommend that the patient's physiological status be carefully evaluated prior to the institution of medication, so that side effects can be meaningfully interpreted. For example, the pregnant patient may suffer syncope, headache, and constipation *without* medication.

2. Although the fetus cannot be spared the exposure to the agent, it can be spared the bolus effect that administering relatively large doses of medication at infrequent intervals may cause. In order to attain levels and avoid fluctuations that may occur and predispose to toxicity in the mother and fetus, we recommend that the usual frequency of dosage for an agent be increased if compliance will not be forfeited. For example, the minimum effective total dose, if usually given twice daily, would be administered three or four times daily in divided doses. This is of greater importance in the case of agents such as lithium compared to the longer acting antipsychotics and antidepressants. Although stud-

ies have demonstrated that nortriptyline yields similar plasma levels when administered in a single bedtime dose or in a three-times-daily schedule, there is interindividual variability.[174] These findings have not been validated in a pregnant population.

3. Whenever clinically feasible, decrease or discontinue the psychotropic medication 1 to 2 weeks before the expected date of confinement to allow metabolism of the agent prior to birth. This will minimize the load of the drug that the newborn must metabolize at birth. Lithium is an exception that may warrant discontinuation closer to term.

4. Avoid agents that are new on the market. The side effects profile and safety of an agent are determined by clinical experience with the agent. Pregnant and breast-feeding women are not the population with which to gain experience with new agents.

About the complex task of considering treatment strategies for pregnant women with psychiatric disorder, Gelenberg wrote:

> Confronted with this clinical dilemma you will, at times, feel like Ulysses, seeking to navigate the straits between Scylla and Charybdis. But with adequate time, sensitivity, and knowledge, the skilled clinical pilot usually will be able to guide his or her patient through a safe passage.[171]

References

1. Cupit GC, Rotmensch HH: Principles of drug therapy in pregnancy, in Gleicher N (ed): *Principles of Medical Therapy in Pregnancy*. New York, Plenum Press, 1985, pp 77–90.
2. Levy GH: Pharmacokinetics of fetal and neonatal exposure to drugs. *Obstet Gynecol* **58(Suppl):**9S–16S, 1981.
3. Mirkin BL: Drug disposition and therapy in the developing human being. *Pediatr Ann* **5:**542–557, 1976.
4. Chao ST, Juchau MR: Placental drug metabolism, in Johnson EM, Kochhar DM (eds), *Teratogenesis and Reproductive Toxicology*. New York, Springer-Verlag, 1983, pp 31–48.
5. Soyka LF, Bigelow SW: Drug-metabolizing enzymes and their activity in the human fetus, in Stern L (ed): *Drug Use in Pregnancy*. Sydney, Australia, Adis Health Science Press, 1984, pp 17–44.
6. Finster M, Mark LC: Placental transfer of drugs and their distribution in fetal tissue, in Brodie BB, Gillette JR (ed): *Basic Concepts in Biochemical Pharmacology*. New York, Springer-Verlag, Berlin/Heidelberg, 1971, pp 276–285.
7. American Medical Association: Drug interactions and adverse drug reactions, in: *AMA Drug Evaluations*. Chicago, 1983, pp 31–44.
8. Wilson JG: Current status of teratology. General principles and mechanisms derived from animal studies, in Wilson JG, Fraser FC (eds): *Handbook of Teratology, General Principles and Etiology*, Vol. 1. New York, Plenum Press, 1977, pp 47–74.
9. Vorhees CV, Butcher, RE: Behavioral teratogenicity, in Snell K (ed): *Developmental Toxicology*. New York, Praeger, 1982, pp 249–298.
10. Werboff J, Gottlieb JS: Drugs in pregnancy: Behavioral teratology. *Obstet Gynaec Survey* **18:**420–423, 1963.
11. Coyle I, Wayner MJ, Singer G: Behavioral teratogenesis: A critical evaluation. *Pharmac Biochem Behav* **4:**191–200, 1976, 1976.
12. Hutchings DE: Behavioral teratology: A new frontier in neurobehavioral research, in Johnson EM, Kochhar DM (eds): *Teratogenesis and Reproductive Toxicology*. New York, Springer-Verlag, 1983, pp 207–235.
13. Brent RL: Methods of evaluating the alleged teratogenicity of environmental agents, in: Prevention of Physical and Mental Congenital Defects, Part C: Basic and Medical Science, Education, and Future Strategies. New York, Alan R. Liss, 1985, pp 191–195.
14. Cordero JF, Oakley GP: Drug exposure during pregnancy: Some epidemiologic considerations. *Clin Obstet Gynecol* **26:**418–428, 1983.
15. Bracken MB: Methodological issues in the epidemiologic investigation of drug-induced congenital malfor-

mations, in Bracken MB (ed): *Perinatal Epidemiology*. New York, Oxford University Press, 1984, pp 423–449.

16. FDA Drug Bulletin, Sept., pp 22–23, 1979.
17. Briggs GG, Bodendorfer TW, Freeman RK, et al: *Drugs in Pregnancy and Lactation: A Reference Guide to Fetal and Neonatal Risk*. Baltimore, Williams & Wilkins, 1983.
18. Gutheil TG: Improving patient compliance: Psychodynamics in drug prescribing. *Drug Ther Hosp*, July, pp 35–40, 1977.
19. Mogul KM: Psychological considerations in the use of psychotropic drugs with women patients. *Hosp Comm Psychiatry* 36:1080–1085, 1985.
20. Hillard JR, Hillard PJA: Early diagnosis of pregnancy in a patient receiving antipsychotic medication. *Am J Psychiatry* 138:9–10, 1981.
21. Davis JM, Janicak P, Chang S, et al: Recent advances in the pharmacologic treatment of the schizophrenic disorders, in Grinspoon L (ed): *Psychiatry Update. The American Psychiatric Association Annual Review*. Washington, D.C., American Psychiatric Press, 1982, pp 178–228.
22. Edlund MJ, Craig TJ: Antipsychotic drug use and birth defects: An epidemiologic reassessment. *Compr Psychiatry* 25:32–37, 1984.
23. Milkovich L, van den Berg BJ: An evaluation of the teratogenicity of certain antinauseant drugs. *Am J Obstet Gynecol* 125:244–248, 1976.
24. Kris EB: Children born to mothers maintained on pharmacotherapy during pregnancy and postpartum. *Recent Adv Biol Psychiatr* 4:180–187, 1961.
25. Kris EB: Children of mothers maintained on pharmacotherapy during pregnancy and postpartum. *Curr Ther Res* 7:785–789, 1965.
26. Sobel DE: Fetal damage due to ECT, insulin coma, chlorpromazine, or reserpine. *Arch Gen Psychiatry* 2:606–611, 1960.
27. Slone D, Siskind V, Heinonen OP: Antenatal exposure to the phenothiazines in relation to congenital malformations, perinatal mortality rate, birth weight, and intelligence quotient score. *Am J Obstet Gynecol* 128:486–488, 1977.
28. Rumeau-Rouquette C, Goujard J, Huel G: Possible teratogenic effect of phenothiazines in human beings. *Teratology* 15:57–64, 1976.
29. Hall G: A case of phocomelia of the upper limbs. *Med J Aust* 1:449–450, 1963.
30. Moriarty AJ, Nance MR: Trifluoperazine and pregnancy. *Med J Aust* 88:375–376, 1963.
31. Rawlings WJ, Ferguson F, Maddison TG: Phenmetrazine and trifluoperazine. *Med J Aust* 1:370, 1963.
32. Heinonen OP, Slone D, Shapiro S: *Birth Defects in Pregnancy*. Littleton, Publishing Sciences Group, 1977.
33. Scanlan FJ: The use of thioridazine (Melleril) [*sic*] during the first trimester. *Med J Aust* 1:1271–1272, 1972.
34. Cleary MF: Fluphenazine decanoate during pregnancy. *Am J Psychiatry* 134:815–816, 1977.
35. Donaldson GL, Bury RG: Multiple congenital abnormalities in a newborn boy associated with maternal use of fluphenazine enanthate and other drugs during pregnancy. *Acta Paediatr Scand* 71:335–338, 1982.
36. Kopelman AE, McCullar FW: Limb malformations following maternal use of haloperidol. *JAMA* 231:62–64, 1975.
37. Hanson JW, Oakley GP: Haloperidol and limb deformity. *JAMA* 231:26, 1975.
38. van Waes A, van de Velde E: Safety evaluation of haloperidol in the treatment of hyperemesis gravidarum. *J Clin Pharmacol* 9:224–227, 1969.
39. Donaldson JO: Control of chorea gravidarum with haloperidol. *Obstet Gynecol* 59:381–382, 1982.
40. Patterson JF: Treatment of chorea gravidarum with haloperidol. *Southern Med J* 72:1220–1221, 1979.
41. Hammond JE, Toseland PA: Placental transfer of chlorpromazine. *Arch Dis Child* 45:139–140, 1970.
42. Scokel PW, Jones WN: Infant jaundice after phenothiazine drugs for labor: An enigma. *Obstet Gynecol* 20:124–127, 1962.
43. Falterman CG, Richardson J: Small left colon syndrome associated with maternal ingestion of psychotropic drugs. *J Pediatr* 97:308–310, 1980.
44. Levy W, Wisniewski K: Chlorpromazine causing extrapyramidal dysfunction. *NY State J Med* 74:684–685, 1974.
45. O'Connor M, Johnson GH, James DI: Intrauterine effect of phenothiazines. *Med J Aust* 1:416–417, 1981.

46. Hill RM, Desmond MM, Kay JJ: Extrapyramidal dysfunction in an infant of a schizophrenic mother. *J Pediatr* **69**:589–595, 1966.

47. Desmond M, Rudolph AJ, Hill RM, et al: Behavioral alterations in infants born to mothers on psychoactive medication during pregnancy, in Farrell G (ed): *Congenital Mental Retardation*. Austin, Univ of Texas Press, 1969, pp 235–241.

48. Madsen JR, Campbell A, Baldessarini RJ: Effects of prenatal treatment of rats with haloperidol due to altered drug distribution in neonatal brain. *Neuropharmacology* **20**:931–939, 1981.

49. Whalley LJ, Blain PG, Prime JK: Haloperidol secreted in breast milk. *Br Med J* **282**:1746–1747, 1981.

50. Stewart RB, Karas B, Springer PK: Haloperidol excretion in human milk. *Am J Psychiatry* **137**:849–850, 1980.

51. Kris EB, Carmichael DM: Chlorpromazine maintenance therapy during pregnancy and confinement. *Psychiatric Q* **31**:690–695, 1957.

52. Herson MH, Barlow DH: *Single Case Experimental Designs. Strategies for Studying Behavioral Change.* New York, Pergamon Press, 1976.

53. Brown WA: *Psychological Care during Pregnancy and the Postpartum Period.* New York, Raven Press, 1979.

54. Kargas GA, Kargas SA, Bruyere HJ Jr, et al: Perinatal mortality due to interaction of dephenhydramine and temazepam, letter to editor. *N Engl J Med* **313**:14–17, 1985.

55. Saxen I: Cleft palate and maternal dephenhydramine intake. *The Lancet* **1**:407–408, 1974.

56. Parkin DE: Probable benadryl withdrawal manifestations in a newborn infant. *J Pediatr* **85**:580, 1974.

57. O'Brien TE: Excretion of drugs in human milk. *Am J Hosp Pharm* **31**:844–854, 1974.

58. Cole JO, Schatzberg AF: Antidepressant drug therapy, in Grinspoon L (ed): *Psychiatry Update. The American Psychiatric Association Annual Review.* Washington, D.C., American Psychiatric Press, 1983, pp 472–490.

59. Perel JM: Tricyclic antidepressant plasma levels, pharmacokinetics, and clinical outcome, in Grinspoon L (ed): *Psychiatry Update. The American Psychiatric Association Annual Review.* Washington, D.C., American Psychiatric Press, 1983, pp 490–511.

60. Edwards JG: Antidepressants and convulsions. *The Lancet,* December 22/29, 1979, pp 1368–1369.

61. McBride WG: Limb deformities associated with iminodibenzyl hydrochloride. *Med J Aust* **1**:492, 1972.

62. Australian Drug Evaluation Committee, Tricyclic antidepressants and limb reduction deformities. *Med J Aust* **1**:768–769, 1973.

63. Morrow AW: Limb deformities associated with iminodebenzyl hydrochloride. *Med J Aust* **1**:658–659, 1972.

64. Crombie DL, Pinsent RJ, Fleming D: Imipramine in pregnancy. *Br Med J* **1**:745, 1972.

65. Kuenssberg EV, Knox JDE: Imipramine in pregnancy. *Br Med J* **2**:292, 1972.

66. Scanlon FJ: Use of antidepressant drugs during the first trimester. *Med J Aust* **2**:1077, 1969.

67. Sim M: Imipramine and pregnancy. *Br Med J* **2**:745, 1972.

68. Rachelefsky GS, Flynt JW Jr, Ebbin A, et al: Possible teratogenicity of tricyclic antidepressants. *The Lancet* **1**:838, 72.

69. Banister P, DeFoe C, Smith ESO, et al: Possible teratogenicity of tricyclic antidepressants. *The Lancet* **1**:838–839, 1972.

70. Bracken MB, Holford TR: Exposure to prescribed drugs in pregnancy and association with congenital malformations. *Obstet Gynecol* **58**:336–343, 1981.

71. Eggermont E, Raveschat J, Deneve V, et al: The adverse influence of imipramine on the adaption of the newborn infant to extrauterine life. *Acta Paediatr Belg* **26**:197–204, 1972.

72. Webster PAC: Withdrawal symptoms in neonates associated with maternal antidepressant therapy. *The Lancet* **2**:318–319, 1973.

73. Gualtieri CT, Staye J: Withdrawal symptoms after abrupt cessation of amitriptyline in an 8-year-old boy. *Am J Psychiatry* **136**:457–458, 1979.

74. Petti TA, Law W: Abrupt cessation of high-dose imipramine treatment in children. *JAMA* **246**:768–769, 1981.

75. Law W, Petti TA, Kazdin AE: Withdrawal symptoms after graduated cessation of imipramine in children. *Am J Psychiatry* **138**:647–650, 1981.

76. Dilsaver SC, Kronfol Z, Sackellares JC, et al: Antidepressant withdrawal syndromes: Evidence supporting the cholinergic overdrive hypothesis. *J Clin Psychopharmacology* **3**:157–164, 1983.

77. Shearer WT, Schreiner RL, Marshall RE: Urinary retention in a neonate secondary to maternal ingestion of nortriptyline. *J Pediatr* **81**:570–572, 1972.

78. Sjoqvist F, Bergfors PG, Borga O, et al: Plasma disappearance of nortriptyline in a newborn infant following placental transfer from an intoxicated mother: Evidence for drug metabolism. *J Pediatr* **80**:496–500, 1972.

79. Sovner R, Orsulak PJ: Excretion of imipramine and desipramine in human breast milk. *Am J Psychiatry* **136**:451–452, 1979.

80. Erickson SH, Smith GH, Heidrich F: Tricyclics and breast-feeding. Letters to the editor. *Am J Psychiatry* **136**:1483, 1979.

81. Orsulak R, Sovner PJ: Drs. Orsulak and Sovner reply. Letters to the editor. *Am J Psychiatry* **136**:1483, 1979.

82. Bader TF, Newman K: Amitriptyline in human breast milk and the nursing infant's serum. *Am J Psychiatry* **137**:855–856, 1980.

83. Ananth J: The effects in the neonate from psychotropic agents excreted through breast-feeding. *Am J Psychiatry* **135**:801–805, 1978.

84. Brixen-Rasmussen L, Halgrener J, Jorgensen A: Amitriptyline and nortriptyline excretion in human breast milk. *Psychopharmacology* **76**:94–95, 1982.

85. Verbeeck RK, Ross SG, McKenna EA: Excretion of trazodone in breast milk. *Br J Clin Pharmacol* **22**:367–370, 1986.

86. Kane FJ: Postpartum disorders, in Kaplan HI, Sadock BJ (eds): *Comprehensive Textbook of Psychiatry IV*. Baltimore, Williams & Wilkins, 1985, pp 1238–1242.

87. Hamilton JA: Guidelines for therapeutic management of postpartum disorders, in Inwood DG: *Recent Advances in Postpartum Psychiatric Disorders*. Washington, D.C., American Psychiatric Press, 1985, pp 83–96.

88. Oates M: The role of electroconvulsive therapy in the treatment of postnatal mental illness, in Cox JL, Kumar R, Margison FR et al: *Current Approaches. Puerperal Mental Illness*. Southampton, England, Duphar Laboratories Limited, 1986, pp 1–12.

89. Frank E, Kupfer DG, Jacob M, et al: Pregnancy-related affective episodes among women with recurrent depression. *Am J Psychiatry* **144**:288–293, 1987.

90. Schou M, Amdisen A, Streenstrup OR: Lithium and pregnancy—II, Hazards to women given lithium during pregnancy and delivery. *Br Med J* **2**:137–138, 1973.

91. Weinstein MR: Lithium treatment of women during pregnancy and in the post-delivery period, in Johnson FN (ed): *Handbook of Lithium Therapy*. Lancaster, England, MTP Press, 1980, pp 421–429.

92. Schou M: Practical problems of lithium maintenance treatment, in Kemali D, Racagni G (eds): *Chronic Treatments in Neuropsychiatry*. New York, Raven Press, 1985, pp 131–138.

93. Calabrese JR, Gulledge AD: Psychotropics during pregnancy and lactation: A review. *Psychosomatics* **26**:413–426, 1985.

94. Linden S, Rich CL. The use of lithium during pregnancy and lactation. *J Clin Psychiatry* **44**:358–361, 1983.

95. Nora JJ, Nora AH, Towes WH. Lithium, Ebstein's anomaly, and other congenital heart defects. *The Lancet* **2**:594–595, 1974.

96. Weinstein MR, Goldfield MD: Cardiovascular malformations with lithium use during pregnancy. *Am J Psychiatry* **132**:529–531, 1975.

97. Behrman RE, Vaughan VC (eds): *Nelson's Textbook of Pediatrics*. Philadelphia, WB Saunders, 1983, pp 1136–1137.

98. Giuliani ER, Fuster V, Brandenburg RO, et al: Ebstein's anomaly: The clinical features and natural history of Ebstein's anomaly of the tricuspid valve. *Mayo Clin Proc* **54**:163–173, 1970.

99. Danielson GK, Fuster V: Surgical repair of Ebstein's anomaly. *Ann Surg* **196**:499–503, 1982.

100. Anderson KR, Zuberbuhler JR, Anderson RH, et al: Morphologic spectrum of Ebstein's anomaly of the heart: A review. *Mayo Clin Proc* **54**:174–180, 1979.

101. Wilson JG, Fraser FC (eds): *Handbook of Teratology, General Principles and Etiology*. New York, Plenum Press, 1977.

102. Long WA, Willis PW: Maternal lithium and neonatal Ebstein's anomaly: Evaluation with cross-sectional echocardiography. *Am J Perinatol* **1**:182–184, 1984.

103. Allan LD, Desai G, Tynan MJ: Prenatal echocardiographic screening for Ebstein's anomaly for mothers on lithium therapy. *The Lancet*, October 16, 1982, pp 875–876.

104. Kallen B, Tandberg A: Lithium and pregnancy. A cohort study on manic-depressive women. *Acta Psychiatr Scand* **68:**134–139, 1983.

105. Schou M: What happened later to the lithium babies? A follow-up study of children born without malformations. *Acta Psychiatr Scand* **54:**193–197, 1976.

106. Goodwin FK, Roy-Byrne P: Treatment of bipolar disorders, in Hales RE, Frances AJ (eds): *Psychiatry Update. The American Psychiatric Association Annual Review.* Washington, D.C., American Psychiatric Press, 1987, pp 81–107.

107. Jamison KR: Psychotherapeutic issues and suicide prevention in the treatment of bipolar disorders, in Hales RE, Frances AJ (eds): *Psychiatry Update. The American Psychiatric Association Annual Review.* Washington, D.C., American Psychiatric Press, 1987, pp 108–124.

108. Consensus Development Panel: Mood disorders: pharmacologic prevention of recurrences. NIMH/NIH consensus development panel statement. *Am J Psychiatry* **142:**469–476, 1985.

109. Gelenberg AJ: When a woman taking lithium wants to have a baby. *Biol Ther Psychiatr* **6:**19–20, 1983.

110. Morrell P, Sutherland GR, Buamah PK, et al: Lithium toxicity in a neonate. *Arch Dis Child* **58:**538–539, 1983.

111. Karlsson K, Lindstedt G, Lundberg PA, et al: Transplacental lithium poisoning: Reversible inhibition of fetal thyroid. *The Lancet* **1:**1295, 1975.

112. Stevens D, Burman D, Midwinter A: Transplacental lithium poisoning: Reversible inhibition of fetal thyroid. *The Lancet* **1:**1295, 1974.

113. Wilson N, Forfar JC, Godman MJ: Atrial flutter in the newborn resulting from maternal lithium ingestion. *Arch Dis Child* **58:**538–549, 1983.

114. Mizrahi EM, Hobbs JF, Goldsmith DI: Nephrogenic diabetes insipidus in transplacental lithium intoxication. *J Pediatr* **94:**493–495, 1979.

115. MacKay AVP, Loose R, Glen AIM: Labour on lithium. *Br Med J,* April 10, 1976, p 878.

116. Tunnessen WW Jr, Hertz CG: Toxic effects of lithium in newborn infants: A commentary. *J Pediatr* **81:**804–807, 1972.

117. Sykes PA, Quarrie J, Alexander FW: Lithium carbonate and breast-feeding. *Br Med J* **2:**1299, 1976.

118. Schou M, Amdisen A: Lithium and pregnancy—III, Lithium ingestion by children breast-fed by women on lithium treatment. *Br Med J* **2:**138, 1973.

119. Berlin CM: Pharmacologic considerations of drug use in the lactating mother. *Obstet Gynecol* **58(Suppl):**17S–23S, 1981.

120. Targum SD, Davenport VB, Webster MJ: Postpartum mania in bipolar manic-depressive patients withdrawn from lithium carbonate. *J Nerv Ment Dis* **167:**572–574, 1979.

121. Post RM, Uhde TW: Clinical approaches to treatment resistant bipolar illness, in Hales RE, Frances AJ (eds): *Psychiatry Update. American Psychiatric Association Annual Review.* Washington, D.C., American Psychiatric Press, 1987, pp 125–150.

122. NIH Consensus Conference: Electroconvulsive therapy. *JAMA* **254:**2103–2108, 1985.

123. Repke JT, Berger NG: Electroconvulsive therapy in pregnancy. *Obstet Gynecol* **63(Suppl):**39S–41S, 1984.

124. Varan LR, Gillieson MS, Skene DS, et al: ECT in an acutely psychotic pregnant woman with actively aggressive (homicidal) impulses. *Can J Psychiatry* **30:**363–367, 1985.

125. Wise MG, Ward SC, Townsend-Parchman W, Gilstrap LC, et al: Case report of ECT during high-risk pregnancy. *Am J Psychiatry* **141:**99–101, 1984.

126. Levine R, Frost EAM: Arterial blood-gas analyses during electroconvulsive therapy in a parturient. *Anesth Analg* **54:**203–205, 1975.

127. Impastato DJ, Gabriel AR, Lardaro HH: Electric and insulin shock therapy during pregnancy. *Dis Nerv Syst* **25:**542–546, 1964.

128. Sobel DE: Fetal damage due to ECT insulin coma, chlorpromazine and reserpine. *Arch Gen Psych* **2:**603–611, 1960.

129. Fink M: Convulsive and drug therapies of depression. *Ann Rev Med* **32:**405–412, 1981.

130. Ostheimer G, Warren TM: Obstetric analgesia and anesthesia, in Stern L (ed): *Drug Use in Pregnancy.* Sydney, Australia, Adis Health Science Press, 1984, pp 216–269.

131. Remick RA, Maruice WL: ECT in pregnancy. *Am J Psychiatry* **135:**761–762, 1978.

132. Foldes FF: Enzymes of acetylcholine metabolism, in Foldes FF (ed): *Enzymes in Anesthesiology.* New York, Springer-Verlag, 1978, pp 101–144.

133. Kalow W, Gunn DR: The relation between dose of succinylcholine and duration of apnea in man. *J Pharmacol Exper Ther* **120**:203–214, 1957.

134. Weis WF, Muller FO, Lyell H, et al: Materno-fetal cholinesterase inhibitor poisoning. *Anesth Analg* **62**:233–235, 1983.

135. Moya F, Kvisselgaard N: The placental transmission of succinylcholine. *Anesthesiology* **22**:1–10, 1961.

136. Owens WD, Zeitlin GL: Hypoventilation in a newborn following administration of succinylcholine to the mother. *Anesth Analg* **54**:38–39, 1975.

137. Zbella EA, Gleicher N: Disorders of metal and metalloproteins, in Gleicher N (ed): *Principles of Medical Therapy in Pregnancy*. New York, Plenum, Press, 1985.

138. Brodie MJ, Moore MR, Thompson GG, et al: Pregnancy and the acute porphyrias. *Br J Obstet Gynecol* **84**:726–731, 1977.

139. Forssman H: Follow-up study of sixteen children whose mothers were given electric convulsive therapy during gestation. *Acta Psychiatr Neurol Scand* **30**:437–441, 1955.

140. Brockington IF, Winokur G, Dean C: Puerperal psychosis, in Brockington IF, Kumar R (eds): *Motherhood and Mental Illness*. London, Academic Press, 1980, pp 37–69.

141. Frank JD: The psychotherapy of anxiety, in: *Psychiatry Update. American Psychiatric Association Annual Review*. Washington, DC, American Psychiatric Press, 1984, pp 418–426.

142. Benson H: The relaxation response and the treatment of anxiety, in: *Psychiatry Update. American Psychiatric Association Annual Review*. Washington, DC, American Psychiatric Press, 1984, pp 440–448.

143. Mavissakalian M: Exposure treatment of agoraphobia, in: *Psychiatry Update. American Psychiatric Association Annual Review*. Washington, DC, American Psychiatric Press, 1984, pp 448–460.

144. Kanto JH: Use of benzodiazepines during pregnancy, labour and lactation, with particular reference to pharmacokinetic considerations. *Drugs* **23**:354–380, 1982.

145. Mandelli M, Morselli PL, Nordio S, et al: Placental transfer of diazepam and its disposition in the newborn. *Clin Pharmacol Ther* **17**:564–572, 1975.

146. Moore RG, McBride WG: The disposition kinetics of diazepam in pregnant women at parturition. *Europ J Clin Pharmacol* **13**:275–284, 1978.

147. Byck R: Drugs and the treatment of psychiatric disorders, in Goodman LS, Gilman A (eds): *The Pharmacological Basis of Therapeutics*. New York, Macmillan Publishing Co, 1975, pp 152–299.

148. Kangas L, Erkkola R, Kanto J, et al: Transfer of free and conjugated oxazepam across the human placenta. *Eur J Clin Pharmacol* **17**:301–304, 1980.

149. Whitelaw AGL, Cummings AJ, McFadyen IF: Effect of maternal lorazepam on the neonate. *Br Med J* **282**:1106–1108, 1981.

150. Hauri PJ, Sateia MJ: Nonpharmacological treatment of sleep disorders, in Hales RE, Francès AJ (eds): *Psychiatry Update. American Psychiatric Association Annual Review*. Washington, DC, American Psychiatric Press, 1985, pp 361–394.

151. Mendelson WB: Pharmacological treatment of insomnia, in Hales RE, Frances AJ (eds): *Psychiatry Update. American Psychiatric Association Annual Review*. Washington, D.C., American Psychiatric Press, 1985, pp 379–394.

152. Milkovich L, van den Berg BJ: Effects of prenatal meprobamate and chlordiazepoxide hydrochloride on human embryonic and fetal development. *N Engl J Med* **291**:1268–1271, 1974.

153. Hartz SC, Heinonen OP, Shapiro S, Siskind V, Slone D: Antenatal exposure to meprobamate and chlordiazepoxide in relation to malformations, mental development, and childhood mortality. *N Engl J Med* **292**:726–728, 1975.

154. Safra JM, Oakley GP: Association between cleft lip with or without cleft palate and prenatal exposure to diazepam. *The Lancet* **2**:478–480, 1980.

155. Rosenberg L, Mitchell AA, Parsells JL, et al: Lack of relation of oral clefts to diazepam use during pregnancy. *N Engl J Med* **309**:1282–1285, 1983.

156. deHaan J, Van Bemmel JH, Stolte LAM, et al: Quantitative evaluation of fetal heart rate patterns. *Europ J Obstet Gynecol* **3**:103–110, 1971.

157. Yeh SY, Paul RIT, Cordero L, et al: A study of diazepam during labor. *Obstet Gynecol* **43**:363–373, 1974.

158. van Geijn HP, Jongsma HW, Doesburg WH, et al: The effect of diazepam administration during pregnancy or labor on the heart rate variability of the newborn infant. *Eur J Obstet Gynecol Reprod Biol* **10**:187–201, 1980.

159. Cree JE, Meyer J, Hailey DM: Diazepam in labour: Its metabolism and effect on the clinical condition and thermogenesis of the newborn. *Br Med J* **4**:251–255, 1973.
160. Gillberg C: "Floppy infant syndrome" and maternal diazepam. *The Lancet* **2**:244, 1977.
161. Speight AN: Floppy-infant syndrome and maternal diazepam and/or nitrazepam. *The Lancet* **1**:878, 1977.
162. Volpe JJ: Teratogenic effects of drugs and passive addiction, in Volpe JJ (ed): *Neurology of the Newborn*. Philadelphia, WB Saunders Co., 1981, pp 601–635.
163. Rementeria JL, Bhatt K: Withdrawal symptoms in neonates from intrauterine exposure to diazepam. *J Pediatr* **90**:123–126, 1977.
164. Mazzi E: Possible neonatal diazepam withdrawal: A case report. *Am J Obstet Gynecol* **129**:586–587, 1977.
165. Athinarayanan P, Pierog SH, Nigam S, et al: Chlordiazepoxide withdrawal in the neonate. *Am J Obstet Gynecol* **124**:212–213, 1976.
166. Erkkola R, Kanto J: Diazepam and breast-feeding. *The Lancet* **2**:1235–1236, 1972.
167. Patrick MJ, Tilstone WJ, Reavey P: Diazepam and breast-feeding. *The Lancet* **1**:542–543, 1972.
168. Kumar R: Neurotic disorders in childbearing women, in Brockington IF, Kumar R (eds): *Motherhood and Mental Illness*. London, Academic Press, 1982, pp 71–118.
169. Perel JM, Glassman AH: unpublished data.
170. Nurnberg GH, Prudic J: Guidelines for treatment of psychosis during pregnancy. *Hosp Comm Psych* **35**:67–71, 1984.
171. Gelenberg AJ: Pregnancy, psychotropic drugs, and psychiatric disorders. *Psychosomatics* **27**:216–217, 1986.
172. Margison F, Brockington IF: Psychiatric mother and baby units, in Brockington IF, Kumar R (eds): *Motherhood and Mental Illness*. London, Academic Press, 1982, pp 223–238.
173. Kaplan MM: Thyroid disease in pregnancy, in Gleicher N (ed): *Principles of Medical Therapy in Pregnancy*. New York, Plenum Press, 1985, pp 192–211.
174. Ziegler VE, Knesevich JW, Wylie LT, et al: Sampling time, dosage schedule, and nortriptyline plasma levels. *Arch Gen Psychiatry* **34**:613–615, 1977.

13

The Effect of Prenatal Exposure to Alcohol and Other Drugs

NANCY L. DAY, PATRICIA A. COBLE, AND MARIE D. BLOOM

Alcohol Abuse

Studies of Outcome in Alcoholic Women

Epidemiological evidence gathered in recent years has confirmed earlier case reports of a relationship between alcoholism, alcohol use during pregnancy, and poorer pregnancy outcome. Findings, reported originally by Lemoine, Harrousseau, and Borteyru[1] have been corroborated in several different clinical settings, and a cluster of infant characteristics related to maternal alcoholism has been termed the fetal alcohol syndrome (FAS). Cardinal features of the syndrome include (1) growth deficiency in both the prenatal and postnatal periods, (2) central nervous system anomalies such as microcephaly, mental retardation, and irritability, and (3) craniofacial anomalies including short palpebral fissures, frontonasal alterations, thin upper vermillion border, flat midface, and hypoplastic maxilla and/or mandible.[2] The presence of only some of these features is denoted as fetal alcohol effects or FAE.

The risk of an alcoholic woman having a FAS child is about one-third.[3] There are to date, few, if any, cases of FAS in the literature without a history of chronic alcoholism in the mother. The implication of this is that the full syndrome must be the end result of the interaction of the rather complex factors that exist in a woman who has such a history and may not be the simple result of alcohol use. Olegard et al.[4] found that the offspring of alcoholic mothers who stopped drinking early in pregnancy (5–12 weeks) were not below general population growth norms at birth but that infants of women who stopped later during pregnancy or who continued to drink were smaller.

Nancy L. Day, Patricia A. Coble, and Marie D. Bloom • Department of Psychiatry, Western Psychiatric Institute and Clinic, University of Pittsburgh, Pittsburgh, PA 15213.

A higher rate of other problematic outcomes of pregnancy has also been reported for alcoholic women. Sokol, Miller, and Reed[5] studied 204 alcoholic women and found significantly increased rates of problems during pregnancy, labor, and delivery. During labor, there was an increased risk of premature separation of the placenta, intra-amniotic infection, and maternal fever. Greater fetal distress and neonatal depression were noted. The babies had decreased birth weight and an increased rate of congenital anomalies. Findings of lower birth weight in offspring of alcoholic women have been reported by other investigators as well.[6,7]

In the neonatal period, infants with FAS are often characterized as tremulous, irritable, and hyperactive. It is not known whether these infants are exhibiting signs of neonatal withdrawal as argued by Cole et al.[8] or whether this represents abnormalities of the central nervous system.

Reports of follow-up assessments have been largely limited to case series of children diagnosed at birth as fetal alcohol syndrome and series of children whose mothers were identified as alcoholic. Sample sizes in general have been small and sample selection biased representing, in the main, populations selected from clinics or institutions. In general, these follow-up studies have found that children with FAS are small for their age and have lower IQ scores. Most are mentally retarded although the range is from severely retarded to near normal.[9] Children with FAS have been reported to have a multitude of subsequent behavioral problems including stereotyped behaviors, irritability, hyperactivity, tremulousness, and hyperdistractibility.[4,10–13] Steinhauser, Nester, and Spohr[14] reported on children identified as FAS who were matched with a group of healthy children. They found high rates of complications during the neonatal period, including feeding problems and failure to thrive. Motor and speech development were more often delayed in the FAS group, and behavioral problems were reported. These children had reduced vocabulary, more speech and hearing impairments, and strabismus. Using the Bayley exam as a measure of development, Golden et al.[15] also found that children with FAS do less well at 12 months on measures of both mental and physical development than do their matched controls.

Streissguth, Barr, Martin, and Herman[16] found an increased incidence of impaired intellectual functioning in children of alcoholic mothers, even in the absence of FAS. However, the extent to which CNS abnormalities contribute to these problems as opposed to disordered children-rearing environments remains to be determined.

A case series of 17 children with FAS ranging in age from 9 months to 21 years were studied by Streissguth, Herman, and Smith.[12] Most of these children were in the borderline to mildly retarded range, although some were profoundly mentally retarded. Their IQ scores had remained mostly stable over time, although there was a tendency for the IQ scores of children who were diagnosed at older ages to improve over time. These findings may reflect differences in the course of development in more severely affected children (i.e., diagnosed early) compared to those who are less affected (diagnosed later). An additional report from Streissguth et al.[17] noted that 10 years after the first identification of the initial 11 children with FAS, these children still remained small in size and had IQ scores ranging from 20 to 86. Two of the 11 cases and 3 of the mothers had died in the interim.[3]

Drinking Practices during Pregnancy

In response to the finding of a high rate of abnormal pregnancy outcomes among alcoholic women, investigators turned to studies of drinking during pregnancy to assess directly the effects of alcohol ingestion. These studies that measure drinking practices of pregnant women rather than looking at women with diagnosed alcoholism have produced mixed results. In one of the first prospective studies, Hanson, Streissguth, and Smith[18] interviewed women in the fifth month of pregnancy. Infants of women who drank heavily (> 1 oz absolute alcohol daily or five or more drinks on an occasion) were compared to the next infant born to a mother who was a rare or infrequent drinker. They found that the level of prepregnancy drinking was correlated with a higher rate of fetal alcohol syndrome but reported first trimester drinking was not. This first trimester use was interpreted as the effect of drinking before the mother was aware of her pregnancy. Little[19] interviewed 263 women in their fourth and eighth month of pregnancy and found that birth weight was affected by alcohol use prior to pregnancy and late in pregnancy but not by first-trimester alcohol use. Using a similar study design, Tennes and Blackard[20] found no relationship between alcohol consumption and signs of either the fetal alcohol syndrome or decreased birth weight, though alcohol use during pregnancy did explain a small proportion (2%) of the variance in gestational age.

Kaminski, Rumeau, and Schwartz[21] assessed first-trimester drinking in a large collaborative study and found a higher rate of stillbirths (particularly related to abruptio placenta), small for gestational-age babies, and decreased birth and placental weight among babies whose mothers averaged three or more drinks per day during the first trimester.

On the other hand, a retrospective study of alcohol use and pregnancy outcome among women interviewed in the Boston City Hospital after delivery found no relationship between alcohol use during pregnancy and abnormal infant outcome when confounding factors such as smoking, maternal weight gain, maternal illness, race, and other drug use were controlled.[22] A small but significant inverse relationship was found between alcohol use prior to pregnancy and gestational age.

A subset of this population attending the Boston City Hospital prenatal clinic was interviewed at first prenatal visit. Two separate reports[23,24] have found a relationship between prenatal reports of alcohol use and negative pregnancy outcome. Significant associations were found for growth retardation and congenital abnormalities for the women who drank heavily (1.5 drinks per day throughout the pregnancy and 5+ on occasion). Infants born to women who reduced their heavy drinking by the third trimester had higher rates of congenital anomalies, but the babies were not growth retarded.[24]

In summary, results of studies of drinking practices during pregnancy are inconsistent. A relationship between heavy alcohol use and decreased birth weight has been reported, though in some cases the relationship is to drinking prior to pregnancy[18,19]; in others to drinking during early pregnancy,[21,25,26] and in still others, to drinking during later pregnancy.[19,24] An increased rate of congenital malformations was noted among children of heavy drinkers in some studies[18,22,24] but not others.[20-22] A relationship between prepregnancy drinking and gestational age was noted in one study,[22] gestational age and drinking during pregnancy in another,[20] and in a third, no relationship was found.[21]

There are a number of methodological caveats that must be considered when comparing these studies. First, the measurement of alcohol use varied across studies. Not only were different scales for measurement used, but the time of measurement during pregnancy varied also. Although short-term reporting of alcohol use has been shown to be relatively reliable,[26,27] recall over longer periods of time is less reliable. Two recent analyses have demonstrated that recall over the first trimester and recall of first-trimester use from time periods of 3 and 5 months is not highly reliable, and further, it varies among different levels of drinking.[28,29] In the latter two reports, heavy drinkers and abstainers were the most reliable reporters. Also, women who drink heavily are different; they are more likely to use other substances and to be of lower socioeconomic status, thus confounding the analysis of the results.

Behavioral Assessments of Neonates

Behavioral assessments during the immediate neonatal period in one study indicated three factors on the Brazelton Neonatal Behavioral Assessment Scale (BNBAS) that differentiated infants of heavy-drinking mothers from controls after accounting for confounding factors: (1) infants of heavy-drinking women were less able to habituate to aversive stimuli; (2) these infants exhibited low arousal to social stimuli; and (3) they exhibited more frequent state changes.[30] Naturalistic observations of these same newborns showed that infants of heavier drinking mothers had more tremors, increased time in nonalert states, and less vigorous body activity. They exhibited more hand-to-mouth activity, an increased amount of time spent with the head oriented to the left (an atypical position for newborns), and weaker sucking. A test of one newborn with the full fetal alcohol syndrome demonstrated these same patterns.[31] A study on a different sample of infants reported behavioral effects among infants whose mothers consumed alcohol at even lower levels, finding that the exposed infants were more placid at Day 3.[32]

In contrast, however, a recent study of 395 infants whose mothers were interviewed at the fourth and seventh prenatal months and at delivery found no effect of alcohol use on behavioral assessment using the BNBAS when confounding variables were controlled.[33]

In this same study, a relationship between alcohol exposure during pregnancy and abnormalities on neurophysiological status has been reported when confounding variables such as other drugs, tobacco, infant sex, and demographic factors were controlled for. First-trimester alcohol use was significantly associated with differences in sleep state, arousal, and body movements, and infants exposed to alcohol had fewer small body movements in the third trimester. These effects were found in the absence of any of the morphologic features of the fetal alcohol syndrome.[34] Havlicek, Childiaeva, and Chernick[35] reported that infants of alcoholic mothers had more difficulty reaching quiet sleep and were more easily disturbed during sleep, and similar findings have been reported for infants of mothers who drank heavily throughout pregnancy.

Rosett, Snyder, Sander et al.[36] evaluated 31 infants using a bassinet sleep monitor. Fourteen were children of heavy drinkers, 8 were offspring of heavy drinkers who had reduced by late pregnancy, and 9 were controls. Children of mothers with sustained heavy drinking slept less than the children of ex-heavy drinkers and had poorer quality sleep compared to the controls. Sleep was more restless and more of the quiet times were interrupted by awake periods. Small sample size made it impossible in this study to control for confounding factors, but the results do parallel those of Scher et al.[34]

Issues Relating to Long-Term Outcome in Offspring

An important unanswered question about the effects of drinking during pregnancy is whether the use of alcohol and/or the sequelae of that exposure as measured in the immediate neonatal period might predict later developmental delays. To date, we have limited information on which to base an answer to this question.

There have been few studies relating drinking patterns during pregnancy to the long-term effect on the offspring. Streissguth, Barr, Martin, and Herman[16] assessed the relationship of children's developmental status at 8 months of age to women's average use of alcohol per day prior to pregnancy recognition (AAP). There was a significant inverse relationship between AAP and the motor and mental scores measured by the Bayley exam at 8 months. However, average daily volume of alcohol at the fifth month of pregnancy did not predict infant status at 8 months of age. In contrast, Gusella and Fried[37] reported that drinking during pregnancy, but not drinking level prior to pregnancy, predicted poorer performance on the Bayley mental scale.

A longer term report of the relationship between drinking practices and outcome beyond the first year showed that at age 4, children of mothers who had an average daily volume of one or more drinks during pregnancy had decreased attention span, were more likely to be fidgety, and were less likely to comply with parental demands.[38] Prenatal exposure to alcohol has also been reported to be associated with behavioral and cognitive problems. In particular, it has been reported that alcohol use during pregnancy is related to problems with attention and impulsivity, hyperactivity, and learning disorders.[39–41]

Summary and Conclusions

Several studies point to important prenatal effects of maternal alcoholism. In the neonatal period, these include, of course, fetal alcohol syndrome as well as combinations of the characteristics that constitute the fetal alcohol effect. In general, the degree of mental retardation seen in these children is correlated with severity of morphological malformations. Even in the absence of morphological abnormalities, however, neurological and behavioral differences are noted. In terms of predictive validity, infants with FAS diagnosed at birth are more often retarded in mental and motor abilities, and these problems seem to show relatively little improvement over time. In addition, there are behavioral abnormalities manifested by these children. The variability in IQ coupled with the wide range of scores on behavioral measures demonstrates that there is a spectrum of severity even within the diagnostic rubric of the fetal alcohol syndrome.

Studies of alcohol consumption in the absence of alcoholism have given confusing results. Although fetal alcohol syndrome is found only in offspring of alcoholic mothers, children born to heavy-drinking women do have a number of fetal alcohol effects. The inconsistency of the effects may be a result of differential exposure, exposure at different times during pregnancy, or methodological problems with identification and measure or inadequate control for risk factors that co-vary with alcohol consumption. It does seem evident, however, that heavy alcohol use during pregnancy, although not leading to FAS, does have deleterious effects, and in the absence of an accurate measure of a safe level of use during pregnancy, women ought to be warned of a potential risk.

There have been too few studies to assess accurately the effect of drinking on development beyond the neonatal period. Studies showed infants of heavy-drinking mothers to be developmentally delayed at 8 months of age.[16] These delays were directly related to the level of maternal drinking. Similar findings were reported at 13 months by Gusella and Fried.[37] Measurement at 4 years of age showed that children of mothers who drank daily during pregnancy were more often hyperactive and distractible. Although these studies await replication, the few findings do parallel those reported for children of chronically alcoholic mothers.

Thus, although we have evidence that alcoholic women will experience more problem pregnancies, more problems with pregnancy outcome including a probability of having a child with fetal alcohol syndrome, as well as an increased risk of fetal alcohol effects, a number of questions remain to be answered. We do not yet know what it is about alcoholism that leads to the complete expression of FAS, nor do we know why some alcoholic women, and not others, have affected children. Children who are affected with FAS do exhibit multiple problems as they progress in both their mental and physical development.

Children of women who drink heavily during pregnancy also are affected, though the effect is considerably less than that seen among offspring of alcoholic women. The consequences of heavy drinking are not yet reliably documented but seem to represent the lower end of a continuum of effects seen in the offspring of alcoholics. If this is true, then one might hypothesize that the alcohol exposure is the major underlying cause of FAE and FAS, with other factors, such as chronicity of use and biological effects of alcohol on the mother contributing to the full expression of the fetal alcohol syndrome.

The Effect of Tobacco Use during Pregnancy

Tobacco is a commonly used drug during pregnancy, with studies reporting that substantial portions, and in lower socioeconomic-status cohorts, even majorities of women smoke during their pregnancies. Adverse effects of cigarette smoking during pregnancy include an increased risk of reproductive loss, fetal mortality, preterm birth, and neonatal death. Reported effects on the neonate include fetal growth deficits reflected by lower mean birth weight, shorter length, smaller head and chest circumferences, and a number of problems of adaptation in the neonatal period.[42]

In 1957, Simpson[43] reported that babies born to women who smoked during pregnancy were an average of 200 g lighter than babies born to comparable women who did not smoke. Since this report, over 45 studies have confirmed this finding. The majority of these studies found that maternal smoking independently reduces birth weight regardless of the other determinants of birth weight such as maternal nutrition, gestational age, gravidity, maternal weight gain, and race. The relative risk of low birth weight, defined as births under 2500 g, for smokers versus nonsmokers ranges from 1.5 to 2.5.[44]

The majority of studies that examined the association between maternal smoking and prematurity have found that maternal smoking is not a significant predictor of gestational age,[45,46] although some have reported an association with prematurity, mediated mostly by placenta previa and abruptio placentae.[47] Thus, with the exception of these problems, maternal smoking affects low birth weight through intrauterine growth retardation rather than decreased gestation.

Studies have demonstrated an increased rate of spontaneous abortions for smokers versus nonsmokers.[46,48,49] An increase in perinatal mortality associated with maternal smoking has often been associated with antepartum hemorrhage or abruptio placentae.[50,51] Excess neonatal deaths have been associated with immaturity, asphyxia, atelectasis, and with respiratory distress syndrome.[50,52]

Findings of association between maternal smoking and congential malformations are mixed. Several studies have found that the incidence of congential malformations was lower for smokers than for nonsmokers.[50,51] However, a significant positive association between cardiac malformations and maternal smoking was shown by Fedrick.[53]

The Effect of Marijuana Use during Pregnancy

Given the prevalence of marijuana use in the childbearing age group, it is surprising that so little is known about its potential teratogenic effects. The reports, using human populations, that are in the literature are inconclusive and often conflicting. The most comprehensive studies of the effect of marijuana use during pregnancy on infant outcome have been those of Fried. This prospective study used a volunteer sample from obstetrical practices in Ottawa, Canada. In general, the women were middle class, although the marijuana users were of lower social class than the nonusers. Fried reports that the infants of women who used marijuana at the rate of five or more "joints" per week throughout their pregnancy were more likely to be premature[54] and exhibited more tremors and startles and altered visual responsiveness on the Brazelton Neonatal Behavioral Assessment Scale.[55] These infants, however, were not smaller than infants of nonusers and had no more minor physical anomalies. This is in contrast to an earlier report by Hingson, Alpert, Day, et al.[22] that reported that infants who were exposed to marijuana during pregnancy were smaller and had more physical anomalies. Linn et al.[56] in a large cohort interviewed at delivery found that there were no significant relationships between marijuana use during pregnancy and either growth or morphological changes. Tennes,[57] also, in a prospective study of marijuana use among young women in Denver reported that this exposure was not correlated with growth or morphological abnormalities. The one exception to this was that the infants exposed to marijuana were significantly shorter at birth. They also exhibited increased rates of tremulousness, altered visual responses, and high-pitched cries. A recent study by Hatch and Bracken[58] reported that infants exposed to marijuana during pregnancy were smaller at birth. However, this relationship existed only among white mothers and did not hold true for black women.

The Effect of Other Drug Use during Pregnancy

The specific effects of use of other illicit drugs during pregnancy are extremely difficult to assess. Research to date has presented mostly reports of case series or studies of women in treatment for substance abuse. These women not only represent a highly selected population but also are most likely to be multidrug users, including alcohol and tobacco as well as other illicit or "street" drugs. In addition, the environment of these women is often disordered, with financial problems and a life-style that generally signifies a higher risk for problems. And the fact that these drugs are purchased on the street in the absence of quality control means that often contaminants are added to the drugs.

Cocaine

Several recent papers have reported that cocaine use during pregnancy can cause adverse pregnancy outcomes. Chasnoff et al.[59] studied four groups of women. One group used only cocaine during pregnancy; another used cocaine plus narcotics. These two groups were compared to two control groups—one that used narcotics in the past and were being maintained on methadone and a final group that was drug-free. The cocaine-exposed infants were not significantly smaller than other infants, nor were they more likely to be premature. However, they did exhibit differences on the Brazelton Neonatal Assessment Scale, including a greater degree of tremulousness and startle responses and differences in the interactive state organization clusters. It was also reported that four of the cocaine-using women in this cohort had onset of labor with abruptio placentae immediately after an intravenous self-injection of cocaine. Cocaine users also reported a higher rate of spontaneous abortions.

Heroin and Methadone

There is now a substantial literature on the effect of heroin and methadone use during pregnancy on the newborn. Major findings include low birth weight with 50% small for gestational age and withdrawal in a majority of the infants.[60] Most of the literature on the effects of these substances are reports of case series and lack appropriate controls for confounding variables. Chasnoff et al.[61] have reported on a prospective study of women who conceived while using heroin but who were switched to methadone, a group of polydrug abusers, and nondrug users. The infants born to methadone-maintained mothers were significantly smaller than the nonexposed group and had significantly smaller head circumferences compared to the polydrug-abusing group. These infants also exhibited more depression of interactive behaviors and state controls. The infants of the polydrug-abusing women were midway between the methadone-exposed infants and the normal controls in growth and in behavior.

The most marked effect of maternal opiate use is the neonatal abstinence syndrome, or the withdrawal experienced by infants born to opiate- and methadone-using mothers. Symptoms of withdrawal include tremulousness, irritability, hyperactivity, sleep and feeding problems, and a high-pitched cry. The narcotics that are reported to cause these symptoms are heroin, methadone, meperidine, morphine, codeine, pentazocine and propoxyphene. Symptoms of withdrawal can be present at birth or begin as late as 10 days after delivery, depending on the drug used, and may last for 4 to 6 months.[62]

There are few prospective reports of the long-term development of these children. In the first year of life, these infants are more likely to have poor motor coordination, high activity level, and poor attention.[63] These problems seem to remain through early childhood as Wilson et al.[64] reported that children exposed to heroin and Lodge[65] reported that children exposed prenatally to methadone were hyperactive and had difficulties with impulse control. Interpretation of all of these studies is problematic, however, because of the lack of adequate sample size, inaccurate measurement of exposure, biased sample selection, polydrug abuse, and the failure to control for the psychosocial environment of the mother and the child.

References

1. Lemoine P, Harousseau H, Borteyru J, et al: Children of alcoholic parents. Abnormalities observed in 127 cases. *Quest Med* **21:**476–482, 1968.
2. Eckardt M, Harford T, Kaelber C, et al: Health hazards associated with alcohol consumption. *JAMA* **246:**648–666, 1981.
3. Landesman-Dwyer, S: Maternal drinking and pregnancy outcome. *App Res Mental Retard* **3:**241–263, 1982.
4. Olegard R, Sabel K, Aronsson, M, et al: Effects on the child of alcohol abuse during pregnancy. *Acta Paediatr Scand Suppl* **275:**112–121, 1979.
5. Sokol R, Miller S, Reed G: Alcohol abuse during pregnancy: An epidemiological study. Alcohol: *Clin Exp Res* **4:**135–145, 1980.
6. Little R, Streissguth A, Barr H, et al: Decreased birth weight in infants of alcoholic women who abstained during pregnancy. *J Pediatr* **96:**974–977, 1980.
7. Hollstedt C, Dahlgren L, Rydberg U: Alcoholic women in fertile age treated at an alcohol clinic. *Acta Psychiatr Scand* **67:**195–204, 1983.
8. Coles CD, Smith IE, Fernhoff P, et al: Neonatal ethanol withdrawal: Characteristics in clinically normal, nondysmorphic neonates. *J of Ped* **105:**445–451, 1984.
9. Landesman-Dwyer S: The relationship of children's behavior to maternal alcohol consumption, in Abel, EL: Fetal Alcohol Syndrome: Human Studies. Boca Raton, Florida, CRC Press, Inc., 1982, p. 127.
10. Majewski F: Studies on alcohol embryopathy. *Fortschritte der Medizin* **96:**2207–2213, 1978.
11. Majewski F: The damaging effect of alcohol on offspring. *Nervenarzt,* **49:**410–416, 1978.
12. Streissguth A, Herman C, Smith D: Stability of intelligence in the fetal alcohol syndrome: A preliminary report. *Alcohol Clin Exp Res* **2:**165–170, 1978.
13. Shaywitz S, Cohen D, Shaywitz B: Behavior and learning difficulties in children of normal intelligence born to alcoholic mothers. *J Ped* **96:**978–982, 1980.
14. Steinhauser H, Nester V, Spohr H: Development and psychopathology of children with the fetal alcohol syndrome. *J Dev Behav Ped* **3:**49–54, 1982.
15. Golden M, Montare A, Bridger W: Maternal alcohol use and infant development. *Pediatr* **70:**931–934, 1982.
16. Streissguth A, Barr H, Martin D, et al: Effects of maternal alcohol, nicotine and caffeine use during pregnancy on infant mental and motor development at eight months. *Alcohol Clin Exp Res* **4:**152–164, 1980.
17. Streissguth AP, Claren SK, Jones KL: A 10-year follow-up of the first children described as having "fetal alcohol syndrome." *Alcohol Clin Exp Res* **8:**21, 1984.
18. Hanson J, Streissguth A, Smith D: The effects of moderate alcohol consumption during pregnancy on fetal growth and morphogenesis. *J. Ped* **92:**457–460, 1978.
19. Little R: Moderate alcohol use during pregnancy and decreased infant birth weight. *Am J Public Hlth* **67:**1154–1156, 1957.
20. Tennes K, Blackard C: Maternal alcohol consumption, birth weight and minor physical anomalies. *Am J Obstet Gynecol* **138:**774–780, 1980.
21. Kaminski M, Rumeau C, Schwartz D, Alcohol consumption in pregnant women and the outcome of pregnancy. *Alcohol Clin Exp Res* **2:**155–163, 1978.
22. Hingson R, Alpert J, Day N, et al: Effects of maternal drinking and marijuana use on fetal growth and development. *Pedatr* **70:**539–546, 1982.
23. Ouellette R, Rosett H, Rosman N, et al: Adverse effects on offspring of maternal alcohol abuse during pregnancy. *New Engl J Med,* **297:**528–530, 1977.
24. Rosett H, Weiner L, Lee A, et al: Patterns of alcohol consumption and fetal development. *Obstet Gynecol* **61:**539–546, 1983.
25. Kuzma J, Sokol R: Maternal drinking behavior and decreased intrauterine growth. *Alcohol Clin Exp Res* **6:**396–402, 1982.
26. Mau G, Netter P: Kaffee und Alkoholkonsum. Risikofaktoren in der Schwangerschaft: *Geburtsch u Frauenheilk* **34:**1018–1022, 1974.
27. Streissguth AP, Martin DC, Buffington VE: Identifying heavy drinkers: A comparison of eight alcohol

scores obtained in the same sample, in Seixas FA (ed): *Currents in Alcoholism,* Vol. 2. New York, Grune & Stratton, 1977, p. 395.

28. Day N, Robles N, Richardson G, et al: Accuracy of the measurement of alcohol use in the first trimester of pregnancy. Unpublished paper, 1987.

29. Robles N, Day N: Recall of alcohol consumption during pregnancy. Unpublished paper, 1987.

30. Streissguth A, Barr H, Martin D: Maternal alcohol use and neonatal habituation assessed with the Brazelton Scale. *Child Dev* **545:**1109–1118, 1983.

31. Landesman-Dwyer S, Keller LS, Streissguth AP: Naturalistic observations of newborns: Effects of maternal alcohol intake. *Alcohol Clin Exp Res* **2:**171–177, 1978.

32. Jacobson SW, Fein GG, Jacobson JL et al: Neonatal correlates of prenatal exposure to smoking, caffeine, and alcohol. *Inf Behav and Dev* **7:**253–265, 1984.

33. Richardson G, Day N: Alcohol use during pregnancy and neonatal outcome. Paper presented at the International Conference on Infant Studies, Los Angeles, April 1986.

34. Scher M, Richardson G, Coble P, et al: The effects of prenatal alcohol and marijuana exposure: Disturbance in neonatal sleep cycling and arousal. Unpublished report, 1987.

35. Havlicek V, Childiaeva R, Chernick V: EEG frequency spectrum characteristics of sleep states in infants of alcoholic mothers. *Neuropediatrie* **8:**360–373, 1977.

36. Rosett H, Sander L, Snyder P, et al: Effect of maternal drinking on neonate state regulation. *Dev Med Child Neurol* **21:**464–473, 1979.

37. Gusella J, Fried P: Effects of maternal social drinking and smoking on offspring at 13 months. *Neurobehav Tox Terat* **6:**13–17, 1981.

38. Landesman-Dwyer S, Ragozin A, Little R: Behavioral correlates of prenatal alcohol exposure: A four-year follow-up study. *Neurobehav Tox Terat* **3:**187–193, 1981.

39. Shaywitz SE, Cohen DJ, Shaywitz BA: Behavior and learning difficulties in children of normal intelligence born to alcoholic mothers. *J Ped* **96:**978–982, 1980.

40. Streissguth AP, Barr HM, Parrish-Johnson JC, et al: Attention and distraction at seven years related to maternal drinking during pregnancy. *Alcohol Clin Exp Res* **9:**66, 1985.

41. Streissguth AP, Martin DC, Barr HM, et al: Intrauterine alcohol and nicotine exposure: Attention and reaction time in 4-year-old children. *Dev Psych* **20:**533–541, 1984.

42. U.S. Department of Health and Human Service: *The Health Consequences of Smoking for Women.* Rockville, Public Health Services, 1979.

43. Simpson, WJ: A preliminary report on cigarette smoking and the incidence of prematurity. *Am J Obstet Gynecol* **73:**808–815, 1957.

44. Meyer, MB: Reply to Rush. *Am J Obstet Gynecol* **135:**282–284, 1979.

45. Bailey, RR: The effect of maternal smoking on infant birth weight. *N Zealand Med J* **71:**293–294, 1971.

46. Kullander, S, Kaellen, B: A prospective study of smoking and pregnancy. *Acta Psychiatr Scand* **50:**83–94, 1971.

47. Meyer MB, Tonascia JA: Maternal smoking, pregnancy complications and perinatal mortality. *Am J Obstet Gynecol* **128:**494–502, 1977.

48. Hollingsworth DR, Moser RJ, Carlsen JW, Thompson KT: Abnormal adolescent primiparous pregnancy: Association of race, human chorionic somatotropin production, and smoking. *Am J Obstet Gynecol* **126:**230–237, 1976.

49. O'Lane, JM: Some fetal effects of maternal cigarette smoking. *Obstet Gynecol* **22:**181–184, 1963.

50. Andrews J, McGarry JM: A community study of smoking in pregnancy. *J Obstet Gynecol Br Com* **79:**1057–1073, 1972.

51. Goujard J, Rumean C, Schwartz D: Smoking during pregnancy, stillbirth and abruptio placentae. *Biomedicine* **23:**20–22, 1975.

52. Comstock GW, Shah FK, Meyer MB, Abbey H: Low birthweight and neonatal mortality rate related to maternal smoking on socio-economic status. *Am J Obstet Gynecol* **111:**53–59, 1971.

53. Fedrick J: Factors associated with low birthweight of infants delivered at term. *Brit J Obstet Gynecol* **85:**1–7, 1978.

54. Fried PA: Marijuana use by pregnant women and effects on offspring: An update. *Neurobehav Tox Terat* **4:**451–454, 1982.

55. Fried PA, Buckingham M, Von Kulmiz P: Marijuana use during pregnancy and perinatal risk factors. *Am J Obstet Gynecol* **146:**992–994, 1983.

56. Linn S, Schoenbaum S, Monson R, et al: The association of marijuana use with outcome of pregnancy. *Am J Pub Hlth* **73**:1161–1164, 1983.

57. Tennes K, Avitable N, Blackard C, et al: Marijuana: Prenatal and postnatal exposure in the human, in: *Current Research on the Consequences of Maternal Drug Abuse,* Research Monograph Series, No. 59, Rockville, MD, National Institute on Drug Abuse, 1985.

58. Hatch EE, Bracken MB: Effect of marijuana use in pregnancy on fetal growth. *Am J Epidemiol* **124**:986–993, 1986.

59. Chasnoff IJ, Burns WJ, Schnoll SH: Cocaine use in pregnancy. *New Engl J Med* **313**:666–669, 1985.

60. Householder J, Hatcher R, Burns W: Infants born to narcotic-addicted mothers. *Psych Bull* **92**:453–468, 1982.

61. Chasnoff IJ, Hatcher R, Burns WJ: Polydrug- and methadone-addicted newborns: A continuum of impairment? *Pediatr* **7**:210–213, 1982.

62. American Academy of Pediatrics, Committee on Drugs: Neonatal drug withdrawal. *Pediatr* **72**:895–901, 1983.

63. Bernstein V, Jeremy RJ, Hans SL, Marcus J: A longitudinal study of offspring born to methadone-maintained women. II. Dyadic interaction and infant behavior at 4 months. *Am J Drug Alc Abuse* **10**:161–193, 1984.

64. Wilson GS, McCreary R, Kean J, et al: The development of preschool children of heroin-addicted mothers: A controlled study. *Pediatr* **63**:135–141, 1979.

65. Lodge A: Developmental findings with infants born to mothers on methadone maintenance: A preliminary report, in: *Symposium on Comprehensive Health Care for Addicted Families and Their Children.* Rockville, MD, National Institute on Drug Abuse. May 20–21, 1976, p 79.

14

Principles of Genetic Counseling for Psychiatric Liaisons

ANN P. WALKER AND M. ANNE SPENCE

Introduction

Medical genetics is a specialty that draws from and, increasingly, influences virtually every other branch of medicine and many of the basic sciences. Our growing understanding of the genetic basis not only of a few relatively rare diseases but of numerous birth defects and many of the common ills of mankind has led to an explosion of knowledge about the human genome that has far-reaching implications for diagnosis, treatment, and prevention.

The rapidity of the advancement of our knowledge of genetics and the technology that has arisen from it have caught the public's attention. Nearly every day, the media report mapping of a gene whose location previously was unknown, debates the social and ethical implications of revolutionary reproductive technologies, discusses ''gene therapy,'' describes a newly discovered basis for a particular malformation or disease, or argues the propriety of applying certain prenatal diagnostic techniques and fetal interventions. This flood of information often is received with excitement and awe but also with unrealistic expectations, confusion, and anxiety not only by the lay public but by medical professionals as well.

Simultaneously, changes have occurred in our society that have resulted in individuals taking a more active role in their own health care and reproductive decisions. Couples who become pregnant are forced to confront the fact that their own exposures and

Ann P. Walker • Division of Human Genetics, Department of Pediatrics, University of California at Irvine, Irvine, CA 92717.   **M. Anne Spence** • Division of Medical Genetics, Departments of Psychiatry and Biomathematics, School of Medicine, University of California at Los Angeles, Los Angeles, CA 90024.

health behavior may affect or have affected the well-being of their unborn child. Although these concerns may be unfounded, they often are a source of anxiety to patients and of confusion to their physicians.

Reproductive behavior itself has changed. New technologies have become available to aid infertile couples who, in the past, would have remained childless. Advances that have made it possible to detect numerous fetal anomalies have increased the willingness of couples at increased risk because of age, health history, or ethnic background to undertake pregnancy.

The increased complexity of medical care, the frequent lack of an ongoing relationship with a single trusted care provider, the inherent difficulty of truly eliciting patients' concerns or of communicating complicated technical information in the brief time often alloted for most medical interactions, and the litigiousness of today's society, make health professionals vulnerable. When patients deem that they should have been informed of reproductive risk or that such risk was incorrectly assessed and that they were not made aware of reproductive options that may have been available, they may (appropriately) feel that a tort has occurred.

The mental health professional working in a reproductive medicine setting has both the opportunity and the obligation to ascertain when a woman or couple may benefit from genetic evaluation and counseling. Conversely, genetic counselors may need to work with colleagues in psychiatry, psychology, or social work in providing support to patients and families overwhelmed by the occurrence or impact of a birth defect or genetic disease.

The first part of this chapter is intended to help the mental health worker recognize situations in which a genetic referral may be appropriate, to understand what this type of evaluation and counseling may involve, and to appreciate the types of situations in which geneticists may rely on *their* expertise. The latter part of this chapter will describe our nascent understanding of the genetic contribution to certain psychoses and affective disorders. Mental health professionals are in a unique position to identify families that may augment this knowledge. They also are the ones who most frequently will have to respond to queries from patients confused and concerned by the implications of new developments in this area.

Reasons to Refer for Genetic Counseling

Often with a pregnancy, and particularly one that has been marred by a miscarriage, stillbirth, or birth of a child with a congenital malformation, parents express concern over issues in their own or their family's medical history. Much of the time, these concerns have nothing to do with the event that has occurred, but they may indeed represent a causative factor, or they may signal a reproductive or even a personal health risk of an unrelated nature. Because pregnancy itself raises fear and an untoward pregnancy outcome may result in guilt or blame laying, a couple may voice their concerns about their health history to a mental health professional. Whether or not this happens, a careful family medical history should be obtained, not only to identify risk factors that may be of significance but also to elicit issues that the mother, or couple, may have implicated as causative. Individuals or couples may benefit from further genetic evaluation if:

1. They, or someone in their family, has had a birth defect.
2. There is a family history of mental retardation or a known genetic disease (for example, cystic fibrosis, Down's syndrome or muscular dystrophy).*
3. There is significant family history of mental illness or of later-onset neurodegenerative disorders (such as Huntington's, Wilson's, or Alzheimer's disease).
4. Several family members have had the same type of cancer.
5. A child in the family has been stillborn or has died in infancy or early childhood for unknown reasons.
6. A child or young adult in the family is unusual or delayed in his or her sexual development.
7. There is short stature (particularly disproportionate short stature) or excessively tall stature in the patient or in a close relative.
8. A prospective parent is known to be a "carrier" for a genetic disorder or a chromosome rearrangement.
9. The couple comes from an ethnic group that is more likely to have certain genetic conditions such as sickle-cell anemia (Blacks and couples of Mediterranean origin), thalassemia (those of Mediterranean or Oriental descent), or Tay-Sachs disease (Jews of Eastern European origin).
10. A woman is 35 or older, or a man is 55 or older and the couple is pregnant or considering pregnancy.
11. The couple has had difficulty in conceiving or carrying a pregnancy to term (particularly if there have been two or more early miscarriages).
12. The couple is blood-related (for example, as first cousins).
13. The mother has a chronic condition (such as certain genetic diseases, diabetes, or epilepsy) that may increase fetal risk.
14. The couple is concerned because they have been exposed to chemicals, radiation, infections, medications, drugs, or alcohol.
15. A fetal abnormality is found or suspected during pregnancy (for example, through ultrasound, maternal serum alphafetoprotein screening, or other diagnostic studies).

When issues such as these are identified in the history, discussion with a medical geneticist or genetic counselor may help to clarify whether referral is indicated. If so, the genetics professionals can be alerted to psychosocial matters that may help them in dealing with the patient. Similarly, the mental health worker can be apprised of the type of evaluation that will be necessary. Together, they can decide how the referral should be presented to the patient in order to minimize the additional anxiety such a referral may create and to maximize the likelihood that it will be acted upon. It is important for the mental health professional to establish a working relationship with the nearest center providing genetic services.†

*A catalog, *Mendelian Inheritance in Man*,[1] lists diseases known or suspected to be inherited on the basis of single genes and their probable modes of inheritance. These, as well as chromosomal and multifactorial conditions, are described in *Principles and Practice of Medical Genetics*.[2]

†A national directory of centers providing comprehensive genetics services is available from the U.S. Department of Health and Human Services.[3]

Depending on the indication, the extent of a genetic evaluation may range from a simple blood test to an exhaustive review of medical records with specialized examinations and testing of many family members. Genetic counseling is an integral component of any such consultation and involves gathering information about family history and psychosocial issues and identifying the individual's or couple's specific concerns. Once a diagnosis has been established, information is provided regarding the probability that the disorder may recur, the outlook and treatment for affected individuals, and the reproductive options available to those family members who may have a higher chance of developing the condition themselves or of having an affected child.

Because of its far-reaching implications, this information may be provided in increments, over a period of time, so that the family has time to review and assimilate it. Throughout the process, the geneticist may work with a mental health professional to help the family make effective use of all resources that are available for financial or emotional support. If subsequent reproduction is an issue, the genetics professional will help the couple arrive at a course of action most consistent with their values, needs and beliefs. Options may include taking the genetic risk, utilizing prenatal diagnosis (which in the majority of cases provides reassurance that the fetus is *un*affected), relying on artificial insemination or inovulation, adopting, or refraining from childbearing. A decision to follow any of these courses obviously can have long-lasting repercussions, so supportive genetic counseling may continue over a period of years. Sometimes reproductive decisions will need to be reconsidered if new means of diagnosis or management become available or if personal circumstances change.

Prenatal Diagnosis

Prenatal diagnosis is an aspect of genetic evaluation and counseling that presents unique considerations. A variety of methods, including ultrasound, amniocentesis, and more recently, chorion villus sampling, make it possible to image the fetus or to obtain fetally derived tissues that can be tested for numerous genetic disorders.* Up until recently, these types of diagnostic procedures have been utilized primarily by couples known to be at increased risk because of their age, their reproductive or family history, or their identification through carrier-testing programs. Most of these couples have had genetic counseling prior to deciding to have prenatal diagnosis.

Recently, though, prenatal diagnosis is being much more broadly applied. In many states, maternal serum alphafetoprotein-screening programs have been established to identify fetuses at a higher risk for neural tube defects and other malformations or certain chromosome defects. Once the province only of university or other tertiary medical centers, fetal diagnostic use of ultrasound and amniocentesis by private obstetricians and laboratories has grown tremendously. Often, diagnosis of an anomaly may be made fortuitously in the fetus of a couple not previously thought to be at risk.

Ideally, counseling should be provided regarding the risks, benefits, and limitations of the procedures and the significance of possible findings *prior* to prenatal diagnosis.

---

*A good overview of prenatal diagnosis indications and techniques can be found in *Clinical Genetics Handbook*.[4]

Such counseling also should explore the couple's feelings about the pregnancy and thoughts about their course of action should an abnormality be found. It is important that the couple fully understand the implications and consequences of opting for *any* fetal diagnostic procedures. Unfortunately, office ultrasound examination and maternal blood testing is often presented as a routine part of prenatal care, with the result that a suspicion of fetal abnormality may be raised with little or no forewarning.

With or without prior counseling, discovery of a fetal anomaly is a major crisis for the prospective parents. In many cases, they themselves have had no prior experience with the condition. Furthermore, the limitations of the diagnostic techniques may make it impossible to ascertain with certainty or to predict accurately the severity of the problem. Because the diagnosis may not be made or suspected until the fourth or fifth month of pregnancy, time may be too limited for a lengthy deliberation about whether or not to continue the pregnancy. Also, by this time, friends and family are aware of the pregnancy, fetal movement usually has been felt, and both parents probably have heard the heartbeat and observed the baby on ultrasound. Even for a couple with prior knowledge of a high genetic risk who has defended themselves from involvement with the pregnancy as much as possible, it is inevitable that significant bonding already has occurred. Regardless of whether the couple elects to terminate or continue the pregnancy, they are likely to need considerable support over the coming months or even years.

General Genetic Counseling Issues

Other situations arise in medical genetics that may require the expertise of the mental health professional. Among these are the birth of a child with a previously *un*diagnosed birth defect or genetic disease. Here, the family may be helped to surmount the trauma of the newborn period only to become dysfunctional later on as relationships are stressed by the unanticipated and ongoing physical, emotional, and financial demands of a handicapped child. In other families, an older child who is mentally retarded may become a significant management problem. Or a parent or spouse may be affected with a genetically transmitted neurodegenerative disorder, raising fears for one's own or one's children's future health, concerns about long-term care, and fear of separation or abandonment. In still other couples, discovery of significant genetic reproductive risk or infertility can lead to anxiety, guilt, depression, and recrimination. Any of these situations would challenge the reserves of the most psychologically healthy individual or family. In one that is emotionally fragile to start with or battered by years of confronting a genetic risk or disease, the consequences can be devastating.

Specific Mental Health Counseling Issues

The genetic counseling issue most likely to be directed to the psychiatric liaison regards recurrence risk for a behavioral condition known to exist either in a previous child (such as autism) or in a parent or other relative (such as bipolar affective disorder). Here the expertise of the mental health professional is often needed to establish or evaluate the appropriateness of the purported diagnosis before genetic counseling can be provided.

This is because clinically similar (or even identical) conditions may be inherited in different ways (each with a different recurrence risk) or may result entirely from non-genetic factors. This phenomenon is known as "genetic heterogeneity."

With the large number of behavioral disorders, the rapidity with which understanding of the genetic basis for these conditions is changing, and the difficulty of determining the relative contribution of environment and heredity, there is no single adequate clinical reference that the mental health worker can use to determine the chances that such a condition will recur in a family. For this reason, assessment of genetic risk and provision of this information to the patient or family is best done in cooperation with a geneticist. However, familiarity with genetic terminology and patterns of inheritance will help the mental health professional in discussing cases with the geneticist and patients and their families. Several references listed at the end of the chapter provide good reviews of medical genetics concepts.[2,4,5]

Behavioral conditions, from a genetic standpoint, fall into three categories: (1) those that appear to occur sporadically—with no greater incidence of recurrence in the family than in the general population; (2) those for which a hereditary component is suspected because the incidence within certain families is higher than in the general population; and (3) those in which a responsible contributing genetic mechanism has actually been established, either by demonstration of a chromosome abnormality or by identification of an individual gene or genes that can be tracked through families in ways consistent with recognized patterns of inheritance. In a few conditions, such as Wilson's disease, the actual pathogenetic mechanism causing symptoms is understood but even for disorders in which the mode of inheritance and recurrence risk are well-established, the actual mutation and its biochemical effects usually remain to be discovered.

Occasionally, a family will request information regarding risk for recurrence of a disorder that has occurred in a single individual in the family. If the condition is one that has not been shown to recur in *other* families, the case is termed "sporadic" and the chances for recurrence are no higher than in the general population, that is, the population incidence can be quoted as the recurrence risk. However, families are more likely to express concern about recurrence of conditions such as alcoholism, for which they have observed a familial liability. The role of genetic factors in alcoholism has been clearly demonstrated in mice,[6] as has its familial nature in humans.[7] Consequently, in this case, the population frequency can no longer be used in counseling a family in which there are one or more affected individuals. On the other hand, no specific responsible gene or genes for alcoholism has yet been identified,[8] so it is also inappropriate to base recurrence risks on known patterns of inheritance.

Unfortunately, in this and other conditions for which there is little or no information as to exact etiology, counseling must be based on "empiric" risk figures, that is, those derived from observation of large numbers of similarly affected families. Among difficulties inherent in the use of empirical data are the fact that these data represent an *average* risk; the risk may in fact be zero in some families and considerably higher in others. Second, data may not be available for a given family's specific situation. For example, although the risk for the son of an alcoholic to become alcoholic has been estimated to be 18%,[7] comparable data may be unavailable for a case in which both parents, both sibs, and the man's spouse are alcoholic. Obviously, use of empirical data must be tempered by clinical judgment.

For disorders in which the hereditary nature is well-recognized, the counseling may be straightforward or (as is more usually the case) quite complex. In a few conditions, such as Huntington's disease, the transmission of the trait is completely understood. This condition is inherited as an autosomal dominant, meaning that a single mutant gene, not located on the sex-determining (X and Y) chromosomes, causes the trait. An affected individual has a 50% chance of transmitting the disease gene to each of his children. Any child who receives the mutant gene will ultimately develop the condition and have the same 50% chance of passing it on, whereas a child who does not receive the gene will neither develop the trait nor transmit it. In contrast, Wilson's disease, which also results in behavioral changes, is inherited as an autosomal recessive. This type of inheritance requires that the mutation (again, on a chromosome other than the X or Y) be present in *both* members of a gene pair, the one inherited from the mother and the one inherited from the father, for the trait to be expressed. Usually for such a trait, neither parents nor offspring of an affected individual have the condition, although sibs are at a 25% risk. These types of conditions are known as "single-gene" or "Mendelian" disorders, and recurrence risks for various family members can be calculated using established principles.

Even simply inherited disorders can present counseling dilemmas. In many conditions, the clinical picture may differ greatly, even among affected individuals within the same family. The trait may be have a wide variety of manifestations, any one or all of which may be present in an affected individual. Furthermore, severity and age of onset may vary considerably. This sometimes makes it difficult to identify which family members carry the trait, to determine genetic risk, and to give a realistic picture of the possible range and severity of impairment that might result. A case in point is Tourette syndrome, in which the genetic pattern in families may become evident only when symptoms such as tics or obsessive-compulsive behavior are identified in relatives of a more dramatically affected individual.[9]

Unfortunately for genetic counseling, most behavioral traits are probably not even inherited in a simple Mendelian fashion, and the major psychoses clearly are not. It is likely that the behavior traits result from numerous causes, including the action of several different genes. This complexity can be appreciated by examining two disorders: autism, in which very little of the genetics is understood, and the bipolar affective disorders, for which the inheritance is becoming much better known.

For autism, a very rare condition, it is easy to document that the frequency of affected sibs is much greater than the population frequency.[10] However, the condition appears to be genetically heterogeneous. If families with *at least* two children affected with autism are analyzed, autosomal recessive inheritance cannot be ruled out.[11] Such families should be quoted a 25% recurrence risk, despite the fact that not all observations (such as an unequal sex ratio) are consistent with autosomal recessive inheritance. However, for the majority of families who have only one affected child, the *empirical* recurrence risk of only 3%[10] is appropriate. Recently, autism has also been associated with the "fragile X," an often familial chromosomal abnormality that, if identified, carries yet another set of recurrence risks.[12,13] At present, all that is clear about autism is that it can have at least two, and probably several genetic etiologies, and perhaps nongenetic ones as well.

In contrast, at least three different *specific* genes have been identified that can produce bipolar illness. A study of the Amish population identified families in which the gene is located on a region of chromosome 11.[14] But in other families for whom autosomal dominant inheritance is evident, this location for the gene has been ruled out.[15] In the non-Ashkenazi Jewish population in Israel, a gene that produces bipolar disease has been mapped to the X chromosome.[16] However, in most families with bipolar disease, it is not possible to document *any* clear-cut pattern of inheritance, again indicating that the genetics is complex and the condition heterogeneous.

For families in which a specific causative gene has been identified, it has been found using the important technique of genetic linkage analysis. Such studies involve statistical analyses to determine if the disease gene is being transmitted (or is "cosegregating") with another (presumably) unrelated gene or segment of DNA (a "marker") whose chromosomal location *is* known. A consistent association between the marker and the disease state is called "linkage." Demonstration of linkage, when appropriately carried out, indicates that the condition *is* genetic and specifies a relatively precise location for the disease gene. This localization ("mapping") of the gene permits comparison among families and may, in turn, demonstrate that different genes produce the same clinical picture in different families.

Once a gene is mapped, it theoretically becomes possible to detect the presence of the disease gene in a person before symptoms appear—even prenatally. To do this in a given family, DNA usually must be available from individuals known to be definitely affected or definitely unaffected. (Further discussion of the process of linkage and mapping for genetic diseases in general,[17] for psychiatric disorders in particular,[18,19] and the utility of this technique in diagnosis can be found in the references cited.) For conditions such as Huntington's disease, which appear to result from only one mutation, this is relatively simple. But for conditions that are etiologically heterogeneous, such as bipolar affective disorder, each family will have to be evaluated individually to determine which (if any) of several genes is causative. Even in the most apparently straightforward situations, other considerations, such as uncooperative or deceased family members, or uninformative genetic linkage may make diagnosis impossible. Furthermore, it is important to consider the ethical and social implications of providing prenatal or presymptomatic diagnosis of conditions for which there is no cure.

Obviously, it is beyond the scope of this chapter to discuss thoroughly the genetics of mental illness. Moreover, the field is changing so rapidly that such a discussion quickly would become obsolete. It is hoped that the key references at the chapter's end will point the way for the mental health professional who wishes to further explore this dynamic area and will facilitate establishing a dialogue with genetics professionals. We have reached a point in our knowledge of behavior illnesses where close collaboration between the two disciplines is essential in order that each can continue to serve its patients well.

References

1. McKusick VA: *Mendelian Inheritance in Man*, 7th ed Baltimore, The Johns Hopkins University Press, 1986.
2. Emery AE, Rimoin DL: *Principles and Practice of Medical Genetics*, Vol 1 and 2. Edinburgh, Churchill Livingstone, 1983.

3. U.S. Department of Health and Human Services: *Comprehensive Clinical Genetic Services Centers—A National Directory.* DHHS Publication No HRS-D-MC 86-1, Washington, DC, 1985.

4. Berini RY, Kahn E (eds): *Clinical Genetics Handbook.* Oradel, New Jersey, National Genetics Foundation, Inc., Medical Economics Books, 1987.

5. Thompson JS, Thompson MW: *Genetics in Medicine,* 3rd ed. Philadelphia, WB Saunders and Co, 1979.

6. Fuller JL, Collins RL: Ethanol consumption and preference in mice: A genetic analysis. *Ann NY Acad Sci* **197**:42–48, 1972.

7. Schuckit MA: Genetic and clinical implications of alcoholism and affective disorder. *Am J Psychiatry* **143**:140–147, 1986.

8. Donovan JM: An etiologic model of alcoholism. *Am J Psychiatry* **143**:1–11, 1986.

9. Comings DE, Comings BG: Tourette syndrome: Clinical and psychological aspects of 250 cases. *Am J Hum Genet* **37**:435–450, 1985.

10. Smalley SL, Asarnow RF, Spence MA: Autism and genetics: A decade of research. Archives of Psychiatry (in press) 1988.

11. Ritvo ER, Spence MA, Freeman BJ, et al: Evidence for autosomal recessive inheritance in 46 families with multiple incidences of autism. *Am J Psychiatry* **142**:187–192, 1985.

12. Spence MA, Ritvo ER, Marazita ML, et al: Gene mapping studies with the syndrome of autism. *Behav Genet* **15**:1–13, 1985.

13. Opitz JM, Sutherland GR: Conference report: International workshop on the fragile X and X-linked mental retardation. *Am J Med Genet* **17**:5–94, 1984.

14. Egeland JA, Gerhard DS, Pauls DL, et al: Bipolar affective disorders linked to DNA markers on chromosome 11. *Nature* **325**:783–806, 1987.

15. Detera-Wadleigh SD, Berrettini WH, Goldin LR, et al: Close linkage of c-Harvey-ras-1 and the insulin gene to affective disorder is ruled out in three North American pedigrees. *Nature* **325**:806–808, 1987.

16. Baron M, Risch N, Hamburger R, et al: Genetic linkage between X chromosome markers and bipolar affective illness. *Nature:* **326**:289–292, 1987.

17. Sparkes RS, Spence MA, Mohandas T, et al: Human gene mapping, genetic linkage, and clinical applications. *Ann of Intern Med* **93**:469–479, 1980.

18. Hodge SE, Spence MA, Crandall BF, et al: Huntington disease: Linkage analysis with age-of-onset corrections. *Am J Med Genet* **5**:247–254, 1980.

19. Spence MA: Linkage methods in psychiatric disorders, in Gershon ES, Matthysse S, Breakefield XO, et al (eds).: *Genetic Research Strategies for Psychobiology and Psychiatry.* Pacific Grove, CA, The Boxwood Press, 1981, p. 295.

IV

Areas of Special Concern

15

Variations

MARGARET F. JENSVOLD

Introduction

In *The World According to Garp*,[1] a feminist mother selects a stud and proceeds to raise her offspring in a fatherless world. This delightful book, published in 1976, raised the reader's consciousness about reproductive options, motivations for their use, and potential for abuse or good in individuals' lives and in the greater whole of society. Today, many new reproductive options are available, with more on the horizon.

How is the mental health professional to help the patient who is making choices or dealing with the increasing array of reproductive options? The consultation/liaison psychiatrist will be asked to render opinions in cases for which no outcome studies are available. In most cases, short- and long-term psychological and social effects of the new reproductive technologies are not known. The object of this chapter is to point out current trends and to suggest guidelines for the consultation/liaison psychiatrist working with cases on the frontiers of the burgeoning reproductive technologies. For simplicity, I will divide the subject matter into four categories: first, developments complicating genetic, gestational, and social parenting; second, prenatal diagnosis and counseling and genetic engineering; third, legal trends; and finally, implications of the preceding for mental health professionals.

Developments Complicating Genetic, Gestational, and Social Parenting

It is more true now than at any other time in history that the genetic mother, gestational mother, and social mother need not be the same person. They could be two or

Margaret F. Jensvold • Biological Psychiatry Branch, National Institute of Mental Health, National Institutes of Health, Bethesda, MD 20892.

even three different women. The genetic and social fathers need not be the same. Up to five persons could be involved as parents[2] (see Table 1).

The situation becomes even more complicated when considering grandparents' rights, as in the Baby M. case[3] in which the parents of the surrogate mother, Mary Beth Whitehead's, filed suit for grandparents' custody rights, requesting that the judge allow them visitation regardless of which set of parents was granted custody of the child. As there are 2 sets of grandparents for every "parent" involved, there may be up to 10 sets of "grandparents" for one child. Although it would be highly unlikely that all of these sets of "grandparents" would claim rights, this point illustrates the high degree of complexity that can evolve among family lines.

The fact that family lineage and social parenting may be discontinuous is not new. Adoption, artificial insemination by donor (AID), and "blended" families have been around for some time. However, the advent of newer technologies, including in vitro fertilization with and without embryo washing (IVF and IVF-ET), surrogate mothering, and gamete intrafallopian transfer (GIFT) (all of which are currently in use) increase the complexity of possibilities and further complicate issues related to "Who is the mother?" "Who is the father?" "Who has the rights and responsibilities of raising the child, once born?" "Who bears responsibilities for decisions made during pregnancy that would affect intrauterine conditions of the fetus and medical status of the gestational mother?" "Who has what rights of access to the child after birth?"

Motivations for participating as a donor in such situations are complex and varied as illustrated by some recent cases. A British judge awarded custody of a child to the

Table 1. Reproductive Variations

No.	Genetic parents	Fertilization processs	Gestational mother	Social patterns
1.	$\male_C + \male_C$	Natural	C	C + C
2.	$\female_C + \male_C$	AIH	C	C + C
3.	$\female_C + \male_C$	IVF	C	C + C
4.	$\female_C + \male_D$	AID	C	C + C
5a.	$\female_D + \male_C$	IVF	C	C + C
5b.	$\female_D + \male_C$	AI + embryo flushing	C	C + C
6.	$\female_D + \male_C$	AI	D	C + C
7a.	$\female_C + \male_C$	Natural or AI with embryo flushing	D	C + C
7b.	$\female_C + \male_C$	IVF	D	C + C
8.	$\female_D + \male_D$	Natural, AI, or IVF	D	C + C
9.	$\female_C + \male_D$	IVF	C	C + C
10.	$\female_1 + \male_2$	IVF or Natural/AI/with embryo flushing	3	4 + 5

Abbreviations: ♀ = female; ♂ = male; D = donor; C = member of couple seeking a child; AID = artificial insemination by donor; AIH = artificial insemination by husband; and IVF = in vitro fertilization.

Modified from Capron, AM, The new reproductive possibilities: Seeking a moral basis for concerted action in a pluralistic society. *Law, Medicine and Health Care* 12:192–198, 1984. Reprinted with permission.

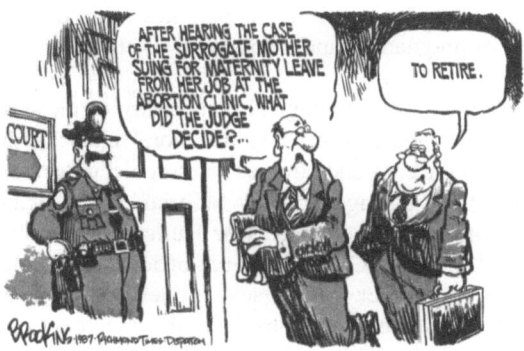

Figure 1. "Surrogate Mother." From *Richmond Times-Dispatch*. Reprinted with permission.

surrogate mother who had reneged on the contract. Shortly thereafter, she filed suit for the biological father, a physician, to pay child support. A 48-year-old woman in South Africa served as surrogate mother bearing triplets for her daughter, the genetic mother. One readily understands the judge's reaction in the Brookins cartoon shown here. (see Figure 1.)

Possible future technologies include (1) the likely implantation of a fertilized ovum into the uterus of another woman, so that the genetic and rearing mother, but not the gestational mother, are the same; or (2) the less likely, but possible, future development of an extracorporeal placenta such that the fertilized egg can develop free of the intrauterine environment. These and other future developments raise additional questions regarding the responsibilities and rights of those raising the developing fetus and child, particularly with respect to any damage to the fetus. Obviously, the legal complications are immense and the psychological and societal ramifications are almost entirely unknown.

The American College of Obstetricians and Gynecologists (ACOG) guidelines for physicians, "Ethical Issues in Surrogate Motherhood," outlines ethical issues shared by surrogate motherhood and the more commonly accepted procedure of AID, then emphasizes that special ethical issues complicate the surrogate arrangement,[4] and recommends proceeding slowly.

Similarly, surrogate mothering could be expected to share certain psychological factors in common with adoption (e.g., the desire by the child to seek out and communicate with the genetic parents, and an increased tendency for the child to feel rejected or discarded and to have self-esteem issues), or artificial insemination by donor (AID) (also seeking out the genetic parent; and in some cultures, for example, Australia, dealing with being legally labeled as an illegitimate child, with its resultant self-esteem effects).

Other psychological factors could be expected to be different (e.g., the surrogate mother's bonding to the child during gestation and struggling with awareness that she had deliberately contracted even before conception to give up the child at birth).

Certain technologies have inherently more complicated psychological ramifications than others. For instance, the sperm donor who contributes genetic material but is involved for only 15 minutes and whose identity is never known is very different from the surrogate mother who contributes not only genetic material but is intimately involved throughout the gestational period, who may experience more or less discomfort or even medical complications of pregnancy, and who is very likely to develop a strong affiliation to the child.

In addition to the inherent psychological complexity of these reproductive options, pronunciations by religious bodies regarding the moral unacceptability of certain procedures create additional concerns and stresses for some couples considering those techniques. On March 10, 1987, during the Baby M. trial, the Vatican released a 40-page document entitled, "Instruction on Respect for Human Life in Its Origin and on the Dignity of Procreation," in which Catholic church officials condemned procreative techniques resulting in conception other than by sexual intercourse between married persons. It called upon Catholic physicians to be conscientious objectors to IVF, surrogate motherhood, and AID but accepted AIH and GIFT.[5] Talmudic scholars argue that by Jewish law, surrogate mothering contracts should not exist in the first place and that existing ones are unenforceable for a number of reasons, two of which are that under Jewish law a contract can be written only on an object that exists and that there is a religious prohibition against artificial insemination except in extreme cases.[6] Thus Catholic and Jewish persons may experience anguish and guilt not only about their own infertility but about whether or not to avail themselves of existing reproductive technologies in light of religious condemnation.

Few studies have examined motivations for the outcome of use of reproductive technologies. Parker[7,8] interviewed 275 prospective surrogate mothers and found that motivations for becoming a surrogate mother included liking pregnancy and birthing without child rearing; better economic opportunities; enjoying being pregnant and getting attention; mastering guilt from other pregnancies that resulted in abortion or adoption; and pleasure similar to that which organ donors feel from giving the gift of life. One Australian study[9] of psychosocial follow-up of parents and children conceived by AID found that 84% of parents planned not to tell their offspring of their AID origins. The authors hypothesized that this might change if pending litigation would change AID children from illegitimate to legitimate status, underscoring the effect of cultural factors upon psychological status. The large majority of parents did go on to have another AID child, indicating overall satisfaction with the procedure.

Prenatal Diagnosis and Counseling and Genetic Engineering

Technological advances such as ultrasound, amniocentesis, and chorionic villi biopsy have made prenatal diagnosis possible, resulting in a whole new field—genetic counseling. Most university and many nonuniversity obstetric services have some genetic counseling facility. Prenatal testing becomes more relevant as interventions such as intrauterine surgery and abortion for genetic reasons become readily available.

These advances impact radically upon the parents' experience of a pregnancy, altering some of the normal developmental phases of adjustment to pregnancy and parenting (see Chapter 14). Genetic screening may result in stress ordinarily reserved for the time of delivery and may threaten the self-esteem of parents. Even a stable marriage may be inordinately stressed by the knowledge that a recessive gene disease endangers their fetus and future fetuses but that pregnancy with almost any other partner would result in unaffected fetuses. On the other hand, partners sharing recessive gene defects may serve as a mutual support system because they share the gene. X-linked disease may wreak more emotional havoc with the woman being "punished" for passing the gene along. Whereas parents previously "accepted God's will," now they must decide whether to conceive and whether the fetus will live or die. Many are unprepared for this responsibility.[10] Siblings may be affected, such as the child who hid in the closet when his mother returned from having a therapeutic abortion for genetic reasons.[10]

Abortions following amniocentesis must occur during the second trimester due to limitations of the technology and are more emotionally and physically traumatic than first-trimester abortions because fetal movements have been felt and the pregnancy is apparent to others.[11] The waiting period of up to several weeks for prenatal diagnostic results is typically characterized by a "suspension of commitment to the pregnancy" and postponement of the "integration" stage of pregnancy.[11]

Psychological effects of long waiting periods for results and of late abortions can be expected to improve as chorionic villi testing permits prenatal diagnoses in the first trimester and as more rapid techniques are developed for laboratory testing of the genetic material.[12]

Some of the anxiety typically experienced in the third trimester may now be experienced at the time of the decision to undergo genetic tests. Also, some of the events typically occurring at the time of delivery, such as naming the baby, informing relatives, and celebrating,[11] may now occur at the time of learning the sex and condition of the fetus.

Expansion of obstetric care to include preconception as well as early postconception counseling has been proposed, with the aim of decreasing *medical* problems, for example, diabetic complications.[13] Preconception or early postconception *psychological* counseling for the future parents could also decrease anguish or problems associated with the pregnancy and improve long-term outcome.

A thus far entirely unexplored field for the psychiatric consultant is genetic engineering. For human use the procedure is probably some years away, however, remarkable advances are already being made in animal models. For example, fertility was restored to infertile mice using gene therapy. A hereditary form of infertility was caused by a deletion mutation of about half of the gene coding for the precursor of gonadotropin-releasing hormone (GnRH) and GnRH-associated peptide (GAP) and was corrected by introducing DNA fragments containing the mouse GnRH gene into eggs later implanted into surrogate mothers. Offspring had normal hormonal levels and fertility.[14] In another example, tremors and convulsions in mice carrying the "shiverer" gene mutation were corrected with genetic engineering. Therapeutic genes injected into fertilized shiverer eggs developed into individuals free of the behavior.[15] The technique, called germline gene transplantation, is unacceptable in humans under current biotechnology guidelines, but future developments may be more acceptable. Techniques are currently being developed in sheep for in utero gene transfer.

Genetic engineering almost certainly will raise significant issues in preconception and prenatal counseling. The techniques may ultimately be considered to be a variant of in utero or even preconception surgery. An extension of fetal rights earlier and earlier in pregnancy may raise issues regarding the rights of the "future person" to genetic engineering.

Legal Trends in Reproductive Decision Making

For excellent reviews of significant legal trends impacting upon reproductive decision making, see Chapter 17 and Engelhardt's 1985 paper.[16]

Key court decisions in recent years have articulated "a secular ethics which places the locus of reproductive decision making in the hands of the reproducing couples and ultimately in the hands of the women who could become pregnant,"[16] as opposed to the locus of decision making being with the state. This is most profoundly seen with the legalization of abortion before the point of viability.

However, the ready availability of abortion implies a responsibility for informed decision making regarding whether or not to continue a pregnancy. It creates a moral tension, on the one hand, implying an obligation on the part of health care providers to inform would-be parents so they can avoid the birth of a defective child and, on the other hand, an obligation to impose treatment on behalf of the fetus even against the expressed wishes of the mother to the contrary. The salience of fetal rights increases as in utero fetal surgical procedures become available, such as laser surgery to cure a fetal tumor or placement of shunts into the kidney in utero.[10] There is no conflict of interest between the fetus and parents before viability when parents have an unchallenged right to terminate the pregnancy. The concept of a "future person" has developed in recent years and implies certain rights for the fetus after the point of viability. At what point, the rights of the future person override the rights of the mother is controversial and has been decided differently in different cases.

In summary, the secular ethics articulated by recent court decisions implies increased responsibility for parents and health care givers to provide for conditions minimizing defectiveness of this future person once the point of viability has been reached. Outcomes of this secular process include wrongful life decisions; for example, the physician whose tubal ligation procedure failed, resulting in an unwanted pregnancy, or the physician who failed to inform a woman who had had rubella that many women would choose to abort following rubella.

Many psychological questions are raised:

- What of the child who wins a wrongful life case? How will he or she feel about himself or herself having a "wrongful life"?
- What of the mother for whom cesarean section or in utero surgery is ordered against her will for the benefit of the fetus? How will her affiliative relationship with the child develop? Where will her anger be placed?

Answers to these and related questions are uncertain, but prevention of psychological problems by early intervention is the aim, and follow-up studies are needed. Changes in family legal trends create stresses and expectations for which individuals or systems are often unprepared, requiring adaptation and growth, or causing duress, regression, or psychological decompensation.

Implications for the Psychiatric Consultant

Let us consider a real-life case and its implications for the mental health consultant.

The psychiatric consultant is asked to see a couple who are considering using surrogate mothering or artificial insemination by donor or adoption in order to have a child. They had delayed childbearing. They are still grieving the death of their first and only child who died 9 weeks after birth 6 months ago. The child was born with a debilitating and lethal autosomal recessive neuromuscular illness, indicating that the parents each contributed a gene and that there is a one-in-four chance of any subsequent child having the disease. They cannot currently imagine ever going through this experience again. Furthermore, the wife's sister had a devastating course of bipolar illness and committed suicide a year ago. The couple wonder what chance the wife's offspring will have of having bipolar illness.

This complicated and fascinating real-life case raises many issues for both the consultant and consultees. The issues pertain to biological and gestational parenting and genetic counseling and legal issues.

The consultees' questions include: "How should we decide whether to opt for natural childbirth, with the risk of yet another child dying young of a debilitating illness?"

No means are available for prenatally diagnosing this autosomal recessive illness; therefore abortion for therapeutic reasons based upon prenatal diagnosis is not an option. "Should we decide upon artificial insemination by donor," using the mother's but not the father's genes, making chances of the autosomal recessive illness essentially nil but doing this still with concern regarding a family history of psychiatric illness?

"Or should we decide upon surrogate mothering?", using the father's but not the mother's genes, avoiding the autosomal recessive illness and family history of bipolar illness but with greater expense plus potentially explosive emotional and legal complications as evidenced by the Baby M. case. "Or should we adopt? Which is the best choice for us?" "What are the risks to our future offspring of developing bipolar illness in light of family history in first-degree relatives?" "How much should the risk of psychiatric illness influence our decision to have a child?"

Genetic counseling questions will almost certainly be raised more frequently as genetic markers of psychiatric illness are discovered and the public becomes more aware of genetic causes of psychiatric illness, as with the recent publicity surrounding the finding of a genetic marker for bipolar illness found on chromosome 11 in members of one large family.[17] For the consultant, many questions are raised:

- How did the husband and wife deal with the illness and death of their first child? Did they effectively grieve? How far along are they in the process? Are either of them significantly depressed? What strengths or vulnerabilities have they demonstrated in dealing with this loss? Are they "ready yet" psychologically to start again?
- How has this experience affected their relationship to one another?
- What are their conscious and unconscious motivations for having another child and for considering each of the reproductive options?
- What are their fears regarding each of the reproductive options?
- What are the psychological meanings to this couple of having an unhealthy child? What are their fears of being childless?
- What was the significance to them of the sister's bipolar illness? What are their fears about it? Are they still grieving from her death?

A consultant must also consider the larger moral and legal question: What responsibility does a consulting psychiatrist have to warn parents prior to or shortly after conception of risks of future illness? Will the psychiatrist be held liable for not warning?

The consultant may consider doing grief work for the couple in this example.

In short, the consultant mental health professional must attend to issues of process as well as of content. Conscious as well as unconscious motivations and fears should be looked for and explored. The consultant at times will play an educative role and at times a facilitative role, using standard psychotherapeutic techniques of support, clarification, ventilation, confrontation, and interpretation.

Long-term psychological and psychosocial outcomes of most of the newer technologies are not known, but attention to the needs and outlooks of the individuals involved, the conscious as well as unconscious motivations and fears, process issues and weighing risks and benefits will help the individuals in making their decisions and coping with them. Attention to these issues will help individuals or couples to come to their own decisions about what is right for them and to deal with their losses in a manner that is adaptive and growth oriented, rather than maladaptive or regressive.

At times, the mental health professional may have the opportunity to assist in the development of psychological screening or treatment programs, for example, (1) developing screening programs for couples or individuals considering becoming involved with surrogate motherhood or for couples considering AID; or (2) developing educational or support groups, for example, for infertile couples or for couples going through IVF; or (3) adding a psychological support component to a genetic counseling program (see Chapter 14).

On a broader level, mental health professionals can become involved via ethics committees or legal or political bodies in setting standards for the newer reproductive technologies, insisting that standards be built that will likely optimize the psychological adjustment of the parties involved. For example, the psychiatric consultant might play a role in requiring that potential surrogate mothers be screened regarding their psychological stability, motivations and preparedness to give up the child, or requiring psychological screening and psychological support for couples seeking to embark upon the costly and often emotionally trying process of IVF.

Mitchell and Thompson,[18] in their review of methodological issues in consultation/liaison psychiatry, found a recent shift from descriptive to outcome-oriented research and concluded that the latter should be the direction of the future.

New technologies have been integrated into obstetric care with minimal attention to psychological effects on individuals, families, or society. We would caution against untempered enthusiasm for new procedures as learned in the case of retrolental fibroplasia. Long-range consequences are less examined than the techniques themselves. Without established guidelines, for instance, for surrogate mothering, confusion, frustration, and embarrassment ensue. Offspring are not necessarily at risk of physical harm but of psychosocial harm.[4] There are not yet enough data to draw mental health conclusions about the newer reproductive technologies, but we should follow prospectively and provide services rather than react after the fact. A number of authors argue that at least as important as the new technologies are services for the affected children and families.[11]

Advances in the reproductive technologies make newspaper headlines daily. The Baby M. case occupied our collective consciousness for months and spawned strong opinions among many who hadn't previously held opinions upon the subject.[19] Multiparenting, prenatal diagnosis and interventions, and changing legal trends are altering the character of reproductive decision making. Reproductive advances such as surrogate mothering, in vitro fertilization, and genetic engineering fascinate us precisely because they cut at the core of our very being. They force us to ask questions about ourselves, about the nature of being human, and about the nature of our relationships to one another. How much will we actively shape our progeny even before their conception or birth? Things that once seemed simple no longer are. In this field, we continue the perennial human task—that of coming to know ourselves better.

References

1. Irving J: *The World According to Garp*. New York, Pocket Books, 1976.
2. Capron AM: The new reproductive possibilities: Seeking a moral basis for concerted action in a pluralistic society. *Law, Medicine and Health Care* **12**:192–198, 1984.
3. *White vs Stern:* New Jersey Superior Court, March 30, 1987.
4. Robertson JA: Surrogate mothers: Not so novel after all. *The Hastings Center Report* **13**:28–34, 1983.
5. Woodward KL, Cohn B, Springen K: Rules for making love and babies: Opposing many artificial aids to conception, the Vatican generates heat as well as enlightenment. *Newsweek,* March 23, 1987, pp 42–43.
6. Borden ME: A Jewish look at surrogate mothers. Jewish Chronicle of Pittsburgh, March 30, 1987, p 9.
7. Parker P: Surrogate mothers' motivations: Initial findings. *Am J Psychiatry* **140**:117–118, 1983.
8. Parker P: Surrogate motherhood, psychiatric screening and informed consent, baby selling, and public policy. *Bull Am Acad Psychiatry Law* **12**:21–39, 1984.
9. Leeton J, Backwell J: A preliminary psychosocial follow-up of parents and their children conceived by artificial insemination by donor (AID). *Clin Reprod Fertility* **1**:307–310, 1982.
10. Andrew LB: *New Conceptions: A Consumer's Guide to the Newest Infertility Treatment*. New York, St. Martin's Press, 1984, pp 87–95, 135–145, 182–187, 207–208, 221–223.
11. Beeson D, Douglas R, Lunsford TF: Prenatal diagnosis of fetal disorders (Part II): Issues and implications *Birth* **10**:233–241, 1983.
12. Embury SH, Scharf SJ, Saiki RK, et al: Rapid prenatal diagnosis of sickle cell anemia by a new method of DNA analysis. *New Engl J Med* **11**:656–661, 1987.
13. Hollingsworth DR, Jones OW, Resnik R: Expanded care in obstetrics for the 1980's: Preconception and early postconception counseling. *Am J Obstet Gynecol* **149**:811–814, 1984.
14. Mason AJ, Pitts SL, Nikolics K, et al: The hypogonadal mouse: Reproductive functions restored by gene therapy. *Science* **234**:1372–1378, 1986.
15. Readhead C, Popko B, Takahasni N, et al: Expression of a myelin basic protein gene in transgenic shiverer mice: Correction of the dysmyelinating phenotype. *Cell* **48**:703–712, 1987.
16. Englehardt HT: Current controversies in obstetrics: Wrongful life and forced fetal surgical procedures. *Am J Obstet Gynecol* **151**:313–318, 1985.
17. Egeland JA, Gerhard DS, Pauls DL, et al: Bipolar affective disorders linked to DNA markers on chromosome 11. *Nature* **325**:783–787, 1987.
18. Mitchell WD, Thompson TL: Some methodological issues in consultation/liaison psychiatry research. *Gen Hosp Psychiatry* **7**:66–72, 1985.
19. Fleming AT: Our fascination with Baby M. *New York Times Magazine,* 33, pp 35–36, 87–88, March 29, 1987.

For additional information consult:

1. Richardson JW: The role of a psychiatric consultant to an artificial insemination by donor program. *Psychiatr Ann* **17**:101–105, 1987.
2. Sarrel PM, DeCherney AH: Psychotherapeutic intervention for treatment of couples with secondary infertility. *Fertil Steril* **43**:897–900, 1985.

16

The Current Controversy in Childbirth Care

A Consultant's Viewpoint

RICHARD L. COHEN

Introduction

Because young adults of childbearing age are exposed almost daily to opinions and "data" from the proponents of the various childbirth schools of thought (whether in the electronic and print media or through family and social contacts), there tends to be a sense of uncertainty about what is best for them and their infant-to-be. How they arrive at decisions about what kind of care is most appropriate for them has been discussed in the preceding chapter. Many of the arguments have become so emotionally charged that the mental health consultant may find a more dispassionate (if that is possible) exposition of the issues useful in working with families and caregivers. That is the basic purpose of this chapter. As is often the case, it is best to begin by letting the actors in the "drama" speak for themselves. The following are verbatim excerpts from tape-recorded interviews that I have conducted over the past few years.

Interviews with the Principal Actors

Dr. L. is a 35-year-old neonatologist interviewed in his office at a prestigious university hospital in the northeastern United States. After some description of his daily activities and the excitement he finds in his work, particularly with high risk neonates, the interview moves into the area of discussion of out-of-hospital options for childbirth:

Richard L. Cohen • Department of Psychiatry, Western Psychiatric Institute and Clinic, University of Pittsburgh, Pittsburgh, PA 15213.

Dr. C.:   What is your general reaction to what seems to be a growing interest in out-of-hospital delivery on the part of young parents?

Dr. L.:   I'm unalterably opposed to the whole idea. For me, it represents the epitome of *me*ism.

Dr. C.:   Why do you say that?

Dr. L.:   I think these people are saying, "To hell with what might be some risk for my baby. The only thing that's important to me is my personal experience."

Dr. C.:   Doesn't that seem a bit harsh?

Dr. L.:   Not at all. In my opinion, out-of-hospital deliveries are the last form of child abuse that is legitimate.

Dr. C.:   Do you feel that any of the complaints about high-technology obstetrics and the impersonal care in some hospitals are justified?

Dr. L.:   Sure they are. That's always going to be the case, and I don't think it has anything to do with high technology. Some doctors and nurses just aren't very people oriented in their care. They would be the same way regardless of the level of technology.

Dr. C.:   Is it possible that the growing movement toward high-technology care may become the focus of management itself, a kind of belief system that gets in the way of individualized care?

Dr. L.:   Again, that can happen with any system. One concern I have about the various childbirth education and natural childbirth groups is that they are becoming just as rigid and doctrinaire as some of the traditional obstetricians. What the hell good is that when they are preaching individualized care?

Dr. C.:   Do you think all families and newborns really need high-technology care?

Dr. L.:   Yes. I think everybody should have the advantage of the latest advances of medicine. In fact, I don't think there is any excuse anymore for a normal or custodial newborn nursery. They should all be closed, and the staffs should be combined with the high-risk groups so that all families get one level of extremely expert surveillance and management.

Mrs. J. is a 27-year-old attorney who lives in a large metropolitan area in southern California. She is obviously very thoughtful, very articulate, and very considered in her judgments. At this point in the interview, she describes her reaction to the reading she did during her first pregnancy and then to a hospital tour provided by staff of the university hospital located a short distance from her office. The gynecologist/obstetrician whom she has used since her adolescence is a full-time faculty member on the staff of that hospital. As a result of her experience during her pregnancy, she made a decision to deliver in an out-of-hospital birthing center.

Dr. C.:   What kind of reading were you doing during your pregnancy?

Mrs. J.:   Well, for a long period, I never questioned that the famous university hospital where my obstetrician was on staff wasn't the ideal place to have my baby. The more I read, the more I felt there was real chaos in the field of obstetrics and newborn care. So many contradictory articles and practices. When there are 500 ways to do the same thing, it means to me that nobody knows what to do.

Dr. C.:   Did the hospital provide any classes or orientation for you?

Mrs. J.:   Yes. We were taken on a tour of the hospital. Right away we were told that there were three different places we had to sign permission papers when I came in in labor! My husband would be separated for at least an hour right at the beginning. Then you would have to be examined by a strange resident you never saw before. The labor rooms were obviously constructed to get as many as possible on a floor. Very austere and bare with IVs and monitors and a very uncomfortable little stool without a back for the husband. For me, that was a symbol. Yes, my husband could be there, but they would see to it that he was not comfortable for 10 or 12 hours. They also said once you were in a labor bed you were not allowed out. If you wanted to turn, you had to call an R.N. to get your monitor adjusted.

We went to the delivery room, and it was unbelievably cold. We were told it was kept that way (63 °F) because the staff has to wear gowns and masks and they get too uncomfortable if its warmer than that but not to worry about the baby because they are put into an incubator immediately. Then the R.N. who was touring us said that while he's in that incubator he gets his vitamin K injection. I had never heard of that. She said it was a state law. I later learned that she was an OB nurse. What she was talking about was the screening for PKU. My God, this was a university hospital! Later, we met some of the neonatal nurses. It was clear from the beginning that there was almost no communication between the OB nurses and the neonatal nurses. The OB nurse didn't even know what PKU was when I asked her.

Then we looked at the recovery room with 20 beds in it. There were women coming out of anesthesia moaning and groaning next to little unmarried teenagers who were giving up their babies and scared to death—next to mothers and fathers who were trying very uncomfortably to bond with their new babies.

We went to the new nursery which was built largely with research funds, we were told. It sounded like any excuse possible was used to get the baby into that intensive care unit so it could be studied—like it was too large or too small or too old or too young or there were little squiggles on the monitor tracing—a long list of criteria. It was like a museum—a fishbowl. It meant total separaration from your baby for the first 24 hours whether there was really anything wrong or not.

My husband and I looked at each other and decided right there that this was not for us. We were not going to go through all of this and pay $3000–$4000 to boot.

DR. C.:   So what did you do then?

MRS. J.:   It was very hard to tell my obstetrician that we had made this decision. We've been very close. I had used her as a gynecologist for years. I knew she'd be hurt. I told her I was going to use a midwife program. I received a letter from her which was very angry, very hurt. She also said she would not accept any responsibility for me as a patient until the postpartum period was completely over. She was really washing her hands of me. When you're pregnant, no matter how stable you are, you're kind of emotional and vulnerable, and I was sort of devastated by this because I had secret misgivings about whether I was right to buck the system and getting a letter like that really shook me up. If something went wrong, she would really slam the door in my face.

Mrs. Y. is the president of the board of directors of an alternative birthing center in a large eastern city. Mrs. B. is the nurse–midwife director of that unit. They were interviewed together in order to learn more about the philosophy of their unit and their experience with practicing obstetricians in their metropolitan area.

DR. C.:   What kinds of families come to you for care?

MRS. Y.:   Our clients have read a good bit and have been informed much more than the usual "run of shad" that walks into the nearest clinic or doctor and says, "Here I am. Take over." That is a point of view with which I have very little sympathy. Our clients have an overriding concern about the welfare of their child that forces them to investigate things.

Dr. C.:   Would it help to maintain a better working relationship with obstetrics if you had students and house officers rotating through your program?

Mrs. Y.:   We think it is very important to maintain the privacy and intimacy of the family experience. We will not declare open season for interns and students. They tend to destroy the intimacy of the entire process. Anyway, M.D.s have an exclusive interest in sickness, and they want to do everything that they have learned about sickness to you whether you are sick or not. We say to parents, "You tell us what you want done. You run the show." We are militant only in our belief that people should have options. We are not militant about specifics of our program. We feel we have a tradition of being innovative.

Dr. C.:   You seem to focus your attention on the medical profession. What about nursing?

Mrs. B.:   I think OB nurses ought to be taught low-risk, primary care. They shouldn't be given more skills than that in obstetrics. Then they become like physicians. If you teach them that stuff, then they feel compelled to use those skills whether or not the patient needs them.

Dr. C.:   The kind of one-to-one care you are talking about is extremely expensive these days. Is it realistic to ask hospitals to provide that kind of individualized attention?

Mrs. B.:   Yes, one-to-one care may be expensive, but it's not as expensive as supporting the whole new technology, the medical/industrial complex with its salesmen, P.R. people, and its factories, technicians, etc. You have to remember that there are now about 20,000 obstetricians and gynecologists in the United States. Their current pattern of practice cannot and should not be maintained simply to protect their economic base. They can go on salary just like anybody else and practice gynecology, screen OB patients for risk levels, and practice high-risk obstetric care where it is indicated.

Dr. C.:   Have you really made an active effort to collaborate more closely with obstetricians in this city?

Mrs. B.:   I think obstetrics has a kind of seige mentality now in relation to places like ours, to consumer groups, to insurance companies, regulating bodies, etc. They have pulled up the drawbridge, and it's only the rare obstetrician who is secure enough and courageous enough to stand outside the castle.

Mrs. C. is a master's-level perinatal nursing supervisor in a university hospital. She views herself as a highly skilled, intelligent professional who is delivering a much needed service to parents and babies, and she sees herself at the cutting edge of modern obstetric practice.

Dr. C.:   A good many mothers and childbirth educators seem to be turned off by the way electronic fetal monitoring is being used. Many seem to feel that it has intruded itself into the exciting and personal experience of childbirth.

Mrs. C.:   Mostly, I think that is due either to ignorance or defensiveness on the part of professionals. Lots of prepared childbirth instructors are like old-time obstetricians in some ways. When parents ask what is this fetal monitoring stuff, they do not want to admit that they're really not familiar with the details. They may say, "Oh well, I've been delivering babies for years without it, and I don't have any problems. Who really needs this new-fangled technical stuff." The fact is, when problems start in labor, they are often hard to predict ahead of time, and they come very quickly.

Dr. C.:   What do you think electronic fetal monitoring has contributed to the process?

Mrs. C.:   Before fetal monitoring, you could really only follow the condition of the mother in labor, not how much labor the baby could bear. You know, there are two patients. If they don't allow me to use the monitor, they are tying my hands. Then, I can't really look at how one of my patients [the fetus] is doing. That isn't fair.

Dr. C.: What is your answer to the claim that fetal monitoring has caused a marked increase in the use of cesarean sections?

Mrs. C.: If the C-section rate has gone up because of more appropriate obstetrical care with attention to what the fetus can tolerate early, so what. Maybe we weren't doing enough of them before and allowed too many babies to be damaged.

Dr. C.: I've heard people say that the electronic fetal monitor has become a kind of hardware stand-in for the doctor who really ought to be there in attendance. What's your attitude about that?

Mrs. C.: It's not realistic anymore to ask the MD to be in attendance all through labor and delivery. Those days are gone. But if the MD is to practice "perineal obstetrics," which means "don't call me until the patient is ready," then you must provide the nurse with all the tools available to take care of the maternal-fetal unit. It is not fair to say to the nurse, "You can take care of the mother. However, you'll just have to guess how the baby is doing. But that baby had better turn out good, or I'll want to know why you didn't call me sooner."

To learn something about how a nurse-midwife functioning in an alternative birthing center might react to the preceding comments, I played portions of the tape of that interview (with extreme care at maintaining anonymity) at a staff meeting I attended in an alternative birthing center in a different city. The responses of the nurse–midwife staff to Mrs. C.'s comments are fairly summarized by the comments of Mrs. McM.

Mrs. McM.: The first statement that we couldn't follow the status of the fetus before fetal monitoring is ridiculous. We did and we do. That sounds like somebody who has become completely dependent upon a machine, like Linus on his blanket. I'll bet they do need constant electronic monitoring there in that hospital after everything they do to the women like placing them flat on their backs, giving them pitocin, and overmedicating them. Somehow I get the impression from that tape that she seems critical that professionals like us get "involved" with our patients! We can only assume that she keeps her distance.

Dr. G. is a full-time faculty member in a university hospital and has been practicing obstetrics for over 10 years. He is now an associate professor and enjoys a good reputation among his colleagues and with the house officers and students.

Dr. C.: My impression is that there may be a good bit more heat than light in the current controversy about how to deliver childbirth care. What do you think?

Dr. G.: Part of the problem is that consumers are so much more organized and vocal. One woman has a bad experience with childbirth, goes out and writes a book, gets interviewed on television and, suddenly, thousands of woman are influenced by this. We need to mount a countercampaign of education, but we don't do it.

Dr. C.: Can you be objective about out-of-hospital births?

Dr. G.: I don't know. I try. There is an obstetrician here in town who has assisted at some of these and has even done a few home deliveries. I think these families are getting cheated. What my colleague describes is a situation where you have bad visibility because the lighting is so poor and where you are very nervous about something going wrong and not having the right people or equipment to turn to in an emergency. You are concerned about sanitary conditions and, in one situation where he was working, there were not only seven family members in the room but two of them were small children. I don't have any objection to fathers being present. That often helps. But delivering a baby in a crowd with a couple of scared and confused children there and several older women giving advice— damnit, that's just too many cooks in the kitchen. The bottom line is, if something goes wrong, you're it. Not the grandmother or the labor assistant.

DR. C.:   Don't you see some advantage to having a more natural and homelike environment in which childbirth can take place?

DR. G.:   Yes, of course, there may be some advantages. I think the trade-off of being in a modern hospital with all of the latest advances available to you versus being in a homelike environment is just no contest. So there are some inconveniences and unpleasantness in being a patient in a hospital. Big deal! The stakes are pretty high, and you are only in there for a few days. You can damn well bet I wouldn't let my wife or my daughter try it.

Mrs. K. is a special education teacher also trained in physical therapy. She works in a large rehabilitation institute and recently delivered her first child who is now a healthy and normally developing 2-month-old boy. At this point in the interview, Mrs. K. was discussing a friend of hers who had decided to have her baby at home delivered by a lay midwife.

MRS. K.:   I guess our friendship almost broke up over it. In fact, she is probably still so sore at me that things may never be the same between us.

DR. C.:   What happened between you?

MRS. K.:   You don't work in a place like this for 6 or 7 years without being pretty uptight all through your pregnancy. The ultrasound examination helped, and I don't know what I would have done without my obstetrician who kept reassuring me that everything was okay. You can't believe some of the fantasies that went through my mind in the middle of the night about the baby. I think you are really taking somebody else's life in your hands and playing God a little bit when you don't avail yourself of the most advanced medical care there is during your pregnancy and during your delivery. I know how little it takes for things to go wrong, and I know some of the horrible situations we have here in our program which might have been prevented had a well-trained neonatologist been on the spot when the baby was delivered—or maybe if the mother had had a C-section instead of going through a 28-hour labor. People are just so damn hard-headed and ignorant about these things. I always thought Sylvia [her friend] was a very sharp lady. She's really been suckered in by all this touchy, feely stuff about childbirth.

It may be patently obvious by this time that there is not only a wide variety of viewpoints about what is the most desirable kind of childbirth care, a situation neither unusual nor undesirable, but also that positions have become polarized and many voices have become strident.

Beyond the rhetoric, what we seem to hear on one side is that families who are interested in naturalistic, out-of-hospital childbirth care are concerned only about their own personal experiences and not enough about the welfare of the baby, and that parents who opt for this kind of service are really not as well informed as they claim to be because they are not weighing advantages against disadvantages for themselves and for the baby. What we seem to hear from the other side of the aisle is that obstetricians have become too procedure oriented, that they are approaching pregnancy as an illness instead of a healthy developmental experience, that they have become excessively dependent on technology versus individualized care, and that they are exploiting pregnant families by exposing them to unnecessary tertiary care both for professional reasons and for economic gain.

It is my conviction that the mental health consultant needs to be well informed about the issues in this controversy because many tensions arise in caregiving situations that are unrelated to the basic facts of the clinical picture. They may, in fact, be connected with unresolved turf issues, with unexpressed hostility between caregivers and consumers, or may spring from resentment on the part of professionals toward administrators, policymakers, or regulators who may be perceived as interfering with their best clinical judgment or the welfare of the patient.

It is not the function of the consultant to resolve these matters on a factual or scientific basis. If it were, the poor consultant would be at sea. My own reaction to many of the arguments is that they are often very convincing. I sometimes have found myself agreeing with everyone!

Most of the research aimed at studying efficacy, risk-benefit ratios, or long-term outcome of one form of care versus another is methodologically weak. Much of what is referred to as scientific literature is merely based on anecdotal reports extolling the advantages of one type of care over all others.

The medical/obstetric literature cannot really claim any greater degree of objectivity than literature emerging from nonmedical or alternative health care sources. The oft-quoted example of the perineal shave is the classical case in point. In an effort to reduce child-bed fever, millions of women endured the discomfort and indignity of having their perineal areas shaved while in labor as a result of reports in the obstetric literature around the turn of the century that indicated that the incidence of infection could be greatly reduced by such a procedure. It was not until the 1960s that controlled clinical trials were conducted by Burchell,[1] by Kantor,[2] and others. These indicated that, as long as the area was properly scrubbed, shaving had little or no effect on the actual incidence of infection. Even more recent reports about the relative advantages of procedures that seem to have a more scientific base such as electronic fetal monitoring have been seriously challenged by studies that have attempted to replicate results. The work of Banta and Thacker[3] challenging the use of electronic fetal monitoring except in high-risk situations has caused major controversy among proponents on both sides of the question. Haverkamp's[4,5] studies of electronic fetal monitoring would appear to support the work of Banta and Thacker, yet there are innumerable studies[6-9] that certainly seem to suggest that electronic fetal monitoring has considerable value in evaluating the level of distress of the fetus during labor, and, as such, may be quite useful as a marker for determining at what point more radical intervention (such as cesarean section) may be indicated.

The several publications of Mehl[10-12] that appear to indicate the relative safety, efficacy, and excellent outcome of out-of-hospital birthing approaches have also been criticized because of design flaws and lack of adequate matching with control populations.

Many of the most often-quoted examples from the alternative birthing literature merely represent the viewpoints of the author and large numbers of women who have been interviewed and have had excellent birthing experiences with low-risk pregnancies in the home or out-of-hospital centers. They tend to be unipolar in their judgments and lack adequate balance in their presentation of advantages and disadvantages for one approach over another. The consultant would do well to familiarize himself or herself with the most commonly quoted of these works because they have had a strong influence on consumers and on health providers in the alternative health systems. Most prominent among these are the works of Milinaire,[13] Oakley,[14] Arms,[15] Corea,[16] and Stewart and Stewart.[17,18]

For a more detailed explication of the problems and pitfalls in conducting research in this field, the reader is referred to several excellent publications. For instance, issues that plague clinical investigation in this field are outlined in exhaustive detail in a volume published jointly by the Division of Health Sciences Policy of the Institute of Medicine and the Commission on Life Sciences of the National Research Council. These two bodies appointed a joint committee on assessing alternative birth settings. The report[19] of that group, entitled *Research Issues in the Assessment of Birth Settings* should be required reading for all obstetricians and allied health professionals. It is a humbling and painfully honest document.

Chard and Richards[20] have written very persuasively about the risks of making causal inferences in obstetric practice. Adamson and Gare[21] conclude in a particularly useful paper about the relative merits of home versus hospital births that the present data are too inconclusive to support any position in a convincing manner.

Given the number of confounding variables and the need for evaluating long-term rather than short-term outcome, it is understandable that the field is beset with methodologic boobytraps. The most troubling aspects of these studies is not so much their relatively weak design but rather a surprising and simplistic belief system that suggests that there are one-to-one relationships between a given prenatal or perinatal event and long-term outcome in the child and/or family. Except in the most extreme circumstances, everything we have learned about human development mitigates against such a belief system. For instance, to suggest that a certain period of skin-to-skin contact between baby and mother will result in better long-term relationship between them seems just as unsupportable a position as to suggest that two or three late deceleration curves on a fetal monitoring tracing are indicative of a baby with a seriously impaired central nervous system.

In the concluding chapter, we will consider many of the implications of the dilemma and make some recommendations for mental health professionals who have an interest in contributing to clinical investigation into childbirth care. In the meantime, some conceptual grasp of the underlying conflicts at work in the field is important in carrying out one's everyday clinical tasks.

My own conclusion about the basic issues in this controversy is that they have comparatively little to do with medical versus nonmedical procedures (especially because many of the protagonists on both sides are physicians.) The more dynamic and, therefore, perhaps more relevant issues for the mental health consultant, appear to be very much related to the questions of the following:

1. Locus of control issues that have become intertwined with the feminist movement and with the fact that obstetrics is still basically a male dominated profession, whereas the alternative health system is primarily initiated and managed by women.
2. Economic issues that have pitted the interests of a large and complex medical/scientific/industrial complex against those of consumer and regulatory forces.

3. Philosophical issues that have to do with theoretical constructs of pregnancy as a healthy state versus pregnancy as an at-risk medical condition akin to illness.

If these conclusions are accurate, it becomes quite important for the mental health consultant to be acutely aware of their presence and to factor these questions into any assessment and recommendations because they may be individually or collectively influential in determining both the presenting picture and the conclusions and recommendations of the consultant.

The expert consultant addresses these (often indirectly) and in a manner that facilitates a maximum of emotional comfort for the patient and caregiver.

It must also be obvious from the foregoing that there is a crying need for well-designed, long-term outcome studies that incorporate both biomedical and psychosocial variables. So many of the studies have relied heavily on mortality rates or morbidity rates (such as infection, learning disabilities in the offspring, postpartum psychosis, etc.) that are either so gross or so simplistic that they are not true measures of the overall outcome of a given approach or procedure. What is sorely needed is a series of collaborative studies planned by behavioral scientists and childbirth personnel both in the conventional and alternative birthing systems. These should provide opportunities to study developmental outcome in both the family and child. Such studies are not taking place at this writing, in part because genuine collaboration between the two streams of health care is almost nonexistent.

Although the mental health professional cannot be assigned the role of bringing these two "camps" together, he or she can play a role in identifying the basic issues and in stimulating a more careful and considered examination of the relative merits of all approaches based on long-term outcome. Such studies are probably impossible without the intensive involvement of well-trained mental health professionals.

Thankfully, it is appropriate to end this chapter on a modest optimistic note. A tendency toward the mean appears to be a powerful force in most human behavior, and there are some signs that various schools of thought are beginning to learn important lessons from each other (though not always acknowledging due credit).

On the one hand, there seems to be an increasing inclination on the part of out-of-hospital birthing centers to seek input from obstetricians and pediatricians in screening and monitoring risk levels of their clients and in being immediately available at birth to assess the status of the neonate. In many states, third-party reimbursers such as Blue Cross are beginning to recognize the professional contribution of such centers and to underwrite at least a portion of the cost of care for families. National standards are beginning to surface for professional care in alternative birthing centers, which is always a sign of increasing professionalism and accountability.

There is a growing tendency for the development of programs that better integrate the advantages of the medical model with those of alternative center birthing (e.g., Feinbloom[22]).

In hospitals, there is now emerging a greater acceptance of so-called birthing rooms that are separated from but contiguous to the conventional labor and delivery suites and that are more homelike in their atmosphere. These allow involvement and participation of family members and permit much more decision making on the part of the woman in labor to deliver her baby with more freedom, to move around and assume positions that are comfortable and facilitating to the progress of delivery. One also sees the growing number of consultation and liaison programs in obstetric units and hospitals and the development of classes that are not simply preparation for labor and delivery but focus on preparation for parenting for first-time parents.

There is also a healthy process emerging in which realistic limits for the application of high-technology approaches are being considered by members of the medical community (e.g., Friedman[23]).

These straws in the wind are important because they may presage a trend toward increasing communication and collaboration between various schools of thought with growing opportunities for well-designed research on the efficacy of various service models.

References

1. Burchell RC: Predelivery removal of pubic hair. *Obstet Gynecol* **24**:271–273, 1964.
2. Kantor HI, Rember R, Tabio P: Value of shaving the pudendal-perineal area in delivery. *Obstet Gynecol* **25**:509–512, 1965.
3. Banta HD, Thacker SB: *Costs and Benefits of Electronic Fetal Monitoring: A Review of the Literature.* Washington, D.C., Office of Health, Statistics and Technology, National Center for Health Services Research, 1978.
4. Haverkamp A, et al: The evaluation of continuous fetal heart rate monitoring in high risk pregnancy. *Am J Obstet Gynecol* **125**:310–320, 1976.
5. Haverkamp A, et al: A controlled trial of the differential effects of intrapartum fetal monitoring. *Am J Obstet Gynecol* **134**:399–412, 1979.
6. Kelly VC, Kulkarni D: Experiences with fetal monitoring in a community hospital. *Obstet Gynecol* **41**:818–824, June 1973.
7. Freeman RK: The clinical value of antepartum fetal heart rate monitoring, in Gluck L (ed): *Modern Perinatal Medicine.* Chicago, Yearbook Medical Publishers, 1974, pp 163–178.
8. Liu DTY, Blackwell RJ, Tukel S: The relevance of antenatal and intrapartum fetal heart rate patterns to fetal outcome. *Br J Obstet Gynaecol* **85**:270–277, April 1978.
9. Dalton K, Dawson A, Gough N: Long distance telemetry of fetal heart rate from patients' homes using public telephone network. *Br Med J* May 1983, p 1545.
10. Mehl LE: Complications of home birth. *Birth and Family J* **24**:123–131, 1975.
11. Mehl LE: Statistical outcomes of home delivery: Comparison to similarly selected hospital deliveries. Presented at the First Annual Meeting of the National Association of Parents and Professionals for Safe Alternatives in Childbirth, Washington, DC, May 1976.
12. Mehl LE: Outcomes of elective home births: A series of 1146 cases. *J Reprod Med* **19**:281–290, November 1977.
13. Millinaire C: *BIRTH.* New York: Harmony Books, 1974.
14. Oakley A: Women confined: Towards a sociology of childbirth. New York, Schocken Books, 1980.
15. Arms S: *Immaculate Deception.* Boston, Houghton Mifflin, 1975.
16. Corea G: *The Hidden Malpractice: How American Medicine Mistreats Women.* New York: Jove Books, 1977.
17. Stewart D, Stewart L: *21st Century Obstetrics Now,* Vols 1 and 2. Chapel Hill, NC, NAPSAC, Inc 1977.
18. Stewart D, Stewart L: *Safe Alternatives in Childbirth.* Chapel Hill, NC, NAPSAC, 1977.
19. Institute of Medicine and National Research Council: *Research Issues in the Assessment of Birth Settings.* Washington, DC, National Academy Press, 1982.
20. Chard T, Richards M (eds): *Benefits and Hazards of the New Obstetrics, Clinics in Developmental Medicine,* ed 64. London, William Heinemann Medical Books, 1977.

21. Adamson GD, Gare DJ: Home or hospital births? *JAMA* **243:**1732–1736, 1980.
22. Feinbloom RI: A proposed alliance of midwives and family practitioners in the care of low risk pregnant women. *BIRTH* **13:**109–113, 1986.
23. Friedman, EA: The obstetrician's dilemma: How much fetal monitoring and cesarean section is enough? *New Engl J Med* **315:**641–643, 1986.

17

Professional Responsibility for the Welfare of Potential Life

GEORGE A. HUBER, KATHLEEN R. NEGLEY, AND
LOREN H. ROTH

Introduction

Most physicians who treat women are, from time to time, confronted with pregnant patients whose treatment will affect the welfare of the patient, the fetus, or both. Treatment may or may not be lifesaving for the mother and thereby only indirectly involve the fetus, or the treatment may directly involve the fetus, requiring invasive diagnostic or therapeutic procedures. The patient may or may not agree with either type of treatment. Also, during the course of assessment or treatment, the physician may discover that certain maternal activities are potentially injurious to the fetus, for example, substance abuse or self-mutilation. Finally, there is a growing concern about the care of patients who are not pregnant but who have the potential for becoming so and about new societal trends in surrogate parenting and in vitro fertilization.

The psychiatrist is no exception to these experiences and is perhaps called upon in the most complex of such circumstances because of the specialty's close association with social and legal systems. The psychiatrist's expertise lends itself to consultation in cases regarding psychosocial or ethical/legal issues such as these. Therefore, the purpose of this chapter is to provide an awareness of the complex issues involved to the attending or consulting physician and psychiatrist when there is concern about harm to potential life because of the patient's action or inaction. One evidence of a growing societal concern for potential life and of the movement to ensure fetal rights is the recognition of the fetus' legal existence.

Consequently, the status of the fetus serves as a beginning point, and we begin by

George A. Huber, Kathleen R. Negley, and Loren H. Roth • Department of Psychiatry, Western Psychiatric Institute and Clinic, University of Pittsburgh, Pittsburgh, PA 15213.

summarizing the evolution of the rights bestowed upon the fetus by the courts. This historical base provides the foundation for the discussion of the recent court cases involving the fetus. These court cases have been divided into two sections: (1) competing interests of maternal and fetal rights and (2) medical malpractice. The summary of court cases is followed by a discussion of suggestions to limit physician liability and to optimize professional care for potential life and the patient. The chapter concludes with a glimpse at the issues of the future.

Evolution of Fetal Rights

Beginning with the Romans, Curran traces the history of law as it relates to the human fetus and the rights of women.[1] In Roman law, the fetus was not considered to be a legal entity but rather a part of the woman's body. The concept of "viability" did not exist. Apparently, at that time, there was no liability for injury to the fetus while in utero. The first reference to viability occurred many centuries later in the writings of Sir Edward Coke. Coke observed in 1644 that killing of the fetus in the womb after quickening was a serious misdemeanor but was not murder.

Blackstone, during the eighteenth century, in his analysis of the laws of England, addressed the critical issue involving the applicability of the law to the fetus after quickening.[2] English courts used the work of Blackstone to support the crime of abortion after quickening. According to Curran, it was not until 1803 that English law first recognized abortion after quickening as a felony punishable by death. After 1837, all reference to quickening was removed, and the penalty was reduced to a prison term of 15 years to life.

After the mid-1800s, the English and American legal systems recognized abortion as a crime.[3] However, at about the same time, the idea of therapeutic abortion to protect the life of the mother was beginning its evolution as an exception to the prohibitions against abortion. By the 1940s, the American states had adopted the exception by statute. Contrary to the objections of some religious groups, notably the Roman Catholics, the law was being applied in such a manner to support the contention that the life of the pregnant woman had a higher relative value than the potential life of the fetus.[4] Such application was based upon the concept of medical necessity and that if *both* the lives of the fetus and the mother could not be preserved, the mother's life should prevail.

Even the renowned 1973 abortion decision of the United States Supreme Court in *Roe v. Wade* does not bestow upon the fetus a legal value equal to or greater than the life of the pregnant woman.[5] Jane Roe was unmarried and pregnant. In her home state of Texas, abortions were illegal unless the mother's life was threatened. As Ms. Roe could not afford to travel to another state for an abortion, she filed suit challenging the Texas statute. The district court said that the statute on abortion was void on its face but did not grant the plaintiff an injunction that would have permitted her to receive the abortion. Both Ms. Roe and the state of Texas appealed to the Supreme Court for a determination of the constitutionality of the Texas statute.

The holding of the Supreme Court in *Roe v. Wade* takes into account both the developmental stages of the fetus and protection of the health of the mother. During the first trimester of pregnancy, the mother and her physician may elect abortion if the decision is medically sound and abortion is desired by the mother. In the second trimester, where abortion is more risky to the health of the mother, states may enact public health laws to protect the mother, but not the fetus, if she desires an abortion. Finally, when the mother desires an abortion after fetal viability, states can prohibit abortion except when medical necessity justifies the preservation of life or health of the mother. These rules in effect place the decision-making guidelines in a state of flux as a function of medical progress. The age of fetal viability is being lowered as a function of improved medical technology.[6] Although the court was willing to recognize the right of potential life for the viable fetus, the mother is still granted priority over the potential life of the fetus during the time when there is a question of whether the mother's health or life will benefit from an abortion. In fact, the Supreme Court was more concerned about the dangers of abortion to the mother in the third trimester than about protection of the fetus. Even so, *Roe v. Wade* represents the modern day pivotal point in the American legal system for trends toward recognition and protection of fetal rights. Just recently in 1985, the U.S. Supreme Court in *Thornburgh v. American College of Obstetricians and Gynecologists* again upheld the logic of *Roe v. Wade* despite a legal brief by the Reagan administration urging the overrule of the 1973 decision and shifting of responsibility for legal regulations in this area to the state.[7]

Although the United States courts have not yet consistently articulated the legal rights of the fetus, as a person, several recent court cases, not involving abortion, are instructive from the standpoint of understanding the evolution of fetal rights and the duties of health care professionals to protect them. These cases illustrate two types of court actions: those involving the competing interests of maternal and fetal rights and those involving medical malpractice. Court decisions in these areas begin to define the rights of the fetus and help to prescribe management parameters for the physician or consulting psychiatrist.

Competing Interests of Maternal and Fetal Rights

The interest of the mother versus the fetus has emerged in the courts when medical intervention necessary for the fetus was refused by the mother on the basis of religious reasons. In *Hoerner v. Bertinato*,[8] the New Jersey Juvenile and Domestic Relations Court awarded custody of a fetus to a third party to take effect immediately following birth, for the limited purpose of administering a blood transfusion refused by the mother for religious reasons. In *Raleigh Fitkin-Paul Morgan Memorial Hospital v. Anderson*,[9] the New Jersey Supreme Court ordered a pregnant woman of 8 months to undergo a blood transfusion for the benefit of the unborn child. The physicians involved believed that at some time before giving birth she would hemorrhage severely endangering the life of her fetus and herself. She refused a lifesaving blood transfusion because she was a Jehovah's Witness.

Concerning more invasive procedures of increased risk to the mother, courts are demanding information on the viability of the fetus and the necessity of the invasive procedure to preserve already established life. Two cases illustrate this point. Procedures more intrusive than blood transfusions were ordered by the Georgia Supreme Court in *Jefferson v. Griffin Spalding County Hospital Authority*.[10] In this case, the physicians involved determined that the probability that the child would die if a vaginal birth was attempted was 99%. In addition, it was determined that the mother had a 50% chance of not surviving a vaginal delivery. Both mother and child were given excellent chances of surviving a cesarean section. The mother objected to the surgery on religious grounds. To protect the fetus, the court authorized a sonogram, blood transfusions, and a cesarean section. The state interest in protecting the fetus was balanced against the mother's right of parental autonomy, bodily integrity, and freedom of religion.

In general, court-ordered interventions have occurred only when protecting a viable fetus. In *Taft v. Taft*,[11] the Massachusetts Supreme Judicial Court reversed a lower court's order to require a woman carrying a nonviable fetus to submit to surgery to prevent a miscarriage. In this case, the husband of a 4-month-pregnant woman sought a court order to force his wife to undergo an operation to suture the cervix so that it would hold the pregnancy. The physician involved testified that without the operation, the pregnancy would end in miscarriage. The mother refused the surgery for religious reasons. The Supreme Court noted that no court to date had ordered a pregnant woman to submit to invasive procedures to prevent the miscarriage of a nonviable fetus.

Maternal versus fetal rights also have been an issue before the courts when the mother's mental status and subsequent behavior pose a threat to the life of the unborn child. Soloff, Jewell, and Roth[12] discuss the involuntary commitment by a Pennsylvania Court of Common Pleas of the mother of a viable fetus for the duration of the pregnancy to protect both the unborn child and the mother. In this case, the mother was diagnosed as schizophrenic. She continued to deny a visible pregnancy of 7 months' duration and participated in activities injurious to herself and the fetus. Under the Mental Health Procedures Act in the Commonwealth of Pennsylvania, one is required to provide evidence of danger to self or others within the preceding 30 days and evidence of a high probability of recurrence of danger in the next 30 days if treatment is refused.[13] In this case, commitment may have been possible solely on the basis of the mother's danger to self as defined in the Mental Health Procedures Act.

Finally, the issue of maternal versus fetal rights arises in cases of substance abuse. Several court cases have been discussed in the literature regarding substance-abusing mothers. A criminal charge brought against an addict for endangering her fetus by continuing to use heroin during the last 2 months of pregnancy was dismissed on the basis that the California Penal Code did not include unborn children.[14] In a 1980 Michigan case, a newborn infant's symptoms of narcotics withdrawal initiated a charge of prenatal neglect.[15] The court held that the infant may be properly considered a neglected child due to prenatal maternal drug abuse. In Baltimore, a physician requested a court order from the juvenile division of the Circuit Court to enjoin a woman in her seventh month of pregnancy from using drugs that were dangerous to the fetus. The court ordered the woman to enroll in a drug rehabilitation program and to submit to weekly urinalysis until the baby was born.[16] In a third related case, the parents of a 6-month-old fetus were referred to the child protection services after a psychiatrist concluded that the pregnant woman was a significant hazard to the well-being of her fetus due to repeated drug intoxications, the secretive use of medication, and physical abuse by her husband.[17] In each of these cases, the fetus being afforded protection was viable.

Mackenzie et al. suggest two possible courses of action in such cases: civil commitment of the mother or custody of the fetus under child protection statutes.[17] Civil commitment, in this context, is not to take custody of the fetus but to restrain the mother. This course of action has been discussed previously. The second course of action is to seek custody of the fetus under child protection statutes. The Federal Child Abuse Act[18] authorizes intervention if the child is threatened with harm; the act does not require waiting until injury has occurred. All of the states have mandatory reporting requirements for third parties who observe or have reason to suspect abuse. The major question is whether the unborn is protected under these laws and at what developmental stage: preconception, previable, or viable.

Several issues arise, however, with the cited court actions. The first is the potential conflict between federal law that protects the confidentiality of drug addicts receiving treatment[19] and state laws mandating the reporting of child abuse if the fetus is to be considered protected under these laws. In the Michigan case,[20] the court addressed this conflict and made a judgment that, in this instance, the child's interest outweighed the mother's claim of confidentiality.

If the fetus is protected by the child protection laws, then mandatory reporting of fetal abuse by third parties is required. This requirement would open a liability for the physician if suspected fetal abuse is not reported. In *Landeros v. Flood,*[21] a physician's failure to report the initial abuse of a child made him liable for subsequent abuse of the child. This ruling establishes case-law precedence that a physician failing to report suspected abuse or abuse can be held liable for subsequent abuse.

The last issue deals with intrafamilial torts where the parents may be liable to the child for prenatal injuries. A case such as this was brought before the courts in *Grodin v. Grodin.*[22] In *Grodin v. Grodin,* the Court of Appeals of Michigan upheld the right of a child to present testimony concerning the negligence of his mother in failing to seek proper prenatal care. The court held that the injured child's mother would bear the same liability as a third person.

In conclusion, courts across the nation have intervened to afford protection to a viable fetus in situations involving conflicts in maternal wishes or behavior and the fetus's health and safety. The principles used by the courts in balancing the two interests, mother and fetus, in general follow the reasoning articulated by the U.S. Supreme Court in *Roe v. Wade.* Prior to viability, the mother's interests dominate. After viability, however, the courts attempt to balance the risk to the mother vis-à-vis the risk to the fetus.

Medical Malpractice

The right of the parents, the fetus or child, to sue for medical malpractice has been discussed in the literature in connection with terms such as "wrongful birth," "wrongful life," "wrongful conception," and "wrongful death." A discussion of the definitions of these terms and the applicable recent court decisions will provide a perspective on the status of fetal rights.

In *wrongful birth,* a suit for damages is brought by the parents of a child with alleged injuries from having been "wrongfully" brought into existence. In *wrongful life,* a suit for damages is brought on behalf of the child under these circumstances. These suits arise primarily in response to four scenarios.[23]

- Failure to diagnose a medical condition (e.g., rubella) of the mother that has an effect on fetal health or the failure to advise the mother regarding the effects on fetal health.
- Failure to diagnose pregnancy early enough to allow the woman the choice of an elective abortion even if the child is healthy but unplanned.
- Negligence in the performance of an abortion or sterilization resulting in the birth of a child, whether normal or deformed.
- Negligence in genetic counseling, including failure to advise the mother of the availability of diagnostic techniques (e.g., amniocentesis) or of the risk of bearing a deformed child.

Wrongful birth cases are based on the premise of the parents that if properly advised, they would not have conceived or would have aborted the fetus. The distinction between *wrongful birth* and *wrongful conception* is generally made on the basis of the health of the child. Although the terms overlap in the literature, in general, wrongful conception refers to the action when a healthy but unplanned child is produced, whereas wrongful birth usually involves a child who is abnormal or deformed in some manner. In wrongful life, the child seeks recovery for his or her existence on the premise that it is better not to have been born than to have been born under the circumstances in question.[24]

The Georgia Supreme Court ruled that an action for wrongful conception was no more than a type of malpractice and should be recognized. In *Blash v. Glisson,* a Georgia appellate court ruled that the parents of a child born after an allegedly negligent sterilization procedure could recover expenses for the procedure, pain and suffering, medical complications, costs of delivery, lost wages, and loss of consortium. The cost of rearing the child until the age of 18 years was not found to be recoverable.[25]

Wrongful birth actions are generally well recognized by the courts.[26] For example, the failure to properly determine if a Jewish couple were carriers of Tay-Sachs disease, with the resultant birth of an affected child, was a cause for action.[27] Similarly, failure to diagnose maternal rubella during pregnancy and therefore to warn the mother of the risks of severe congenital defects in the child is a cause for liability when a defective child is born.[28] Wrongful birth liabilities have been established even prior to conception. In *Wells v. Orthopharmaceutical Corp.,* the claim was made and upheld that oral contraceptives taken prior to conception were the proximate cause of birth defects in a subsequently born child. The court found that the corporation negligently failed to warn of an increased risk of birth defects accompanying the use of its product.[29]

Wrongful life actions are not consistently accepted by courts, in part because life itself is regarded as an inherent good and to avoid further stigmatizing of unwanted conditions. They often are rejected in favor of allowing a wrongful birth action on the same incident.[30] Wrongful life actions have been more readily accepted when the statute of limitations for wrongful birth had expired.[31] However, some courts have accepted both wrongful life and wrongful birth actions.[32] Liability exists regardless of the developmental stage of the fetus and cases have been upheld where the negligent act occurred prior to conception.[33] A typical example of preconception negligence is the failure to diagnose a hereditary disease in the first child and, therefore, a failure to inform the parents of the risks of having a second defective child. In *Renslow v. Mennonite Hospital,*[34] for example, a 13-year-old received an inappropriate blood transfusion that caused birth defects in a child born to her 8 years later. The court upheld a wrongful life action for the child.

In all of these case examples, the physician had the responsibility to gather the appropriate information required to make a thorough assessment and accurate diagnosis. In Coplan's view,[35] children with incurable defects such as mental retardation, major structural anomalies, and deafness should be given more than palliative therapy for the defect. These children should be subjected to an intense assessment to determine the underlying etiology and make an accurate diagnosis. If the primary physician is not capable of providing assessment and treatment, then appropriate consultations should be obtained. The physician is required to provide the parents with adequate information regarding the diagnosis to allow them to make informed future procreative decisions.

Although these cases of wrongful birth, wrongful life, and wrongful conception have been recognized by the courts to some degree, much controversy continues to exist as to recoverable damages. Several cases have cited the "benefits rule" in determining recoverable damages. This rule balances the benefits of the parenthood against the damages of the cost of raising a child. Under the benefits rule, recovery has varied from no award of damages to holding the physician liable for all child-rearing costs.[36]

A "wrongful death" action is brought by the deceased person's beneficiaries and alleges that death was attributable to the willful or negligent act of another. Courts today are divided as to whether a fetus rather than a live-born child harmed while in vivo may be the subject of a wrongful death action. In either situation, most courts allow a wrongful death action if the fetus was viable at the time of the death-causing injury.[37] For example, in *Werling v. Sandy et al.*,[38] the Ohio Supreme Court chose to recognize the viable fetus as a person under the wrongful death statute because at the moment of viability the fetus has the capability of meaningful life outside the mother's body. In *Mone v. Greyhound Lines, Inc.*,[39] a Massachusetts Court elaborated on the reasons for its adoption of the viability rule. The court believed that the live-birth rule allowed incongruous results in that injuries serious enough to cause death were not recoverable, whereas less severe injuries that did not cause death were recoverable. The court acknowledged that the live-birth rule is simpler to administer but the viability rule better serves justice. In 1985, the Pennsylvania Supreme Court upheld the right of recovery under wrongful death on behalf of a stillborn child in *Amadio et al. v. Levin et al.* Prior to the Supreme Court's opinion in this case, Pennsylvania courts uniformly required "live birth" prior to a wrongful death action. The reason cited by the court for the reversal was the incongruency in results cited by the Massachusettes courts in *Mone v. Greyhound.*[40] The trend of the courts is to recognize a viable fetus that is subsequently stillborn for a wrongful death action. Still, some courts have required live birth prior to a wrongful death action.[41] Yet others have allowed wrongful death actions to a nonviable fetus.[42]

Suggested Guidelines for Case Management

As the previously cited cases demonstrate, the responsibilities of the physician treating the pregnant patient or even the patient with childbearing potential are very broad. Various elements of the American judicial system have recognized the existence of legal rights before conception, before viability, and without the necessity of the fetus to survive the womb. In addition, they have recognized the existence of legal rights in the viable fetus and in the born infant or child for prebirth harm even if subsequent death follows.

Thus it appears that the fetus or born child may sue and recover for harm occurring during a period that spans preconception to the time of birth. This also means that the parents of the fetus or born child have certain recoverable legal rights on behalf of the fetus or born child as well as on their own behalf.

What does this mean for the treating physician? In addition to the obvious care and concern for the patient, it means that the physician, regardless of specialty, must first be sensitive to whether identified medical problems, courses of recommended treatment, and patient life-style would be harmful to a normal birth and life thereafter should the patient have the potential for becoming pregnant, or in fact be pregnant.

Physicians are held responsible for any negligent acts or substandard care. Increased rights being afforded the fetus as well as new technologies have created new duties for the physician. Some of these new duties include:

- Advising the patient of the possibility of natural failure in birth control methods.
- Thoroughly assessing the history of genetic diseases.
- Advising the patient of the risks of having a deformed child.
- Assessing the risks of treatment on women in general as future childbearers.
- Assessing the woman's life-style (in terms of drug and alcohol abuse) on ability to produce a normal fetus whether pregnant or not.
- Communicating and documenting in a letter and in the medical record of the advice given to a woman as well as the woman's acknowledgment of this advice.
- Assessing any medical condition of a pregnant woman that may have a significant effect on fetal health and advising appropriately.
- Early diagnosis of pregnancy.
- Advising the mother of the availability of amniocentesis when appropriate.
- Assessing the risks of treatment on a pregnant woman and her fetus.
- Thoroughly assessing the mental status of a woman taking into consideration the pregnancy and future motherhood.
- Assessing a woman's competency to comprehend alternative forms of treatment and risks, and, if not competent, having available means of evaluation to declare incompetent.
- Referring cases to a specialist when appropriate.
- Obtaining legal advice in areas of concern.

Within the bounds of reasonable* medical knowledge and available consultive expertise, the treating physician, with diagnosis, possible management, and patient history in hand should draw conclusions about the degree of risk to fetus (potential or existing), normal birth, and life thereafter. Such conclusions and their rationale should be ade-

---

*Reasonable is a term of art used by lawyers and judges. It is a word that is bothersome, to say the least, to physicians because it appears to have no bounds and defies definition. There is some truth to this perception although courts attempt to formulate the word's meaning on a case-by-case basis by relating facts and circumstance with community or national standards. Unfortunately for the treating physician, words such as available and concerning must also be looked at in the context of reasonableness. Common sense, thoroughness, and caring, together, are words that may be helpful to the physician in conceptualizing the legal idea of reasonableness. Although perhaps comforting to some extent, it is still recognized that the more thorough a professional becomes in a given area, the potential exists for a higher level of standards with a corresponding change in the legal meaning of reasonableness. This may certainly be perceived as a catch-22 situation by those in the professions not wed to the idea of striving for perfection.

quately documented in the patient's medical record even if the significance of risk is determined to be minimal or nonexistent. The physician should be careful to separate during documentation the risks associated with his or her recommended treatment from risks associated with other factors such as life-style and treatment provided by others.

Of course, if it is apparent to the treating physician that an initially identified course of case management will pose a concerning degree of risk to the fetus or life thereafter, then alternatives should be considered when feasible. In the past, the balancing of risk of various treatment alternatives with the risk of no treatment involved solely the patient. The balancing process has now been complicated by the additional consideration of the fetus and life thereafter. Today, preconception issues are also becoming important considerations for risk assessment. This means that risk to a potential fetus must be considered when treating all women.

Where recommended patient treatment or discovered patient life-style pose significant risk to the potential offspring of a patient capable of childbearing, the patient should be adequately advised about the risk and alternatives, if any. When permitted by the patient and where applicable, her mate should also be informed about this information. When there is a question of patient competency either because of age or mental capacity, then within the limits of confidentiality constraints, parents, legal guardians, or concerned others, as the case may be, should be advised and asked for decisions regarding treatment. The patient's medical record should at least reflect the fact that advice or information was given, to whom given if in addition to or other than to the patient, and pertinent responses.[43] It should also be noted if the patient is referred to other specialists for assistance in reducing risk to a potential birth.

The physician or consulting psychiatrist needs to be aware of these issues especially when he or she believes that treatment, or lack thereof, may involve significant risk to a potential life, or when treatment involves risks to both patient and potential life, or when the patient disagrees with the physician's advice to protect a potential life. At this point, the expertise of the psychiatrist as a behavioral scientist with a systems orientation can be most helpful in formulating a strategy for problem resolution and/or for sharing information with troubled parents in an effective way.

Any strategy must have as its central objective advising what is best in the long run for the patient and potential life alike. Such an objective should represent the societal and, hopefully, the judicial norm. The strategy will be dependent upon the circumstances of each case and because the variations in factual situations are virtually infinite, it is practical to consider broad guidelines that can be narrowed as the critical facts and issues are identified.

The process of arriving at a strategy should be guided by what is known at the time about the causal relationships between patient treatment, or lack thereof, and harm to potential life. The physician's responsibility for intervention, beyond advice, when life-style issues are involved is also tempered by available scientific knowledge concerning risk as well as legal enactments at the time for physicians to take on responsibilities against the patients' will for the patient and potential life. (Child abuse statutes that include the fetus are an illustration of this last point.)

The physician must initially assess the degree of risk of treatment and of no treatment for both the patient and potential life. If the degree of risk of serious harm for the patient is greater or equal to that of a potential life, then a strategy that leans towards the patient's decision may be feasible, provided the patient is advised of the risk to potential life. This logic follows the Supreme Court's *Roe v. Wade* line of reasoning discussed previously, where the welfare of the mother, even when the fetus is viable, takes priority over a live birth. Where the patient's risks of serious harm are less than the risks of serious harm to potential life or where the patient's decision is unreasonable in light of the circumstances, the physician must consider more forceful solutions. Examples illustrating this situation include blood transfusions to save the fetus, cesarean sections, electroconvulsive therapy, use of antipsychotic drugs, detoxification procedures, and involuntary mental health commitment for purposes of observational self-protection, if not more active treatment.

If time permits, the treating or consulting physician should take advantage of advice obtainable from colleagues independent of the treatment team, from legal counsel, from applicable medical staff or other institutional committees (for example, ethics and quality care assurance committees), and from agencies such as those involved with child protective services or mental health commitment procedures. In many jurisdictions, the judiciary is also available for advisory services.

Continued dialogue with the patient and concerned others, where there are no confidentiality issues, may prove successful in persuading the patient that a change in her position appears more reasonable in protecting herself and a potential life for which she may be responsible. It may also be appropriate to discuss the criminal and civil law implications of her decision. Even when there are apparent confidentiality conflicts, it is prudent to attempt to persuade the patient (or sometimes to proceed without the patient's consent) to inform others, such as the father, of the mother's need for treatment. As in other areas of clinical practice, the imminence of expected harm to the fetus and the level of severity of harm will determine the justification for breaking a patient's confidence. In such circumstances, it is wise to seek consultations and to "think out loud" on the chart documenting the physician's reasoning about why the patient's confidences need to be violated.

The major legal consideration is whether the fetus, in a viable or nonviable state, is considered by the judicial system to be a "person" against whom murder, assault, or battery can be perpetrated, or who is to be protected under child abuse or mental health commitment acts. As can be gleaned from the preceding discussion of history and case law, the recognition of the fetus for this purpose varies among jurisdictions. However, just as the trend is to recognize fetal rights, so it appears that there is a trend to recognize the fetus as a person. The one exception is at the fringe area of preconception where rights have been recognized to exist in a potential future life but where the concept of "person" has yet to be recognized for the sake of statutory protection.

In practical terms, this means that the physician has a duty within reason to protect the fetus as a person and understand that even preconception rights of a potential life exist. Psychiatry offers a means to protect the fetus. Most mental health procedure acts and competency statutes provide alternatives for the physician to consider. Most state mental health procedure acts are concerned about patient harm to self or others. Although the fetus may or may not qualify as an "other" (person), if it can be shown that the patient qualifies for commitment because of harm to self, then it is not necessary to qualify the fetus as an other person, and the fetus, therefore, benefits from the protective medical custody of the patient. Finally, throughout the process of patient assessment and decision making, the physician or consulting psychiatrist should make a judgment about the patient's mental competency to make her own decisions about treatment. When serious questions about such an issue arise, then the physician should consider the appropriateness of initiating incompetency proceedings. The appointment of a guardian for the patient, even for a temporary period of time, may help the physician in arriving at an objective strategy that maximizes benefits to the patient and potential life.

The Future

Ironically though, just when it seems that clarity is on the horizon, new technology and social changes appear to complicate matters. For example, in vitro fertilization and surrogate parenting raise a whole new range of issues for the courts and the physician, especially the consulting psychiatrist. Questions such as the following will need to be confronted:

- Who are the legal parents: the sperm donor, an egg donor, a surrogate who carries the child, or the couple who raise the child?
- What are the physician's obligations in screening a donor for genetic and infectious diseases?
- Who is responsible, financially, for medical decisions and otherwise, for the baby regardless of the baby's condition: the donors, the surrogate carriers, or proposed parents?
- Does a frozen embryo have a right to be born?
- What records should be kept and who should have access to them?
- Does an embryo have the right of inheritance?
- Who has control over genetic material once it is outside the donor's body: the donor, the physician, or the proposed parents?
- What happens to a frozen embryo if the couple die, divorce, or become incompetent?
- Who is the patient?
- What is the status of potential life?
- Who are significant concerned others?

Even with respect to these new dimensions on the horizon, the guidance in this chapter is intended to be generic and global enough to provide the physician and psychiatrist with a rational starting point and framework for working toward meaningful solutions. However, because technology and law in this area are rapidly changing, the physician, by necessity, cannot rely solely upon his or her own intuitive knowledge base. With comprehensive patient information at hand, additional consultation should be actively sought. This is necessary because both a life in being in the form of the patient and a potential life in the form of an abstraction (preconception) or of a fetus are at stake. Optimal care for both depends upon such a sensitive strategy.

References

1. Curran WJ: An historical perspective on the law of personality and status with special regard to the human fetus and the rights of women. *Milbank Memorial Fund Quarterly/Health and Society* **61**:59–61, 1983.
2. Curran WJ: An historical perspective on the law of personality and status with special regard to the human fetus and the rights of women. *Milbank Memorial Fund Quarterly/Health and Society* **61**:61–63, 1983.

3. Curran WJ: An historical perspective on the law of personality and status with special regard to the human fetus and the rights of women. *Milbank Memorial Fund Quarterly/Health and Society* **61**:65–66, 1983.
4. Curran WJ: An historical perspective on the law of personality and status with special regard to the human fetus and the rights of women. *Milbank Memorial Fund Quarterly/Health and Society* **61**:69, 1983.
5. Roe v Wade, 410 US 113, 1973.
6. Callahan D: How technology is reframing the abortion debate. *Hastings Center Report,* February 1986, pp 33–42.
7. Thornburgh v American College of Obstetricians and Gynecologists, No 84-495, 1986.
8. Hoerner v Bertinato, 67 NJ Super 517, 171 A2d 140, 1961.
9. Raleigh Fitkin-Paul Moran Memorial Hospital v Anderson, 42 NJ 421, 201 A2d 537, 1964.
10. Jefferson v Griffin Spalding County Hospital Authority, 247 Ga 86, 274 SE2d 457, 1981.
11. Taft v Taft, 338 Mass 331, 446 NE2d 395, 1983.
12. Soloff P, Jewel S, Roth L: Civil commitment and the rights of the unborn. *American Journal of Psychiatry* **136**:114–115, 1979.
13. Mental Health Procedures Act, 1976, Public Law 817, No 143.
14. Reyes v Superior Court, 75 Cal App 3d, 214, 141 Cal Rptr 912, 1977.
15. Baby X, 97 Mich App III, 293 NW2d 736, 1980.
16. Shaw MW: Conditional prospective rights of the fetus. *The Journal of Legal Medicine,* **5**:63–116, 1984.
17. Mackenzie RB, Collins MN, Popkin ME: A case of fetal abuse? *American Journal of Orthopsychiatry* **52**:699–703, 1982.
18. Public Law 93-247, Subsection 3, 88 Stat 5, codified at 42 US 5102 Supplement V, 1977.
19. 21 USC1175; 42 CFR 213, 1979.
20. Baby X, 97 Mich App III, 293 NW2d 736, 1980.
21. Landeros v Flood, 131 Cal 69, 551 P2d 389, 1976.
22. Grodin v Grodin, 301 NW2d 869, 1980.
23. Feinberg et al: Obstetrics/gynecology and the law. *Health Administration Press,* Michigan, 1984, pp 92–108.
24. Feinberg et al: Obstetrics/gynecology and the law. *Health Administration Press,* Michigan, 1984, pp 92–108.
25. Blash v Glisson, 325 SE2d 607, Ga Ct App, Nov 20, 1984; cert denied, Ga Sup Ct, Jan 30, 1985.
26. Naccash v Burger, 233 Va 491, 290 SE2d 825, 1982. Jorgenson v Meade-Johnson Laboratories, 483 F2d 237, 10th Circuit, 1973; Jacobs v Theimer, 519 SW2d 846, Texas Super 1975; Berman v Allan, 80 NJ 421, 404 A2d 8, 1979.
27. Naccash v Burger, 233 VA 491, 290 SE2d 825, 1982.
28. Jacobs v Theimer, 519 SW2d 846, Texas Super 1975.
29. Wells v Orthopharmaceutical Corp, No C82-1921A, District Court for the Northern District of Georgia, July 29, 1985.
30. Berman v Allan, 80 JN 421, 404 A2d 8, 1979.
31. Procanik v Cillo, 97 NJ 339, 478 A2d 755, 1984; Schroeder v Perkel, 87 NJ 53, 432 A2d 834, 1981.
32. Turpin v Sortini, 31 Cal 3d 220, 182 Cal Rptr 337, 643 P2d 954, 1982.
33. Turpin v Sortini, 31 Cal 3d 220, 182 Cal Rptr 337, 643 P2d 954, 1982; Renslow v Mennonite Hospital, 67 Ill 2d 348, 367 NE2d 1250, 1977, affirming 351 NE2d 870, 1976; Schroeder v Perkel, 87 NJ 53, 432 A2d 834, 1981.
34. Renslow v Mennonite Hospital, 67 Ill 2d 348, 367 NE2d 1250, 1977, affirming 351 NE2d 870, 1976.
35. Coplan J: Wrongful life and wrongful death: New concepts for the pediatrician. *Pediatrics* **75**:65–72, 1985.
36. Feinberg et al: Obstetrics/gynecology and the law. *Health Administration Press,* Michigan, 1984, pp 92–108.
37. Christafogeorges v Brandenburg, 55 Ill 2d 368, 304 NE2d 88, 1973; Vaillancourt v Medical Center Hospital, 425 A2d 92, Vt 1980; Mone v Greyhound lines, Inc, 331 NE2d 916, Mass 1975; Hopkins v McBane, No 10, 697, ND Supreme Court, 1984; Werling v Sandy et al, No 84-814, Ohio Supreme Court, 1985. Summerfield v Superior Court of the State of Arizona, No 17607-SA, Arizona Supreme Court, 1985.
38. Werling v Sandy et al, No 84-814, Ohio Supreme Court, 1985.
39. Mone v Greyhound Lines, Inc, 331 NE2d 916, Mass 1975.
40. Tort recovery granted to stillborn. *Pennsylvania Law Journal-Reporter,* 8, 1985.
41. White v Yup, 85 Nev 527, 458 P2d 617, 1969.

42. Presby v Newport Hospital, 117 RI 177, 365 A2d 748, 1976; Toth v Goree, 65 Mich App 296, 237 NW2d 297, 1975.
43. Roth LH, Appelbaum PS, Lidz CW, et al: Informed consent in psychiatric research, in: *Mental Health Law and Developments in the 1980s*. New York, Guilford Press, 1985.

V

Summary and Conclusions

18

Conclusions and Future Directions

RICHARD L. COHEN

What lessons have we learned from our early efforts at developing consultation and liaison services for childbirth care providers and the populations they serve? A text such as this does not easily lend itself to summarization. Its complexity together with the larger number of, as yet, unanswered questions makes the drawing of conclusions rather presumptuous.

Nevertheless, at least some tentative ideas emerge from the foregoing:

1. *The unique aspect of consultation to childbirth services.* Specialized knowledge and skills must be acquired by the consultant (regardless of his or her basic discipline) in order to carry out effective consultation and liaison to childbirth services. The process of reproduction is a unique human experience, and the care of the patient and her mate is a unique area of professional activity. They present special opportunities and problems to the mental health consultant.

2. *Societal factors in childbirth.* Because so many belief systems and practices are "culture-bound," an understanding of the overall culture and, if relevant, the subculture in which the pregnancy has been conceived and is progressing are of critical importance.

3. *Development as a basic science.* Because pregnancy is fundamentally a normal human process for both the mother and the fetus, a basic understanding of developmental processes and those factors that may beneficially or adversely influence development can form the basis for data collection, for formulation of case dynamics, and for communication with obstetric caregivers.

4. *Significance of the clinical setting.* Familiarity with the variety of childbirth options now available to families and with their specific resources and limitations are essential if recommendations for general care and for specific types of interventions are to be relevant.

5. *Significance of stress in prenatal development.* Familiarity with the emerging

---

Richard L. Cohen • Department of Psychiatry, Western Psychiatric Institute and Clinic, University of Pittsburgh, Pittsburgh, PA 15213.

body of information that places importance not only on the psychosocial impact of stress during pregnancy but, potentially, on the biological development of the fetus provides both a rationale for mental health collaboration in care and a basis for developing long-range public health approaches to prenatal program development.

6. *High technology obstetrical care, advances in reproductive techniques, and bio-medical ethics.* Obstetrics is now confronted with a spectrum of ethical issues ranging from matters of "wrongful birth" to questions of confused and ambiguous custody that inevitably have an impact on family relationships, intergenerational responsibilities, and child and adolescent development. The mental health disciplines, by their very nature, can hardly escape knowledge of and constructive involvement in attempting to find solutions to some of these problems.

7. *Status of relationship between childbirth professions and mental health clinicians.* Working relationships between mental health professionals and childbirth caregivers have not been as active or as mutually supportive as all of the preceding would suggest is necessary. Although some new approaches hold promise for brighter days to come, more thought and more effort must be invested in developing mutually respectful and helpful collaboration between these two broad groups of professionals.

It is not unusual for psychiatrists to blame obstetricians for their apparent lack of interest in the mental health and well-being of their charges. I have been guilty of this indiscretion myself. In fairness, most of psychiatry and its allied disciplines have been equally guilty of ignoring the reproductive cycle as a rich area for study and clinical practice and have shown comparatively little interest in the mental disorders associated with pregnancy and the postpartum. In 1984, a call to arms appeared in the medical news sections of *JAMA*[1] entitled "Rip van Winkle Period Ends for Peripheral Psychiatric Problems." This article highlights the relative lack of investment in these clinical problems during the past 75 years and observes that there are now many signs of an "awakening" to their immediate and long-range importance for the family and, especially, for its offspring.

It is easy to understand why clinical investigators quickly become discouraged with efforts to design research programs in this field. There is an overwhelming temptation to search for one-to-one relationships between a given prenatal event or disorder and the outcome of pregnancy or development in the child. The bewildering array of confounding variables[2] has usually resulted in frustration and in the collection of unmanageable data bases.

Efforts to study the effects of the clinical setting in which care is given and childbirth takes place have been fraught with methodologic deficiencies.[3] This only increases the temptation for clinicians and consumers to jump on bandwagons and to subscribe to undocumented belief systems with almost religious zeal.

The mystique that has surrounded the early reports on infant bonding has only served to impede controlled research.[4] There is, in fact, no clear-cut evidence at this writing that efforts at "bonding" have any lasting effect either on parent–child relationships or on the long-range outcome of child development. Yet the term "bonding" has insinuated itself into the lexicon of daily clinical communication, has been embraced by consumer groups, and now enjoys surprising advocacy among many lay and professional teachers.

One is reminded of the more than 60-year-period during which most perinea were shaved prior to labor and delivery in order to ensure greater cleanliness and to decrease "child bed fever." Millions of women were subjected to this rather untimely and degrading experience on the basis of little or no data. It was not until the 1960s that any controlled studies were carried out and, of course, they did not support the contention that such a procedure had any clinical value whatsoever.[5,6]

We need to find ways to create a mind set among obstetric practitioners and mental health clinicians that conception, pregnancy, and childbirth are part of a continuum and that, barring catastrophe, it is extremely unlikely that any single event can have a major effect one way or the other on outcome.[7,8] Labor and delivery may take 9 hours, but pregnancy takes approximately 9 months. The assignment of magical omnipotence either to an electronic fetal monitor[9] or a bonding procedure[10] is equally ill advised.

Risks of making rapid assessments about the advantages or disadvantages of a particular advance in technology are well documented if one examines the literature of the philosophy of science. As White[11] points out, there was probably no one alive who could have predicted the impact of the invention of gunpowder or of the fireplace or even of eyeglasses when they appeared upon the human scene. Yet, all of these and many more[12] have had an incredible impact on the ways in which we live and work together.

With respect to the potential value of consultation and liaison programs to obstetrics, we can state very little with authority. There have been some useful studies[13-19] of consultation and liaison programs in other medical settings with particular attention to quality-of-life issues to the outcome of treatment when viewed over the long term, and even to the efficiency of care and length of stay in the hospital. One can assume that at least some of these findings can be extrapolated into the childbirth setting, but this has yet to be proved.

A department chairman of obstetrics and gynecology in one of our most prestigious universities said to me while I was on a sabbatical leave studying childbirth services in the United States that he was very concerned that his obstetric colleagues were in so much disfavor now. "They seem to be unloved by the people they want most to love them [their patients]." He seemed concerned about the "mindless application of high technology" and what he viewed as an increasingly "blind reliance" on technology without the application of good, basic obstetric judgment and skills. He went on to say that he considered that the greatest deficiencies in studies of outcome of intervention in various intrapartum problems have to do with the absence of well-designed behavioral studies of both mother and child. He expressed the hope that our fields would see the development of collaborative research projects between obstetricians and behavioral scientists over the next decade.

Even making allowance for the fact that he was being gracious to a professional guest, I chose to take his words at face value. The alternative may be a continued drift in the direction of psychiatric care that ignores the critical importance of reproduction in the life cycle and obstetric care that restricts itself to the pelvic region rather than the whole woman and her developing fetus. This portrait of Orwellian medical care has been painted by many writers (e.g., Corea[20]). It is an unpleasant prospect and can be avoided through a reexamination of interprofessional attitudes and working relationships.

References

1. Ziporyn T: Medical news: "Rip van Winkle period ends for puerperal problems." *JAMA* **251**:2061–2067, 1984.

2. Institute of Medicine, National Research Council: *A Report of a Study by the Committee on Assessing Alternative Birth Settings: Research Issues in the Assessment of Birth Settings.* Washington, DC, National Academy Press, 1982, p 55.
3. Wortman CB, Kelty MC: Research on childbirth settings: The assessment of psychological variables, in Institute of Medicine & National Research Council (eds): *Research Issues in the Assessment of Birth Settings.* Washington, DC, National Academy Press, 1982, p 102.
4. Chess S, Thomas A: Infant bonding: Mystique and reality. *Am J Orthopsychiatry* **52:**213–222, 1982.
5. Burchell RC: Predelivery removal of pubic hair. *Obstet Gynecol* **24:**272–273, 1964.
6. Kantor HI, Rember R, Tabio P: Value of shaving the pudendal-perineal area in delivery preparation. *Obstet Gynecol* **25:**509–512, 1965.
7. Parmelee AH, Haber A: Who is the "risk infant"? *Clin Obstet Gynecol* **16:**376–387, 1973.
8. Buck C, Gregg R, Stavraky, et al: The effect of single prenatal and natal complications upon the development of children of mature birthweight. *Pediatr* **43:**942, 1969.
9. Goodlin RC, Haesslein HC: When is it fetal distress? *Am J Obstet Gynecol* **128:**440–447, 1977.
10. Klaus MH, Kennell JH: *Maternal–Infant Bonding.* St. Louis, C.V. Mosby, 1976.
11. White L: Technology assessment from the stance of a medieval historian. *American Historical Review* **79:**1–13, 1974.
12. Tittnich EM, Brown N: Positive and negative uses of technology in human interactions. *J Children in Contemporary Society* **14:**15–21, 1981.
13. Pincus H: Making the case for consultation-liaison psychiatry: Issues in cost-effectiveness analysis. *Gen Hosp Psychiatry* **6:**173–179, 1984.
14. Mumford E, Schlesinger HJ, Glass GV, et al: A new look at evidence about reduced cost of medical utilization following mental health treatment. *Am J Psychiatry* **141:**1145–1158, 1984.
15. Lyons JS, Hammer JS, Wise TN, et al: Consultation-liaison psychiatry and cost-effectiveness research. *Gen Hosp Psychiatry* **7:**302–308, 1985.
16. Mitchell W, Thompson T: Some methodological issues in consultation-liaison psychiatry research. *General Hospital Psychiatry* **7:**66–72, 1985.
17. Lyons JS, Hammer JS, Strain JJ, et al: The timing of psychiatric consultation in the general hospital and length of hospital stay. *Gen Hosp Psychiatry* **8:**159–162, 1986.
18. Brent DA, Needleman HL: A data-based method for the evaluation of pediatric consultation-liaison activities. Presented at the 30th Annual Meeting of the American Academy of Child Psychiatry, San Francisco, CA, October, 1983.
19. Trent PJ, Houpt JL, Eaton JS (eds): *Consultation Liaison Psychiatry: Evaluating its Effectiveness.* HIMH, Rockville, MD, 1982.
20. Corea G: Childbirth 2000. *Omni Magazine* **1:**48–50, 104–107, 1979.

Index

Abortion, 6
  as felony, 254
  fetal rights and, 236, 254–255, 256, 258, 261
  religious beliefs against, 254
  spontaneous
    fetal rights and, 256
    pathological mourning following, 74
  therapeutic
    fetal rights and, 236
    genetic counseling and, 235
    legalization, 236
    negligence in performance of, 258
Abruptio placentae, 130
Adjustment disorders. *See* Maladaptive syndromes
Adolescents, pregnancy in, 78, 131–134
Adoption, 232, 233
Adrenocorticotropin, in prenatal stress, 30, 31
Affective disorders
  during postpartum period, 40
  during pregnancy, 43, 44, 74–75
Agoraphobia, during pregnancy, 43, 191
Akineton. *See* Biperiden
Alcohol abuse, maternal, 43
  fetal effects, 207–210, 211, 212
  genetic factors, 224
  neonatal effects, 207, 208, 210–212
Alpha-fetoprotein screening programs, 222
Amadio et al v. *Levin et al*, 259
American College of Obstetricians and
    Gynecologists, 7, 14, 86, 233
American College of Obstetricians and
    Gynecologists v. *Thornburgh*, 255
American Society for Psychosomatic Obstetrics
    and Gynecology, 7
Amitriptyline, 177, 178, 179, 180–181
Amnesia, 15–16
Amniocentesis, 222
  abortion following, 235
Amoxapine, 178, 181

Anesthesia, general, 14
Anorexia nervosa, 42
Antidepressant medication, use during pregnancy,
    125–126, 127, 177–182
  behavioral effects, 179
  breast-feeding and, 179–181
  choice of, 177
  neonatal effects, 179
  in postpartum depression management, 181–182
  teratogenicity, 177–179
Antihypertensive drugs, use during pregnancy, 74
Antiparkinson agents, use during pregnancy, 176–
    177
Antipsychotic drugs, use during pregnancy, 170–
    177
  behavioral effects, 173–174
  breast-feeding and, 174–175
  choice of, 171
  in postpartum psychosis management, 175–176
  pregnancy testing and, 170–171
  teratogenicity, 171–174
Anxiety, prenatal, 22–24, 30–31, 41. *See also*
    Stress, prenatal
  fetal outcome effects, 25, 27
  neonatal behavioral effects, 29
  pregnancy outcome effects, 22–24
Anxiety disorders
  benzodiazepine therapy, 191–197
  during pregnancy, 75–76
Anxiety rating, 140
Aretaeus, 14
Artane. *See* Trihexyphenidyl
Artifical insemination by donor (AID), 232, 233,
    234, 237, 238
Atropine, 190
Attitude, maternal
  towards childbirth care services, 92–93
  pregnancy outcome and, 24
Autism, 225

"Baby blues". *See* Depression, postpartum
Baby M case, 232, 234, 237, 239
Barbiturates, use with electroconvulsive therapy, 190–191
Behavioral disturbances. *See also* Teratogenicity, behavioral
  genetic counseling for, 224
  maternal alcohol use-related, 210
  in parents of premature infants, 160
Benadryl. *See* Diphenhydramine
Benzodiazepines
  use during pregnancy, 191–197
  behavioral effects, 195–197
  breast-feeding and, 197
  neonatal effects, 195–197
  teratogenicity, 193–195
  toxic effects, 195–197
  use during puerperium, 197
Benztropine, 176–177
Bereavement, fetal effects of, 26
Biochemical changes, during pregnancy, 52–54
Biperiden, 176–177
Bipolar affective disorders, 40, 128, 225–226, 237
Birth. *See also* Childbirth
  wrongful, 257–258, 259
Birthing center, out-of-hospital, 13, 87–88, 89–91, 92–96, 97, 98, 99–100, 101, 102, 103, 241–244, 245–248
Birthing room, family-centered in-hospital, 87, 88, 89, 91–92, 93, 94, 95, 96–103, 249–250
Blash v. *Glisson*, 258
Blood flow, uteroplacental, 166, 167
Blood pressure. *See also* Hypertension; Hypotension
  hormonal factors, 27, 30, 31–33
Blood transfusions, legal aspect of, 255, 258, 261
Body image, during pregnancy, 62–63
Bonding, mother–infant, 248, 270, 271
Brain, sexual differentiation, prenatal stress and, 31–33
Breast-feeding
  in neonatal intensive care units (NICU), 159
  during psychopharmacologic agent ingestion, 199
    antidepressants, 179–181
    benzodiazepines, 197
    haloperidol, 174–175
    lithium, 187
Breuer, Josef, 15
Buproprion, 181
Burnout, of nurses, 110, 139

Carbamazepine, 187
Catacholamines, stress and, 27, 31, 32

Celsius, Anders, 14
Central nervous system anomalies, maternal alcohol use-related, 207, 208
Cesarean section, 245, 246, 247
Chamberlens, Pierre, 14
Charcot, Jean Martin, 15
Child bed fever, 14, 247, 270–271
Childbirth
  anxiety related to, 23–24, 25, 27, 29, 30–31, 41
  childbirth care option choice and, 96–99
  historical background, 13–19
  medicalization of, 14–15
  societal factors, 14, 18–19, 269
Childbirth care, information sources, 7–8
Childbirth care options
  birthing centers, out-of-hospital, 13, 87–88, 89–91, 92–96, 97, 98, 99–100, 101, 102, 103, 241–244, 245–248
  birthing rooms, family-centered in-hospital, 87, 88, 89, 91–92, 93, 94, 95, 96–103, 249–250
  current controversy regarding, 5–6, 241–251
  information sources, 7–8
  maternal decision-making regarding, 85–104
    attitudes concerning hospital environment, 92–93
  compromise with mate, 94
  factors influencing, 86–95
  family life attitudes/values, 92
  finances and, 93
  individual responsibility attitudes, 89–92
  marital support deficits, 100
  maternal health concerns, 99–100
  nesting behavior, 100–102
  previous childbearing/childrearing experience and, 96–98
  response to pregnancy, 100–102
    specific procedures, 93–94
Childbirth fever. *See* Child bed fever
Child protection statutes, fetal rights and, 256–257
Child psychiatrists
  historical background, 15–16
  in neonatal intensive care units (NICU), 156, 157–158
Childrearing
  lack of experience in, 140
  parental preparation for, 63, 66, 67, 68, 96–98
    lack of, 140, 141, 144
Chlorazepate, 192
Chlordiazepoxide, 192, 193–194, 196–197
Chlorpromazine, 171–172, 174, 176, 186, 188–189
Chorionic villi sampling, 222, 234, 235
Cigarette smoking, during pregnancy, 212–213

Clinical specialists, 109, 111
Clomipramine, 181
Cocaine use, during pregnancy, 214
Cogentin. *See* Benztropine
Community programs, program consultation to, 145–146
Conception
  alternative methods. *See* Reproductive technology
  wrongful, 258, 259
Congenital malformations. *See also* Genetic counseling; Teratogenicity
  causes, 167
  incidence, 167
  legal aspects regarding, 258
  maternal alcohol use-related, 207, 208, 209
  prenatal stress-related, 21, 24, 26
Consultation, to childbirth services. *See also* Direct case consultation; Interviews; Liaison services
  conceptual model, 3–4, 6–7
  developmental tasks of pregnancy and, 51–70, 107, 111
    assessment model, 52, 54–66
  entrée into the system, 108–111
  general principles, 107–113
  information sources, 7–8
  interaction with hospital staff, 108–111, 112–113
  models, 111–113
    consultation/educational activities with staff, 112–113
    direct case consultation, 111–112
    program consultation and participation, 113
  in neonatal intensive care units (NICU), 158–161
  potential value of, 271
  program consultation, 139–146
    for extramural programs, 145–146
    to out-of-hospital nontraditional services, 145–146
    to special projects and services, 145
    to traditional childbirth services, 139–145
  unique aspect of, 269
Corticotropin-releasing factor, in prenatal stress, 30
Couvade syndrome, 76–77
Craniofacial anomalies, maternal alcohol use-related, 207
Cravings, pathological, 77
Cushing's syndrome, 74

Decision-making
  regarding childbirth care options, 85–104

Decision-making (*Cont.*)
  regarding childbirth care options (*Cont.*)
    attitudes concerning hospital environment, 92–93
    birthing centers, out-of-hospital, 87–88, 89–91, 92–96, 98, 99–100, 101, 102, 103
    birthing rooms, family-centered in-hospital, 87, 88, 91–92, 93, 94, 95, 96–103
    compromise with mate, 94
    factors influencing, 86–95
    family life attitudes/values, 92
    finances and, 93
    individual responsibility attitudes, 89–92
    marital support deficits, 100
    maternal health concerns, 99–100
    nesting behavior, 100–102
    previous childbearing/childrearing experience and, 96–98
      response to pregnancy, 100–102
      specific procedures, 93–94
    reproductive, 236
Delirium, postpartum, 37
Delivery
  anxiety and, 24
  fetal rights regarding, 255–256
Depression
  neonatal, 174
  postpartum, 74–75, 126–127
    electroconvulsive therapy, 181
    hormonal factors, 40, 42
    incidence, 39, 43
    neonatal effects of, 160–161
    nonpsychotic, 75
    pharmacological management, 181–182
    premature infants and, 160–161
    psychotic, 75
    subclinical, 41–42
  during pregnancy, 43, 44, 74
Depression scales, 140
Desipramine, 178, 179–180, 181
Development, as basic science, 269
Developmental crisis, pregnancy as, 4–5
Developmental deficits
  maternal alcohol use-related, 208, 211–212
  maternal drug abuse-related, 214
Developmental tasks, of pregnancy, 51–70, 107, 111
  assessment model, 52, 54–66
    acceptance of pregnancy, 54–57
    affiliation with fetus, 57–60
    preparatory behavior, 60–64
    reality-based perception development, 64–66
Diamine oxidase, 53
Diazepam, 192, 194–196, 197
Diphenhydramine, 176, 193

Direct case consultation, 115–136
  case histories, 117–136
    ability to care for newborn, 135–136
    adolescent pregnancy, 131–134
    emergency psychiatric evaluation, 126–127
    fetal damage, fixed ideas concerning, 122–
      124
    juvenile offender, 133–134
    lithium use, 127–128
    no current disorder identified, 117–119
    patient-initiated request, 121–122
    postpartum depression, 126–127
    psychotropic medication use, 124–126, 129
    reproductive catastrophe, 130–131
    suicidal risk, 120–121, 130–131
  educational components, 138
  types, 111–112
DNA, 226
Dopamine, in prenatal stress, 27, 31, 32
Doxepin, 178, 181
Drug abuse, maternal, 213–214
  fetal rights and, 256–257
Drugs. See also Psychopharmacologic agents, use
      during pregnancy; names of specific drugs
  fetal metabolism, 167
  placental transfer, 166
Dysgenesis, of central nervous system, 25

Ebstein's anomaly, 183, 184
Eclampsia, organic syndrome and, 76
Educational activities/programs for hospital staff,
      112–113, 138–139
  prenatal, 199
Electroconvulsive therapy (ECT), use during preg-
      nancy, 165, 178, 181, 188–191
  fetal effects, 188–189
  indications for use, 188–191
  medication use during, 189–191
  teratogenicity, 191
  use during puerperium, 191
Embryo washing, 232
Emergency psychiatric evaluation, 126–127
Emotional disorders. See also names of specific
      emotional disorders
  during postpartum period, 39
  during pregnancy, 39, 144–145
    epidemiology, 39
  reproductive technology-related, 79, 234–235,
      236, 238–239
Emotional factors
  in dystonic labor, 77
  in pregnancy-related mental illness, 76–77
Epinephrine, maternal blood pressure
  effects, 27

Estrogen, levels during pregnancy, 39
Ethics, biomedical. See Legal issues
Exercise, during pregnancy, 25
Extramural programs, program consultation for,
      145–146
Extrapyramidal syndromes, neonatal, 173, 174

False pregnancy. See Pseudocyesis
Fantasy
  concerning fetus, 58–59, 140
  during postpartum period, 64, 65, 66
  during pregnancy, 58–59, 61, 64, 140
Father
  adaptive behavior, 66–67
  assessment interview, 65, 66–67
  couvade syndrome in, 77
  of premature infants, 152, 153–154
Fear reduction techniques, 16
Federal Child Abuse Act, 257
Fetal alcohol syndrome (FAS), 207, 208, 209,
      210, 211, 212
Fetal distress
  maternal alcohol use-related, 208
  maternal anxiety-related, 24
Fetal monitoring, electronic, 244–245, 247, 248
Fetus
  damaged, parental fears concerning, 75–76,
      80–81, 140, 144
  death of. See also Abortion, direct case con-
      sultation for, 130–131
  drug metabolism by, 167
  maternal affiliation with, 57–60
  maternal alcohol use effects, 207–210
  maternal cocaine use effects, 214
  maternal concerns regarding, 96–98
  maternal fantasy concerning, 58–59, 140
  maternal heroin use effects, 214
  maternal hypertension effects, 26
  maternal methadone use effects, 214
  maternal stress effects, 5, 21–25, 27–28, 107–
      108, 269–270
    activity levels and, 27–28
    brain sexual differentiation, 31–33
    fetal outcome, 24–27
    mechanisms, 31–33
    teratological effects, 21–24, 26
  maternal tobacco use effects, 212–213
  quickening of, 58–60, 140, 254
  rights of, 253–265
    abortion and, 236
    case management implications, 259–262
    genetic engineering and, 235
    historical background, 254–255
    maternal rights versus, 255–257

Fetus (*Cont.*)
  rights of (*Cont.*)
    medical malpractice and, 257–259
    reproductive technology implications, 253, 262–263
  surgery, *in utero*, 236
"Floppy infant syndrome", 196
Flunitrazepam, 193, 195, 197
Fluphenazine, 172–173
Fragile X chromosome abnormalities, 225
Freud, Sigmund, 15

Galen, 14
Gamete intrafallopian transfer (GIFT), 232, 234
Gastrointestinal tract, during pregnancy, 166
Genetic counseling, 234–235
  negligence in, 258
  for psychiatric liaisons, 219–227, 237–238
    general issues, 223
    prenatal diagnosis, 222–223, 226, 234–235
    reasons for referral, 220–222
    specific mental health issues, 223–226
  support groups and, 238
Genetic engineering, 235
Genetic factors
  in alcoholism, 224
  in pregnancy-related mental illness, 40
Genetic heterogeneity, 224
Germline gene transplantation, 235
Glucocorticoid hormone, in prenatal stress, 30
Glycopyrolate, 190
Gonadotropin-releasing hormone, infertility and, 235
Gonadotropin-releasing hormone associated peptide, infertility, and, 235
Grodin v. *Grodin*, 257

Halodol. *See* Haloperidol
Haloperidol, 173, 174–175
Health concerns, maternal, 99–100, 141
  regarding, fetus, 96–98, 122–124
Hemorrhage, postpartum, 24
Heroin, use during pregnancy, 214
Hippocrates, 14
Histaminase, 53
Hoerner v. *Bertinato*, 255
Hormonal changes, during pregnancy, 52–54. *See also* names of individual hormones
Hormonal factors. *See also* names of individual hormones
  in postpartum depression, 40, 42
  in pregnancy-related mental illness, 39–40
  in prenatal stress, 27, 30, 31–33
Hospices, 13

Hospitalization, of psychotic patients, 38, 198–199
Huntington's disease, 225, 226
Hyperemesis gravidarum, 76, 77
  definition, 42
  incidence, 42
  psychotropic medication use and, 124–126
Hypertension
  fetal effects of, 26
  stress and, 26, 27
Hyperthermia, 25
Hypotension, orthostatic, 166
Hypothyroidism, 74
Hysteria, 15

Identity crisis, 80, 81
Illegitimacy, 233, 234
Imipramine, 177–178, 179–180
Infant bonding, 270, 271, 248
Infertility
  functional, 77
  gene therapy for, 235
Intergenerational conflicts, 80, 81
International Childbirth Education Association, 7–8, 86
Interviews
  regarding developmental tasks of pregnancy, 52, 54–68
    formulation of information, 67–68
    organization of information, 67–68
  direct case consultation, 115–136
  prenatal screening, 139–145
    regarding developmental tasks of pregnancy, 52, 54–68
  as staff educational activity, 138
In vitro fertilization, 232, 234, 238, 239
Isocarboxazid, 181

Jaundice, neonatal, 173
Jefferson v. *Griffin Spalding County Hospital Authority*, 255–256
Juvenile offenders, pregnancy of, 133–134

Labor
  of alcoholic women, 208
  anxiety and, 22, 23, 24
  dystonic, 77
  emotional factors in, 77
  lithium therapy during, 182
  prolonged, 77
Laboratory values, during pregnancy, 53, 54
Lamaze method, 90
Landeros v. *Flood*, 257

Legal issues
  in childbirth care, 6
  fetal rights, 254–265
    abortion and, 236
    case management and, 259–262
    genetic engineering and, 235
    historical background, 254–255
    maternal rights versus, 255–257
    medical malpractice and, 257–259
    reproductive technology implications, 253,
      262–263
  in reproductive decision-making, 236
Liaison services
  conceptual model, 3–4, 6–7
  educational activities, 112–113, 138–139
  general principles, 107–113
  information sources, 7–8
  models, 111–113
    consultation/educational activities with staff,
      112–113
    direct case consultation, 111–112
    program consultation and participation, 113
  in neonatal intensive care units (NICU), 158–
    161
  potential value of, 271
Life, wrongful, 257–258, 259
Life events, 140
Linkage, genetic, 226
Lister, Joseph, 14
Lithium, use during pregnancy, 127–128, 182–
    188
  breast-feeding and, 187
  neonatal effects, 186–187
  pharmacological considerations, 182–183
  during puerperium, 187
  recommendations for use, 185–186
  teratogenicity, 183–185
Locus of control, 60–64, 248
Lorazepam, 193, 195, 197

Maladaptive syndromes, 41, 54–55, 76, 101–102,
    141–145
  case examples, 141–143
  risk factors, 144–145
Malpractice, 6, 257–259
Mania, during postpartum period, 187
Manic-depressive disorder, during postpartum pe-
    riod, 40
Maprotiline, 178
Marijuana use, during pregnancy, 213
Masturbation, 15
"Maternity blues". See Depression, postpartum
Mellaril. See Thioridazine
Mendelian disorders, 225

Mental health profession, obstetrics
  historical relationship with, 13–19
Mental health professionals. See also Child psy-
    chiatrists; Psychiatrists
  interaction with obstetrical staff, 108–111, 112–
    113, 270–271
Mental illness. See also specific types of mental
    illness
  genetic counseling and, 223–226, 237–238
  during postpartum period, 43, 44, 71–76, 81
    epidemiology of, 37, 38–40, 41–42, 43, 44
    risk factors, 38–39
    treatment guidelines, 198–200
  during pregnancy, 71–84
    adjustment disorders, 41–42
    adverse interaction with pregnancy, 78–79,
      73
    alternate conceptualization, 79–81
    classification, 71–73, 38
    emotional factors related, 76–77, 73
    epidemiology, 37–47
    historical background, 37–39
    major psychiatric disorders, 43–44, 73–76
    normal psychological reactions and, 41
    psychiatric hospitalization rates, 38
    psychological factors, 40
    psychophysiologic conditions, 42–43
    risk factors, 41, 144–145
    stress-related, 76–77, 73
    stress summation theory, 40
    subclinical states, 41–42
    theories of causation, 39–40
    treatment guidelines, 198–200
Mental retardation, maternal alcohol use-related,
    211
Meprobamate, 193–194
Methadone, use during pregnancy, 214
Midwives, 14, 243, 244
Milk fever, 37
Monoamine oxidase inhibitors, 178
Morbidity, neonatal, prenatal stress effects, 29–
    30
"Morning sickness", 42. See also Hyperemesis
    gravidarum
Mortality
  fetal. See also Abortion direct case consultation
    for, 130–131
  neonatal, in neonatal intensive care units
    (NICU), 151
Mother
  genetic, 231–232, 233–234
  gestational, 231–232
  of premature infants, 152–154
  social, 231–232
  surrogate, 232–234, 237, 238, 239, 262–263

Mother–child relationship
  bonding in, 248, 270, 271
  prenatal stress effects, 28–29
Motherhood, normal psychological reactions, 41
Mourning, pathological, 74, 130–131, 153, 160, 162

Natural childbirth classes, 90
Neonatal abstinence syndrome. *See* Neonatal withdrawal syndrome
Neonatal intensive care unit (NICU)
  acute care, 162
  breast-feeding in, 159
  psychiatric services, 151–164
    child psychiatrist's services, 161–163
    consultation–liaison model, 158–161
    nurses and, 151, 154, 156, 157–158, 159, 161, 162
    lack of parental visiting and, 160–161
    paramedical staff, 162
    parental assessment of infant, 161
    parents and, 152–154, 155–157, 158, 159–161, 162, 163
    physicians and, 154, 156, 157, 159, 160, 162
    psychiatrist's problems/rewards, 155–158
    psychiatrist's role, 154–155
    stress sources and, 152–154, 160
    support groups, 151, 162
  size, 159
  transitional care, 162
Neonatal withdrawal syndrome, 176, 179, 196–197, 214
Neonate
  activity levels, prenatal stress effects, 28–29
  bonding, 248, 270, 271
  maternal alcohol use effects, 207, 208, 210–212
  maternal depression effects, 160–161
  maternal psychopharmacologic agent use effects, 173–176, 185, 186–187, 195–197
Nesting behavior, 60–64, 76, 100–102
Nitrazepam, 193
Norepinephrine
  maternal blood pressure effects, 27
  in prenatal stress, 27, 31, 32
Nortriptyline, 177, 178, 179, 181, 200
Nurses
  burnout, 110, 139
  educational activities for, 112–113, 138, 139
  interaction with mental health professionals, 109
  in neonatal intensive care units (NICU), 151, 154, 156, 157–158, 159, 161, 162
  in out-of-hospital birthing centers, 243, 244, 245
  stress experienced by, 110

Nurse-midwives, in out-of-hospital birthing centers, 243, 244, 245
Nymphomania, 15

Obsessive neurosis, during pregnancy, 43
Obstetrical nurse practitioners, 109
Obstetrical staff. *See also* Nurses; Physicians
  educational programs for, 112–113, 138–139
  female, 110–111
  mental health consultants interaction with, 108–111, 112–113
Obstetricians. *See* Physicians
Obstetrics. *See also* Childbirth care options
  development of, 14–15
  information sources in, 7–8
  relationship with mental health professions, 13–19
Older women, first pregnancy, 78
Organic syndrome, during pregnancy, 76
Out-of-hospital nontraditional services. *See also* Birthing centers, out-of-hospital
  program consultation to, 145–146
Oxazepam, 192–193, 195

Parasympatholytics, 176–177
Parenthood, developmental tasks of pregnancy and, 51–70
Parents. *See also* Father; Mother
  childrearing preparation by, 63, 66, 67, 68, 96–98, 140, 141, 144
  of premature infants, 152–154, 155–157, 158, 159–161, 162, 163
Perineal shave, 247, 270–271
Permitil. *See* Fluphenazine
Perphenazine, 172
Peurperal fever, 37. *See also* Child bed fever
Peurperium. *See* Postpartum period
Phenelzine, 181
Phenothiazines, 171–172
Physicians
  attitudes towards out-of-hospital childbirth options, 241–242, 243, 245–246
  childbirth care involvement, historical background, 14
  fetal rights responsibility of, 253–265
  interaction with mental health professionals, 109–111, 112–113, 270, 271
  in neonatal intensive care units (NICU), 154, 156, 157, 159, 160, 162
  primary, as psychiatrist, 3
  stress experienced by, 6
Physiologic changes, during pregnancy, 52–54, 166
Pica, 77

Placenta
  extracorporeal, 233
  medication transfer by, 166
Polyamine oxidase, 53
Postpartum blues syndrome. *See* Depression,
    postpartum
Postpartum period
  benzodiazepine use during, 197
  electroconvulsive therapy during, 191
  hemorrhage during, 24
  mania during, 187
  mental illness during, 43, 44, 71–76, 81
    epidemiology of, 37, 38–40, 41–42, 43, 44
    risk factors, 38–39
    treatment guidelines, 198–200
  mental symptoms during, 22–23
  psychiatric disorders during, 43, 44
  psychosis during, 175–176
Preconception, fetal rights regarding, 257, 258,
    259, 260–261
Preconception counseling, 235. *See also* Genetic
    counseling
Pre-eclampsia, 23–24, 76
Pregnancy
  acceptance of, 54–57
  alcohol use during, 207, 208, 209–212
  biochemical changes during, 52–54
  as developmental crisis, 4–5
  first, 4
  hormonal changes during, 52–54
  laboratory values during, 53, 54
  maladaptation to, 41, 54–55, 76, 101–102
  maternal response to, 100–102
  nonacceptance of, 54–55
  normal psychological reactions in, 41
  in older women, 78
  physiologic changes during, 52–54, 166
  simulated, 43. *See also* Pseudocyesis
Pregnancy outcome
  of alcoholic women, 207, 210, 211, 212
  maternal stress effects, 22–24
Pregnancy testing, antipsychotic agents' effects
    on, 170–171
Premature birth. *See also* Neonatal intensive care
    unit (NICU)
  maternal marijuana use-related, 213
  maternal tobacco use-related, 212
  psychological factors, 24
  repeated, 76
Prenatal diagnosis, 222–223, 226, 234–235
Progesterone, levels during pregnancy, 39
Program consultation, 139–146
  for extramural programs, 145–146
  to out-of-hospital nontraditional services, 145–
    146

Program consultation (*Cont.*)
  to special services and projects, 145
  to traditional childbirth services, 139–145
Prolixin. *See* Fluphenazine
Protriptyline, 177–178, 181
Pseudocholinesterase deficiency, 190
Pseudocyesis, 42–43, 76–77
Pseudopregnancy, 43. *See also* Hyperemesis
    gravidarum
Psychiatric illness. *See* Mental illness
Psychiatrists. *See also* Child psychiatrists
  in neonatal intensive care units (NICU), 154–
    163
  problems/rewards, 155–158
  role, 154–155
  primary physician as, 3
  reproductive cycle research by, 270–271
Psychiatry, relationship with obstetrics, 13–19
Psychodynamic theory, 15
Psychological factors, in pregnancy-related mental
    illness, 40
Psychopharmacologic agents, use during pregnan-
    cy, 165–206
  antidepressants, 177–182, 199
    behavioral effects, 179
    breast-feeding and, 179–181
    choice of, 177
    neonatal effects, 179
    in postpartum depression management, 181–
      182
    teratogenicity, 177–179
  antiparkinson agents, 176–177
  antipsychotic agents, 199
    behavioral effects, 173–174
    breast-feeding and, 174–175
    choice of, 171
    neonatal effects, 173–176
    in postpartum psychosis management, 175–
      176
    pregnancy testing effects, 170–171
  benzodiazepines, 191–197
    behavioral effects, 195–197
    breast-feeding and, 197
    neonatal effects, 195–197
    teratogenicity, 193–195
    use during puerperium, 197
  carbamazepine, 188
  diphenhydramine, 176
  fetal metabolism and, 167
  lithium, 127–128, 182–187, 188, 199, 200
    behavioral effects, 185
    breast-feeding and, 187
    neonatal effects, 185, 186–187
    recommendations regarding use, 185–
      186

Psychopharmacologic agents (*Cont.*)
  lithium (*Cont.*)
    teratogenicity, 183–185
    use during puerperium, 187
  physiologic changes during pregnancy and, 166
  placental medication transfer and, 166
  teratogenicity, 167–170, 171–173, 177–179, 183–185, 193–195
  treatment recommendations, 198–200
Psychoprophylaxis, 16
Psychosis. *See also* Mental illness
  during postpartum period, 175–176
Psychosomatic medicine, 3
Psychoteratology, 168. *See also* Teratogenicity
Psychotropic medication, use during pregnancy, 124–126, 129. *See also* Psychopharmacologic agents, use during pregnancy
  hyperemesis gravidarum and, 124–126

Quickening, of fetus
  abortion following, 254
  mothers' response to, 58–60, 140

Raleigh Fitkin-Paul Morgan Memorial Hospital v. Anderson, 255
Reality perception, parental, 64–66
Referrals
  for genetic counseling, 220–222
  for psychiatric consultation, 138–139
Renslow v. Mennonite Hospital, 258
Reproductive catastrophe. *See also* Abortion
  direct case consultation for, 130–131
Reproductive technology, 231–240
  emotional disorders related to, 79, 234–235, 236, 238–239
  ethical implications, 270
  genetic counseling, 219–227, 234–235, 237–238
  legal issues, 236, 253, 260, 262–263
  parenting types and, 231–234
  prenatal diagnosis, 222–223, 226, 234–235
  psychiatric consultation implications, 237–239
Reproductive variations. *See* Reproductive technology
Rights
  of fetus, 235, 236, 253–265
    abortion and, 236
    case management implications, 259–262
    genetic engineering and, 235
    historical background, 254–255
    maternal rights versus, 255–257
    medical malpractice and, 257–259

Rights (*Cont.*)
  of fetus (*Cont.*)
    reproductive technology implications, 253, 262–263
  maternal, 255–257
Roe v. Wade, 254–255, 257

Schizophrenia
  during postpartum period, 40
  during pregnancy, 44, 73
    antipsychotic agent therapy, 171
    fetal rights and, 256
    prophylactic medication, 175
Schizophreniform disorders, during pregnancy, 73
Screening interviews. *See* Interviews, prenatal screening
Semmelweis, Ignaz Philippe, 14
Sepsis, 14
Sexual differentiation, of brain, 31–33
Social workers, interaction with mental health consultants, 108, 109, 111, 139
Societal factors, in childbirth, 14, 18–19, 269
Special services, program consultation to, 145
Spousal relationship, assessment, 61, 62–64
Stelazine. *See* Trifluoperazine
Sterility. *See* Infertility
Stillbirth, pathological mourning following, 74
Stress
  definition, 21
  in neonatal intensive care units (NICU), 152–154, 160
  of obstetrical staff, 6, 110
  prenatal, 5, 21–35, 107–108, 269–270
    brain sexual differentiation effects, 31–33
    fetal activity effects, 27–28
    fetal outcome effects, 24–27
    hormonal factors, 27, 30, 31–33
    maladaptive response, 76
    mechanisms, 31–33
    mental illness and, 76–78
    neonatal activity effects, 28–29
    pregnancy outcome effects, 22–24
    teratological effects, 21–24, 26
Stress summation theory, of pregnancy-related mental illness, 40
Succinylcholine, use with electroconvulsive therapy, 190, 191
Suicidal risk/attempts, during pregnancy
  direct case consultation for, 120–121, 130–131
  incidence, 74
Support groups
  genetic counseling-related, 238
  for parents of premature infants, 151, 162

Support systems
  deficits in, 74, 80, 100
  kinship, deficits in, 100
  marital, deficits in, 100
  parental, 61–62, 66, 68
Surgery, fetal, *in utero*, 236
Surrogate mothering, 232–234, 237, 238, 239
  legal issues, 262–263
Systemic lupus erythematosus, 129

Tachycardia, fetal, 25, 26
Taft v. *Taft*, 256
Temazepam, 193
Teratogencity
  behavioral, 167, 168, 169
    antidepressant-related, 179, 180
    antipsychotic agent-related, 173–174
    benzodiazepine-related, 176
    diphenhydramine-related, 176
    electroconvulsive therapy-related, 191
  dose-response curves, 168, 169
  epidemiologic studies in, 169–170
  morphological
    antidepressant-related, 177–179, 188
    antiparkinson agent-related, 176–177
    antipsychotic agent-related, 171–173, 188
    benzodiazepine-related, 193–195
    carbamazine-related, 188
    definition, 167
    diphenhydramine-related, 176
    factors in, 167–168
    lithium-related, 183–185, 186–187, 188
  teratogenic potential categories, 170
Teratology. *See* Teratogenicity
Testosterone, brain sexual differentiation effects,
    31–32
Thalidomide, 168, 178

Thioridazine, 172
Thorazine. *See* Chlorpromazine
Thornburgh v. *American College of Obstetricians
    and Gynecologists*, 255
Tobacco use, during pregnancy, 212–213
Tourette syndrome, 225
Toxic syndrome
  during postpartum period, 37
  during pregnancy, 76
Tranylcypromine, 178, 181
Trazodone, 178, 181
Tricyclic antidepressants, 177–178
Trifluoperazine, 172
Triflupromazine, 172
Trihexyphenidyl, 176–177
Trilafon. *See* Perphenazine
Trimipramine, 178
Trophoblast, implantation, 54

Ultrasound
  genetic counseling applications, 234
  prenatal diagnostic applications, 222, 223
Unipolar illness, 40

Vesprin. *See* Triflupromazine
Vulnerable child syndrome, 76, 122–124

Wells v. *Orthopharmaceutical Corp.*, 258
Werling v. *Greyhound*, 259
Whitehead, Mary Beth, 232
Wilson's disease, 224, 225
Work, during pregnancy, 61
Wrongful birth, 6, 257–258, 259
Wrongful conception, 258, 259
Wrongful life, 257–258, 259